# Modified-Release
# Drug Delivery Technology

# DRUGS AND THE PHARMACEUTICAL SCIENCES
## A Series of Textbooks and Monographs

Executive Editor

**James Swarbrick**
*PharmaceuTech, Inc.*
*Pinehurst, North Carolina*

## Advisory Board

# Modified-Release Drug Delivery Technology

## Second Edition

### Volume 1

edited by

## Michael J. Rathbone
*InterAg*
*Hamilton, New Zealand*

## Jonathan Hadgraft
*University of London*
*London, UK*

## Michael S. Roberts
*University of Queensland*
*Brisbane, Australia*

## Majella E. Lane
*University of London*
*London, UK*

**informa**
healthcare

New York   London

Informa Healthcare USA, Inc.
52 Vanderbilt Avenue
New York, NY 10017

International Standard Book Number-10: 1-4200-4435-4 (v. 1: Hardcover)
International Standard Book Number-13: 978-1-4200-4435-5 (v. 1: Hardcover)
International Standard Book Number-10: 1-4200-5355-8 (v. 2: Hardcover)
International Standard Book Number-13: 978-1-4200-5355-5 (v. 2: Hardcover)

---

**Library of Congress Cataloging-in-Publication Data**

---

Modified-release drug delivery technology/edited by
Michael J. Rathbone . . . [et al.]. - - 2nd ed.
    v. < 1- > ; cm. - - (Drugs and the pharmaceutical sciences ; v. 183, etc.)
    Includes bibliographical references and index.
    ISBN-13: 978-1-4200-4435-5 (hb : alk. paper)
    ISBN-10: 1-4200-4435-4 (hb : alk. paper) 1. Controlled release technology. 2. Controlled
release preparations. I. Rathbone, Michael J., 1957- II. Series.
    [DNLM: 1. Delayed-Action Preparations. 2. Drug Delivery Systems. 3. Technology,
Pharmaceutical. W1 DR893B v. 183 2008 / QV 785 M692 2008]
    RS201. C64M63 2008
    615'.6–dc22

2007047360

---

For Corporate Sales and Reprint Permissions call 212-520-2700 or write to:
Sales Department, 52 Vanderbilt Avenue, 16th floor, New York, NY 10017.

**Visit the Informa web site at**
**www.informa.com**

**and the Informa Healthcare Web site at**
**www.informahealthcare.com**

*To my son Thomas*

—Michael J. Rathbone

# Preface

Optimizing drug therapy through delivery-system design is an ever-expanding area of pharmaceutical research. The first edition of *Modified-Release Drug Delivery Technology* remains the most comprehensive compilation of information on individual modified-release drug delivery systems. However, it must be recognized that this area is very dynamic. Therefore, we decided to produce this second edition, which expands and updates the previous collection.

The second edition has been divided into two volumes. Volume 1 addresses oral mucosal, oral, and gastrointestinal tract drug delivery, with targeting to the colonic and rectal sites. Volume 2 covers modified-release drug delivery technologies via injections and implants and the ocular, dermal nasal, vaginal, and pulmonary routes.

In both volumes, we have assumed that the reader is familiar with fundamental controlled-release theories. The volumes are divided into parts covering a particular route for drug delivery that begin with an overview written by a leader or leaders in that field. Each overview covers the anatomical, physiological, and pharmaceutical challenges of formulating a modified-release drug delivery technology for that drug-delivery route. It includes chapters written by experts in each technology that describe specific examples of the different approaches that have been taken to design and develop an innovative modified-release drug delivery system for those routes.

Our challenge in editing this book was to be comprehensive while acknowledging that no single work can expect to describe every modified-release drug delivery technology currently marketed or under development. This is because of both the vast and evolving nature of the field and the lack of available experts who are able to write a comprehensive and authoritative overview on a particular technology, usually because of the proprietary nature of their work. We hope that we have provided a representative selection of the technologies.

In the second edition, we chose to include not only relevant technologies from the first edition, but emerging technologies as well. We also offer insights into user perspectives and address the market requirements, intellectual property challenges, and regulatory requirements associated with the design and development of modified-release drug delivery technologies.

*v*

Volume 1 of *Modified-Release Drug Delivery Technology, Second Edition*, covers drug delivery technologies for the oral mucosal and gastrointestinal tract routes, as well as intellectual property and regulatory issues. Patrea Pabst expertly edits the topic of intellectual property in Part I. Her efforts provide an insightful summary of issues that, when understood and appreciated, add value to any developed modified-release drug delivery technology. Part II focuses on the oral cavity as the site of drug delivery. Sevda Şenel, Michael J. Rathbone, and Indiran Pather, together with invited coauthors, provide an overview of the issues relating to the development of modified-release drug delivery systems for the oral mucosal route. Many of the chapters included in this section describe innovative technologies being developed for specific regions of the oral cavity, including, sublingual, the buccal cavity, gingival, and the periodontal pocket. Rod Walker, the lead author for Part III, considers the oral route. Professor Walker provides an overview of the challenges involved with this popular route for modified-release drug delivery. The introduction to Part III is followed by chapters that provide the reader with insight into the novel and varied approaches, ranging from microparticles to novel manipulations of tableting technologies (including geometric designs and osmotically driven technologies) to three-dimensional printing and the use of lipids. In Part IV, Clive Wilson and Hardik Shah have compiled chapters that describe several diverse approaches that are used to target compounds to various regions of the gastrointestinal tract. Finally, Part V addresses the topic of regulatory issues relating to modified-release drug formulations. Part leader Michael Roberts brings together contributions from Europe, Japan, the United States, Canada, Australia, and New Zealand.

We would like to express our thanks to each of the lead authors for each part, who spent so much time identifying technologies, writing informative overviews, and editing the chapters associated with the routes of drug delivery that are their areas of expertise. We would also like to thank all of the contributors. Their individual, innovative, research activities have contributed significantly to the current modified-release drug delivery technology portfolio that exists today. We thank them for taking the time to share their experiences and work.

*Michael J. Rathbone*
*Jonathan Hadgraft*
*Michael S. Roberts*
*Majella E. Lane*

# Contents

# Contributors

**Christine Andersen**  Egalet a/s, Vaerlose, Denmark

**Jong Bark**  Protherics, PLC, Salt Lake City, Utah, U.S.A.

**Scott D. Barnhart**  ARx, LLC, a Subsidiary of Adhesives Research, Inc., Glen Rock, Pennsylvania, U.S.A.

**Abdul W. Basit**  The School of Pharmacy, University of London, London, U.K.

**Daniel Bar-Shalom**  Egalet a/s, Vaerlose, Denmark

**Andrew Bartholomaeus**  Drug Safety Evaluation Branch, Therapeutic Goods Administration, Canberra, ACT, Australia

**Brain J. Bellhouse**  Medical Engineering Unit, University of Oxford, Oxford, U.K.

**A. Bernkop-Schnürch**  Department of Pharmaceutical Technology, Leopold-Franzens University Innsbruck, Innsbruck, Austria

**Jörg Breitenbach**  SOLIQS Drug Delivery Unit, Abbott GmbH & Co. KG, Ludwigshafen, Germany

**Bianca Brögmann**  Degussa Pharma Polymers GmbH, Darmstadt, Germany

**Catherine Castan**  Flamel Technologies, Vénisieux, France

**George Costigan**  Medical Engineering Unit, University of Oxford, Oxford, U.K.

**David C. Coughlan**  Merrion Pharmaceuticals PLC, Trinity College Dublin, Dublin, Ireland

**Steve L. Durfee**  Drug Delivery Research, Cephalon Inc., Salt Lake City, Utah, U.S.A.

**Thomas J. Dürig**  Aqualon, a Business Unit of Hercules Incorporated, Hercules Research Center, Wilmington, Delaware, U.S.A.

**Kirk D. Fowers**  Protherics, PLC, Salt Lake City, Utah, U.S.A.

**Sultan Ghani**  Drugs and Health Products, Health Canada, Ottawa, Ontario, Canada

**Florence Guimberteau**   Flamel Technologies, Vénisieux, France

**Janet A. Halliday**   Controlled Therapeutics (Scotland) Limited, East Kilbride, Scotland, U.K.

**Ehab Hamed**   Formulation Development, CIMA LABS INC., Brooklyn Park, Minnesota, U.S.A.

**Aiman H. Hommoss**   Department of Pharmaceutical Technology, Biopharmaceutics, and Nutricosmetics, The Free University of Berlin, Berlin, Germany

**Jette Jacobsen**   Department of Pharmaceutics and Analytical Chemistry, Faculty of Pharmaceutical Sciences, University of Copenhagen, Copenhagen, Denmark

**Cornelia M. Keck**   Department of Pharmaceutical Technology, Biopharmaceutics, and Nutricosmetics, The Free University of Berlin, Berlin, Germany

**Susanne Keitel**   European Directorate for the Quality of Medicines (EDQM), Strasbourg, France

**Richard A. Kendall**   The School of Pharmacy, University of London, London, U.K.

**Janez Kerč**   Lek Pharmaceuticals d.d., Sandoz Development Center Slovenia, Ljubljana, Slovenia

**Peter Klusmann**   Hoffmann-Eitle, Munich, Germany

**B. Kombi**   Remfry & Sagar, New Delhi, India

**Evdokia Korakianiti**   European Medicines Agency (EMEA), London, U.K.

**Roger Kravtzoff**   Flamel Technologies, Vénisieux, France

**David Lee**   Drugs and Health Products, Health Canada, Ottawa, Ontario, Canada

**Thomas W. Leonard**   Merrion Pharmaceuticals LLC, Wilmington, North Carolina, U.S.A.

**Jon Lewis**   SOLIQS Drug Delivery Unit, Abbott GmbH & Co. KG, Ludwigshafen, Germany

**Kenneth Lundstrom**   Flamel Technologies, Vénisieux, France

**Juan A. Mantelle**   Noven Pharmaceuticals, Inc., Miami, Florida, U.S.A.

**Patrick J. Marroum**   Division of Pharmaceutical Evaluation I, Office of Clinical Pharmacology, Center for Drug Evaluation and Research, Food and Drug Administration, Silver Spring, Maryland, U.S.A.

**Emma L. McConnell**   The School of Pharmacy, University of London, London, U.K.

**Rémi Meyrueix**   Flamel Technologies, Vénisieux, France

**Rainer H. Müller**   Department of Pharmaceutical Technology, Biopharmaceutics, and Nutricosmetics, The Free University of Berlin, Berlin, Germany

**Gour Mukherji**   Jubilant Organosys Ltd., Noida, India

**Sudaxshina Murdan**   The School of Pharmacy, University of London, London, U.K.

**Naomi Nagai**   Pharmaceuticals and Medical Devices Evaluation Center, Pharmaceuticals and Medical Devices Agency, Tokyo, Japan

**Jerneja Opara**   Lek Pharmaceuticals d.d., Sandoz Development Center Slovenia, Ljubljana, Slovenia

**Edel O'Toole**   Merrion Pharmaceuticals PLC, Trinity College Dublin, Dublin, Ireland

**Patrea L. Pabst**   Pabst Patent Group LLP, Atlanta, Georgia, U.S.A.

**S. Indiran Pather**   California Northstate College of Pharmacy, Rancho Cordova, California, U.S.A.

**Margrethe Rømer Rassing**   Copenhagen, Denmark

**Michael J. Rathbone**   InterAg, Hamilton, New Zealand

**Ramesh C. Rathi**   Protherics, PLC, Salt Lake City, Utah, U.S.A.

**Michael S. Roberts**   School of Medicine, University of Queensland, Princess Alexandra Hospital, Brisbane, Queensland, Australia

**Steve Robertson**   Controlled Therapeutics (Scotland) Limited, East Kilbride, Scotland, U.K.

**Carolyn Rolls**   Mallesons Stephen Jaques, Melbourne, Victoria, Australia

**Sevda Şenel**   Department of Pharmaceutical Technology, Faculty of Pharmacy, Hacettepe University, Ankara, Turkey

**Hardik K. Shah**   Biovail Technologies (Ireland) Ltd., Dublin, Ireland

**Wilfred Aubrey Soskolne**   Department of Periodontology, Hebrew University-Hadassah Faculty of Dentistry, Jerusalem, Israel

**H. N. E. Stevens** Department of Pharmaceutical Sciences, University of Strathclyde, Glasgow, Scotland

**John A. Tessensohn** Shusaku Yamamoto Patent Law Office, Osaka, Japan

**Satoshi Toyoshima** Pharmaceuticals and Medical Devices Evaluation Center, Pharmaceuticals and Medical Devices Agency, Tokyo, Japan

**George Wade** European Medicines Agency (EMEA), London, U.K.

**R. B. Walker** Faculty of Pharmacy, Rhodes University, Grahamstown, South Africa

**Wang Wang Lee** AstraZeneca, Macclesfield, U.K.

**Neena Washington** Strathclyde Institute of Pharmacy and Biomedical Sciences, Glasgow, Scotland, U.K.

**M. Werle** ThioMatrix GmbH, Research Center Innsbruck, Innsbruck, Austria

**Clive G. Wilson** Strathclyde Institute of Pharmacy and Biomedical Sciences, Glasgow, Scotland, U.K.

**Iris M. Ziegler** Pharmaceutical Development, New Therapeutic Entities, Grünenthal GmbH, Aachen, Germany

## Part I: Intellectual Property Rights

---

# 1

---

# Patent and Other Intellectual Property Rights in Drug Delivery

Patrea L. Pabst

*Pabst Patent Group LLP, Atlanta, Georgia, U.S.A.*

## INTRODUCTION

Advancements in drug delivery technology are often achieved only through a substantial investment of industrial, academic, and governmental resources. Patenting these technological advancements is frequently used to recoup that investment, to create profits that are used in part to develop new or improved products, and to enhance a competitive commercial edge. Other forms of intellectual property protection, such as trade secrets, copyrights, and trademarks may also be used to further protect and exploit drug delivery processes, products, and services.

One of the most frequently asked questions is why we need to go to the trouble and expense of patenting a composition or method. The most common reason is that protecting a new composition or method of manufacture or use provides a means for obtaining the revenue required to develop a new drug or medical treatment. With the cost of developing and obtaining regulatory approval for a new drug approaching $200 million dollars in the United States, patent rights are essential to recovering expenses. For small companies that spend more time raising money then selling products, patents and patent applications represent only tangible assets they can show to potential investors. For universities and other nonprofit research institutions, patents and associated know-how and, in some limited cases, trade secrets can be used to obtain royalties from license agreements, from, in many cases, sponsored research, and from equity in new companies that have been started for the purpose of exploiting the technology.

Patents and other intellectual properties are valued in many different ways. For example, a process for manufacture typically would be licensed for 2% to 3% of the gross selling price of a product of the process. This price would be decreased if multiple licenses had to be obtained to use the process. Patents claiming compositions tend to have a greater market value, e.g., between 5% and 10% of the gross selling price, due to the perception that they are easier to enforce than process patents.

Enforcement, however, is a risky business. A good patent strategy is to obtain patents that claim a product, methods of manufacture, and methods of use, broadly and specifically, so that a patentee is able to assert multiple patents against an alleged infringer. Patents with broad claims generally will be easier to invalidate than more specific patents. Faced with the prospect of fighting several patents, most parties will opt for settlement. The alternative of litigation is extraordinarily expensive for both parties and can result in the patents being invalidated, or the infringer being liable not only for damages for infringement, but also attorney's fees and punitive damages.

## PROPRIETARY RIGHTS IN THE UNITED STATES

The importance of patent protection is clear. To protect and enable innovation, one must seek protection in all areas where the invention will be manufactured, distributed, or used. In the pharmaceutical area, one typically looks to patents to exclude competitors engaged in the manufacture and/or distribution of drugs. It is difficult or impossible to enforce patents *against* patients or the health care providers, and is a disaster in public relations.

Therefore, in determining how and when to patent an innovation, especially in the pharmaceutical area, one focuses on protecting methods of manufacture and novel drugs or drug formulations. Novel chemical entities are far rarer than new formulations. New formulations are typically based on new routes of administration (pulmonary instead of oral, topical instead of systemic); regional instead of systemic delivery; delivery regimes (escalating dosages, delayed release, extended delivery, pulsed release); combinations with other drugs; administration via a new route, form, or dosage to a different class of patients or a different disease or disorder to be treated.

As the following chapters demonstrate, the requirements for patentability and the breadth and enforceability of claims vary dramatically depending upon the country in which protection is sought. The United States has always been "friendlier" to the pharmaceutical industry than a country such as India, which still provides only limited protection despite its own rapidly expanding and powerful generic drug industry. Japan has limited its protection in recent years, making it extremely difficult to obtain broad patents and patents in the absence of detailed working examples.

While creative lawyers in the United States have tried to expand protection of patent rights through the use of patents that define products by their general functional language (a dosage regime or release profile), the European Patent Office has made it clear that such claims do not meet the requirements of European patent law.

Drug screening methods and patents on long product lists obtained from high throughput screening or genomic libraries have become harder to obtain in the United States, and are more expensive, and more difficult to enforce. Trade-secret protection for constantly evolving data bases and drug libraries can provide more cost effective and enforceable protection than is obtainable with patents.

Enforcement actions are extremely expensive, especially in the United States. Typical litigation costs run $3 to $10 million and can be higher. Approximately 60% to 80% of litigations are settled. Creative settlements that provide for the sale of "authorized" generic drugs or that delay entry into competition with the brand owner are, despite opposition by the U.S. Justice Department, increasingly common. Alternative proceedings, especially oppositions or invalidation trials in Europe, Australia, and Japan, are significantly faster and less expensive and are being used to narrow the issues and create incentives to settle prior to litigation in the United States. Absent exclusive rights, however, drug companies cannot ensure the profits required to drive the continued development of new drugs and drug formulations.

In summary, patents and other forms of proprietary protection continue to be of crucial importance to the pharmaceutical industry, even as the apparent scope of protection has narrowed, especially outside of the United States.

## PATENTS

Patents are used to exclude competition, not to "protect" a product. A patent is a limited monopoly granted to an inventor by a government entity in exchange for public disclosure of the invention. The limited monopoly permits the inventor to exclude others from making, using, selling, offering to sell, or importing into a geographical area (such as the United States) the invention, which may be a composition, method of manufacture, or method of use, defined by the claims in the patent, in exchange for teaching the public how to make and use that which is claimed. The patent system is based upon the public policy objective of fostering the collective advancement of technology and science through the sharing of individual achievements. The limited monopoly (limited by geography, by the country or region granting the patent, and in time to a period of years) conferred by a patent provides the incentive for inventors to publicly reveal their technological development.

## PATENTABILITY REQUIREMENTS

Patents have basically the same requirements throughout the world, although, as emphasized in the following sections, they vary in scope and subject matter. In the United States, the requirements for obtaining and asserting a patent are defined by Chapter 35 of the United States Code (U.S.C.). Patents are governed exclusively by federal law.

In the late 1990s, this law in the United States was subject to a considerable number of changes. When the United States entered into the General Agreement on Trade and Tariffs (GATT) in December 1994, major changes in effective U.S. patent term resulted. Ongoing efforts to change the U.S. Patent and Trademark Office from a government agency to a governmental corporation, primarily to avoid further diversion of patent office fees to other government agencies, and harmonization with the Patent Laws of other jurisdictions, has resulted in even more changes to the U.S. patent law.

Further changes to the requirements for obtaining a patent, and in the enforceability of method of medical treatment claims, have resulted from reactionary changes in the laws following unpopular court decisions. This is especially true in the biotechnology area. The late 1990s were known for swift and drastic decisions by the Court of Appeals for the Federal Circuit, invalidating biotechnology patents on the grounds the claims were not enabled by the specifications. Fortunately, more patents have recently been upheld under 35 U.S.C. § 112 based on challenges to enablement and lack of written descriptions, with prior art considerations playing a greater role in validity determinations.

### Patentable Subject Matter

In general, patentable subject matter includes composition, method of manufacture, and method of use (1). Composition may include, for example, biodegradable polymeric microparticles containing a therapeutic agent, or a bioadhesive compound useful for targeted drug delivery within the body. A method of manufacture may be directed to, for example, a process for creating a unique drug delivery device. A method of use may entail a method for the administration of a therapeutic composition, or a surgical implantation of, for example, a synthetic tissue matrix containing implanted isolated cells that secrete insulin.

Although the law provides for patenting of compositions, methods of manufacture, and methods of use, biotechnology can present a problem under U.S. patent law when the subject matter moves away from the realm of the artificial, or "things engineered by the hand of man," to a blend or chimera of "artificial" and "natural" (2). An example is blending cells and a matrix to form a cell-matrix structure that is then implanted into a patient. Then, the matrix degrades to leave only implanted cells, and/or the patient's own tissue grows into an implanted matrix structure, which then degrades. At what point do these materials "become" the patient and not patentable subject matter? Ethical issues may arise because of the overlap between patient material and traditional subject matter, particularly in those cases involving dissociated isolated cells, biodegradable matrices for implantation, polymeric materials for altering cell/cell interaction (such as adhesion or restenosis), and materials for implantation that are designed to remain in the body, such as stainless-steel hip replacements or cryopreserved pig valves.

Outside the United States, methods of treatment for humans or other animals are generally not patentable subject matter. For example, although surgical instruments, drugs, or devices used in surgery are patentable, surgical treatments are not considered patentable subject matter. Therefore, one cannot obtain a patent on a method for surgically treating a patient. Typically, however, while surgical treatment is not patentable, the compositions and methods of manufacture for use in treating patients are patentable subject matter. Claims may be obtained to the composition *per se*, which is to be implanted. In Europe, claims can be obtained to a first, or even a second, use of the material when the material itself is known. However, the patentability is quite limited in individual countries and in the European Patent Office for policy and ethical reasons. Generally, patent offices in Asian countries are far less flexible than the European Patent Office in this matter. As a result, patent attorneys have adopted a number of strategic approaches to obtain protection that is equivalent to the protection available in the United States. For example, one may draft claims directed to methods of manufacture of such materials, as well as to methods of use that are defined by the composition rather than the method of use steps.

## Novelty

The second requirement for patentability is novelty (3). Novelty, in the simplest terms, means that no one, including the applicant, has publicly used or described (orall, in writing, or presented) that which is being claimed before the patent application is filed. In the United States, an exception is made when the publication occurs less than one year before the patent application is filed. The publication can be "removed" as prior art if the applicants are able to demonstrate that, prior to publication, they conceived and diligently reduced to practice what they are claiming.

What constitutes a publication? Generally, a publication is any oral, written, or physical description that conveys to the public that which applicant would like to claim. It may be a talk at the proceedings of a society (including any slides presented), an article in a scientific journal, a grant application that is awarded, a thesis, or even an offer for sale or a press release. A critical requirement is that the publication must be enabling, that is, it must convey to one of ordinary skill in the art how to make and use that which is being claimed. Public use means more than using the composition or method in one's laboratory. However, it can include even a single patient study reported during clinical rounds or at a presentation where a drug company or surgical supply representative is present. In many cases, the courts have had to interpret what it means to be publicly available. A frequent question is when a student's thesis is available as prior art. U.S. courts have held that once the thesis is cataloged, it is publicly available because it has been entered into a computer database so that anyone searching the database will be able to access it (4). Accordingly, the publication date of a thesis is the date on which the thesis is cataloged, not the date on which it is defended or signed by the thesis committee. This rule is not applicable outside of the United States, however, where an earlier date may constitute the date of publication. Slides that are not distributed, but are instead shown at an oral presentation, are considered to be publications, particularly if the meeting is attended by those skilled in the art, who would be able to understand and use the information in the slides.

A disclosure to another party under the terms of a confidentiality agreement is not a publication. Uses that are strictly experimental may not be public disclosures, if, among other aspects, they are designed to determine whether what is to be claimed will work and if other involved parties are clearly informed that the studies are experimental in nature. If something is an announcement that does not enable one of ordinary skill in the art to use or make that which is claimed, then the disclosure is not a publication. For example, an announcement could be a statement made to the press that researchers X and Y have discovered a cure for cancer. Since the announcement does not tell one of ordinary skill in the art how to cure cancer, it is not enabling. However, sufficiency of enablement can be difficult to prove, and standards may change over time. One example is the court case in which the question of whether a publication related to the development of a transdermal patch for delivery of nicotine was enabling (5). The court found that a prior publication referring to transdermal patches for drug delivery mentioned that transdermal patches containing nitroglycerin for the treatment of heart disease could be replaced with nicotine to help patients quit smoking. The court held that the article disclosed or made obvious the transdermal patch for delivery of nicotine claimed by the applicant, because the applicant merely took the transdermal patch described in the article, put nicotine in it, and then demonstrated that the nicotine was delivered and would work exactly as predicted based on delivery of the heart disease drug. Even though there was no information relating to the exact dosage or schedule or to how the drug was to be incorporated into the transdermal patch, the publication was enabling because one of ordinary skill in the art would be able to determine the dosage and how to put the nicotine in the transdermal patch without undue experimentation.

## Nonobviousness or the Inventive Step

The third requirement for patentability is that the claimed method or composition must be nonobvious to those of ordinary skill in the art from what is publicly known (6). This is usually referred to outside of the United States as a requirement for an inventive step. In the 1960s, the U.S. Supreme Court carefully analyzed nonobviousness and the factors to be considered in determining whether that which is claimed is obvious from the prior art (7). This analysis is a fact-based determination, involving not only the elements that are claimed, but also the level of skill in the art and the expectation that the claimed method or composition will perform as predicted, its actual success in the marketplace, the long-felt need for it, and whether there are unexpected results. If there is no better than a 50-50 chance that a particular method will work, and the method does work, it is, arguably, not obvious, although it may be obvious to try. If one tries something and the results are vastly different from what was expected, then the results are not obvious. For example, if one administers two drugs each in the dosage known to yield a particular effect, and the combination yields a substantially greater effect than the sum of the individual effects of each drug , resulting in the ability to use a much lower dosage of each drug than expected, then one would have unexpected results or "synergy." If the prior art teaches away from what the applicant has done, this result would support a finding of nonobviousness. For example, if the prior art states that one cannot administer drugs transdermally using ultrasound except at a very high frequency, then it may be nonobvious if the patent applicant finds that the same or better results are obtained using a very low frequency. Many other considerations factor into whether a claimed composition or method is obvious in view of the prior art.

In May 2007, the U.S. Supreme Court (8) again addressed the issue of obviousness, overturning the general requirements developed by the Court of Appeals for the Federal Circuit (CAFC) over the past 20-plus years. The CAFC had issued a series of decisions in which patents were determined not to be obvious over the prior art if the prior art failed to disclose the claimed elements and the motivation for one skilled in the art to combine the elements as the inventor had done with a reasonable expectation of success. The Supreme Court broadened the prior art that could be used in determining obviousness, and stated that the motivation to combine could be apparent to one skilled in the art and did not have to be explicit in the prior art. This decision has called into question the validity of many issued U.S. patents.

However, the Supreme Court also affirmed their previous decision that nonobviousness can be found when there is long standing but unmet need, commercial success, and/or unexpected results, or any of the other criteria articulated in *Graham v. John Deere Co.* Patents containing data showing greater efficacy, cost efficiency, fewer side effects, or manufacturing benefits should still be valid and enforceable.

## Requirements of 35 U.S.C. §112

To obtain a patent, the patent application (also referred to as the specification) must satisfy the requirements of 35 U.S.C. §112, first paragraph. This part of the statute has three separate requirements: (1) the specification must contain a written description of the invention; (2) the written description must describe the manner and process of making and using the invention; and (3) the specification must describe the best mode contemplated by the inventor of carrying out the invention at the time the invention is filed (9). These three requirements are generally referred to as the written description requirement, the enablement requirement, and the best mode requirement. Although the written description requirement and the enablement requirement are related to each other, the Court of Appeals for the Federal Circuit has repeatedly held that the two requirements are separate and distinct (9).

## Written Description

The purpose of the written description requirement is to "ensure that the scope of the right to exclude, as set forth in the claims, does not overreach the scope of the inventor's contribution to the field of art as described in the patent specification" (9,10). The written description requirement of a patent specification serves a teaching function, as a "quid pro quo" in which the public is given "meaningful disclosure in exchange for being excluded from practicing the invention for a limited period of time" (11). Thus, in the specification the applicant must describe what is being claimed in sufficient detail to "establish that [the applicant] was in possession of the . . . claimed invention, including all of the elements and limitations" (9,12).

In *Univ. of Rochester v. G.D. Searle*, 358 F.3d at 930, the Court of Appeals for the Federal Circuit held that to satisfy the written description requirement, method claims reciting a specific compound or class of compounds must be supported in the patent specification by written disclosure of examples of such compounds or class of compounds. U.S. Patent No. 6,048,850 ("the '850 patent") claimed methods for selectively inhibiting cyclooxygenase COX-2 by administering a nonsteroidal compound that selectively inhibits activity of the PGHS-2 [COX-2] gene product to a human host in need of such treatment. Although the patent specification described methods for screening for compounds that selectively inhibit COX-2, the patent specification did not disclose a single compound that selectively inhibited COX-2. Selective inhibitors of COX-2 were unknown at the time the application resulting in the '850 patent was filed.

On the day the '850 patent issued, the University filed an infringement action against several defendants collectively referred to as Pfizer for the selling the COX-2 inhibitors Celebrex® and Bextra®. Pfizer moved for summary judgment arguing that the '850 patent was invalid for failing to satisfy the written description and enablement requirements. The district court ruled in favor of Pfizer, concluding that the '850 patent disclosed "nothing more than a hoped-for function for an as-yet-to-be-discovered compound, and a research plan for trying to find one" (9: 926–27).

The University appealed to the CAFC which upheld the decision. Although the claims do not require the exact wording as found in the specification to satisfy the written description requirement, the claims must have sufficient written description so that one of ordinary skill in the art would recognize what was claimed (9: 922–23). "Even with the three-dimensional structures of the enzymes such as COX-1 and COX-2 in hand, it may even now not be with in the ordinary skill in the art to predict what compounds might bind to and inhibit them, let alone have been within the purview of one ordinary skill in the art in the 1993–1995 period in which the applications that led to the '850 patent were filed" (9: 925).

## Enablement

To satisfy the enablement requirement, the applicant must describe the invention with appropriate methods and sources of reagents or other materials or equipment, to enable one of ordinary skill in the art to make and use the invention being claimed. This sounds far simpler than it actually is in practice. In many cases, particularly when it is coming out of a university study or a start-up company, the invention that an applicant would like to claim is one that the applicant intends to develop over the next several years, based on a limited amount of data available at the time of filing. Particularly in the case of universities, where the applicant must publish or has submitted grant applications (which in and of themselves constitute prior art once they are awarded), the difficulty is in describing something that has not yet been done. The application must not only describe a specific limited example, but also must describe the various ways in which one intends to practice that which is claimed. Difficulties also arise where an applicant desires to protect the goal (e.g., a release profile), not the specific reagents used in one or two examples of formulations that achieved the desired profile.

The purpose of a patent is to exclude the competition from making and using that which is claimed, not to "protect" a product—a frequent misconception of patents. In order to exclude competition, one must describe and claim not only that which one intends to practice, but that which another party could practice in competition with the patentee. What does this mean in real terms? It means that the applicant for a patent must describe his preferred method, which is known as of the date of filing, the preferred embodiments that he or his company intends to market, as well as any embodiments that a competitor could make and use in competition with the applicant's product.

"Invention" usually consists of two steps, "conception" and "reduction to practice." There are two kinds of reduction to practice: actual and constructive. Constructive reduction to practice means that the applicant has described in the application for patent *how* to make and use what is being claimed, but has not actually made and used it. This may be as simple as stating that although a biodegradable polymer such as polylactic acid-co-glycolic acid is preferred for making a matrix for drug delivery, other biodegradable polymers such as polyorthoesters or polyanhydrides could also be used. It may be less obvious that other drugs may be used when only one example showing reduction to practice of a type of drug is available. The rule of thumb in this case is the level of predictability. Therefore, in stating what kind of drugs one could deliver using the claimed technology, one might list a wide variety of drugs based on the data available with one type of drug. However, delivery of a peptide or a very hydrophobic compound, which usually are viewed as difficult to deliver, may or may not be possible to list based on data obtained with a drug that is "easy" to deliver, such as a sugar or small molecular weight dye. Being too predictive (i.e., engaging in extensive constructive reduction to practice), which includes "nonenabling" or nonenabled technology, may in some cases be a detriment during prosecution of subsequently filed applications, because the examiner may cite the earlier work as making obvious the applicant's subsequent work. (See also concerns regarding prosecution in Japan in subsequent section.) Patent attorneys frequently must play a balancing game in determining how far to go with constructive reduction to practice in order to exclude competitors while not eliminating the applicant's own ability to obtain additional, subsequent patent protection.

## Best Mode

In the United States, there is a requirement to disclose the best mode for practicing that which is claimed at the time of filing the application. No similar requirement exists outside of the United States. Because most applicants file the same application in the United States and outside of the United States, U.S. applicants frequently disclose their best mode in foreign-filed applications. As a result of the American Inventor's Protection Act, U.S. patent applications are now published eighteen months after their earliest priority date unless a request for nonpublication is filed (13). Part of the request for nonpublication includes a certification that the invention disclosed in the application has not been and will not be the subject of an application filed in another country, or under a multilateral international agreement, that requires publication after filing. If the applicant subsequently decides to file the same application in a country that publishes patent applicants, the request for nonpublication must be rescinded before filing the counterpart application or a notice of foreign filing must be submitted to the U.S. Patent Office no later than 45 days after the filing date of the counterpart application to avoid abandonment of the application.

In some circumstances it may be desirable to file a nonpublication request if the patent application will not be filed abroad. In rapidly evolving technologies, e.g., computer software, where a publication of the invention will permit competitors to begin designing around or improving the technology before a patent issues, it may be prudent to forego foreign patent protection and file a nonpublication request. Although an applicant has certain remedies if the claims that ultimately issue in the U.S. patent are substantially the same as the claims in the published patent application, these remedies may not be as commercially valuable as being first to market.

## 35 U.S.C. § 112, Paragraph 4

Recently a relatively unremarkable aspect of Section 112 became the unlikely focus of a patent infringement case concerning the blockbuster drug, Lipitor®. 35 U.S.C. § 112, fourth paragraph provides:

> Subject to the following paragraph, a claim in dependent form shall contain a reference to a claim previously set forth and then specify a further limitation of the subject matter claimed. A claim in dependent form shall be construed to incorporate by reference all the limitations of the claim to which it refers.

35 U.S.C. § 112, fourth paragraph requires that a properly drafted claim further limit the subject matter of the claim from which it depends.

In early 2003, Pfizer filed four complaints against Ranbaxy Pharmaceutical, Inc. ("Ranbaxy") alleging infringement of one or more claims of U.S. Patent No. 4,681,893 ("the '893 patent") and 5,273,995 ("the '995 patent") in response to Ranbaxy's filing of an Abbreviated New Drug Application (ANDA) to market a generic version of Lipitor before the expiration of the '893 and '995 patents (14). Ranbaxy responded that the '893 and '995 patents were invalid, not infringed, and/or unenforceable for various reasons, including anticipation, obviousness, and inequitable conduct.

Prior to trial, Pfizer decided to limit its infringement allegations with respect to the '995 patent solely to claim 6, which claimed atorvastatin calcium (i.e., the hemicalcium salt of atorvastatin acid). Claim 6 and the claims from which it depends (claims 1 and 2) are shown below:

1. Atorvastatin acid or atorvastatin lactone or pharmaceutically acceptable salts thereof.
2. The compound of claim 1, which is atorvastatin acid.
6. The hemicalcium salt of the compound of claim 2.

In its opinion, the U.S. District Court held that the '893 patent was valid and enforceable. With respect to the '995 patent, the Court found that the meaning of claim 6 was clear and unambiguous: the hemicalcium salt of atorvastatin acid. However, the Court recognized that there was a "technical problem in the drafting of claim 6" because it improperly depends from claim 2 (14: 508). Claim 6 depends from claim 2 and is directed to the hemicalcium salt. Claim 2, however, is directed to atorvastatin acid. Claim 6 does not further limit the scope of the subject matter recited in claim 2 from which it depends (14). In fact, claim 6 actually recites different and non-overlapping subject matter. Accordingly, claim 6 violates 35 U.S.C. § 112, fourth paragraph (14).

The District Court, however, understood 35 U.S.C. § 112, fourth paragraph "to be limited to matters of form, rather than matters of substance" and concluded that 35 U.S.C. § 112, fourth paragraph should not be used as the basis for invalidating a dependent claim (14). The CAFC disagreed. The CAFC held that invalidating an improper dependent claim under 35 U.S.C. § 112, fourth paragraph "does not exalt form over substance" and is "consistent with the overall statutory scheme that requires applicants to satisfy certain requirements before obtaining a patent, some of which are more procedural or technical than others" (15). The CAFC went on to note that claim 6 could have been properly drafted as either a dependent or independent claim, but held that a Court "should not rewrite claims to preserved validity" (15). The CAFC did not decide the other defenses raised by Ranbaxy regarding the validity or enforceability of the '995 patent.

A unique aspect of U.S. patent law is that the claims of a patent are analyzed individually with respect to infringement and invalidity (unlike, e.g., under the European Patent Convention in which all claims stand or fall together). Since Pfizer only asserted claim 6 in the litigation, the other claims of the '995 patent are presumed valid in the absence of a Court's ruling to the contrary. In an effort to correct the technical problems in claim 6, Pfizer filed a reissue application with the United States Patent and Trademark Office (USPTO) on January 16, 2007. In its filing, Pfizer rewrote claim 6, as well as the other dependent claims that improperly depended from claim 2 (i.e., claims 4, 5, and 8–10), in independent form. This was one of the suggestions that the CAFC gave in its opinion for correcting claim 6.

## PROVISIONAL APPLICATIONS

Provisional patent applications, while relatively new to the United States, becoming available June 8, 1995, have been utilized for many years in other countries, such as the United Kingdom and Australia. These applications are a mechanism for obtaining a filing date at minimal cost and with fewer requirements for completeness of the application and determination of the inventive entity for a period of one year. The provisional application ceases to exist 12 months after the date of filing. If an application is filed as a provisional application, it can be converted to a standard utility application at anytime during the twelve months period after filing. Alternatively, it can serve as a basis for a claim to priority in a subsequently filed utility application, if the utility application is filed prior to the expiration of the one year life of the provisional application.

Although touted as a great benefit to the small entity or individual applicant, provisional applications have the same requirements for disclosure as a standard utility application. Failure in the provisional application to completely disclose and enable that which is subsequently claimed in an utility application can result in a loss of the claim to priority to the provisional application, if what is claimed is not enabled or supported with written description in the provisional application. Merely filing a journal article manuscript that will be published or presented in order to avoid loss of foreign rights usually will not comply with the enablement and written description requirements, and therefore will not serve as an adequate basis for priority. It is essential that applicants who file provisional applications based on a manuscript augment the description to encompass multiple embodiments of the invention and to provide the basis by which one of ordinary skill in the art can practice that which is ultimately claimed. Application sections that are not required for enablement, which are typically included in a utility application, include the background of the invention, the problems that the claimed invention addresses, and the claims. These sections can be omitted from the provisional application, thus saving time and money in preparing the application. In many cases, fairly standard language can be used to expand or broaden the description in a manuscript in order to meet the enablement requirements, providing a means for those with limited amounts of time or money to protect that which they are disclosing with minimum risk and expenditure.

The World Intellectual Property Organization (WIPO), which implements the provisions of the Patent Cooperative Treaty (PCT) and the European Patent Office, has confirmed that U.S. provisional applications serve as an adequate basis for a claim to priority in corresponding foreign file applications. However, under the Paris Convention, all foreign applications that claim priority from an earlier filed application must still be filed within one year of the U.S. filing date or the filing date of the country in which the first application is originally filed.

## INVENTORSHIP

The U.S. constitution provides that inventors have the exclusive right to their discoveries (16). An application for patent must be made by the inventor, or under certain circumstances (such as when the inventor is dead) by persons on behalf of the inventor (17). When more than one person makes the invention, the inventors are required to file jointly, "even though they did not physically work together or at the same time, each did not make the same type or amount of contribution, or each did not make a contribution to the subject matter of every claim of the patent" (18). A patent may be invalidated if it names one who is not an inventor or if it fails to name an inventor; however, these errors may be corrected if they were not committed with an intention to deceive (19).

In a "nutshell," an inventor is one who conceives and reduces to practice the claimed invention, not at the direction of another. To determine who the inventors are, one must first ascertain that which is claimed. Second, one must determine what is already in the prior art; one is not an inventor if the claimed subject matter is already in the prior art. For example, if one is claiming a polymeric drug delivery device and the claim defines the matrix structure as formed from biodegradable polymer, then this particular element is probably already in the prior art and that element alone would not be the invention of any named inventor upon the application for patent. However, if the polymeric matrix were defined as having a particular structure or shape or composition that has not previously been defined, then the individual (or individuals) who determines that shape or structure or composition would be an inventor. In methods for manufacture, the person who is in the laboratory using the method may or may not be an inventor. If this person has been told by another to go and make composition X using steps A, B, and C, then the person who performs the method is not an inventor—even if there is some optimization of the concentration or selection of reagents or conditions under which they are combined. If, however, that person determines that it is essential to use a concentration ten times greater than what he has been told in order to make it work, then he may be an inventor of the method of use. A patent may name multiple parties as inventors. They do not all have to be inventors of each and every claim that defines the invention. One person may be an inventor of composition claims, another the method of manufacture claims, and yet another the method of use claims. Inventorship may need to be corrected following a restriction requirement or after cancellation or amendment of the claims.

Provisional applications differ from standard utility applications in that there is no requirement to name all, or even the correct, inventors; nor do the inventors have to file a disclaimer of inventorship stating they believe they are the correct inventors of the claimed technology. This is in keeping with the absence of a requirement for having claims defining what applicants think constitutes their invention.

Outside of the United States, patent applications frequently are filed by the assignee rather than by the inventors. Inventorship is not usually a basis for challenging a foreign patent.

## DUTY OF DISCLOSURE

Another unique (although recently Australia, Canada and Israel have implemented similar provisions) requirement of the U.S. patent law is the duty of disclosure, described by Chapter 37 of the Code of Federal Regulations (C.F.R.), § 1.56. Applicants are required to submit to the examiner in the U.S. Patent and Trademark Office ("the Office") copies of all publications or other materials that may be determined by an examiner to be material to examination of the claimed subject matter (19). Failure to cite relevant material prior art to the Patent Office can result in a subsequent finding by a court of appropriate jurisdiction that the patent is invalid for fraud and violation of the duty of disclosure, also referred to as inequitable conduct.

## INEQUITABLE CONDUCT

Inequitable conduct is an affirmative defense to infringement often pled in infringement law suits. Inequitable conduct can occur when an individual associated with the filing and prosecution of a patent application breaches the duty of candor and good faith imposed by the Office. 37 C.F.R. § 1.56 (a). The duty of candor and good faith includes a duty to disclose to the Office all information known to that individual to be material to patentability. "Material to patentability" is defined by the Office as information that is not cumulative to information already of record or being made of record in the application, and

1.  establishes, by itself or in combination with other information, a *prima facie* case of unpatentability of a claim or
2.  refutes, or is inconsistent with, a position the applicant takes in
    (i) opposing an argument of unpatentability relied on by the Office or
    (ii) asserting an argument of patentability (20).

Individuals having the duty of candor and good faith include the patent attorney or agent, the inventors, and every other person who is substantively involved in the preparation or prosecution of the application and who is associated with the inventor, with the assignee or with anyone to whom there is an obligation to assign the application.

The CAFC recently explained that statements or omissions made to the Office during the prosecution of a patent application can be used to invalidate that patent if those statements or omissions are material to the patentability of the invention (21).

Purdue Pharma, L.P. et al. (collectively "Purdue") sued Endo Pharmaceuticals Inc. et al. (collectively "Endo") for patent infringement alleging that Endo infringed Purdue's patents covering an oxycodone formulation. The district court found that Endo's generic version of Purdue's oxycodone product did infringe the claims of U.S. Patent Nos. 5,656,295; 5,508,042; and 5,549,912, but that the patents were unenforceable due to Purdue's inequitable conduct during the prosecution of the patent applications that matured into these patents. On appeal, the CAFC affirmed the finding of inequitable conduct, but on petition for rehearing remanded the case to the district court for additional fact finding relating the issues of materiality and intent. The CAFC noted that "inequitable conduct requires a special kind of balancing, weighing the level of materiality against the weight of the evidence of intent" 438 F.3d at 1126.

During the preparation of Purdue's patent applications the patent attorney wrote:

> It has now been *surprisingly discovered* that the presently claimed controlled release oxycodone formulations acceptably control pain over a substantially narrower, approximately four-fold [range] (10 to 40 mg every 12 hours around-the-clock dosing) in approximately 90% of patients. This is in sharp contrast to the approximately eight-fold range required for approximately 90% of patients for opioid analgesics in general.

438 F.3d at 1127 (emphasis in original and quoting the '912 patent, col. 3, 11. 34–41.) However, Purdue did not have any scientific data to support this statement. Although scientific results are not always required for patentability, the manner in which the invention is described to the Office is very important. Here, Purdue repeatedly argued to the Office that the 4-fold dosage range and more efficient titration process was the "surprising discovery" that distinguished the invention from the prior art. A declaration was even submitted during prosecution further leading one to believe that comparative studies had been conducted. In fact, an inventor testified at trial that the invention was based solely on his insight. Although the trial court agreed that Purdue never explicitly told the Office that clinical trials had been performed, the Court found that Purdue's representations during prosecution of the applications when considered together implied to the Office that the clinical trials had been performed to support the "surprising discovery." The actions by Purdue that resulted in the implication that scientific results supported the date included: referring to the 4-fold range as a "result"; emphasizing the clinical significance of the discovery; comparing the dosage range of controlled release oxycodone to that of other opioid analgesics in concise, quantitative terms (438 F.3d at 1131). Thus, the omission that the invention was predicated on insight was held to be material because the lack of scientific data supporting the discovery was inconsistent with Purdue's statements suggesting otherwise (438 F.3d at 1132).

The fact that Purdue failed to provide scientific proof supporting its "surprising discovery" was not why the Court found inequitable conduct. Inequitable conduct was found by the district court because Purdue failed to tell the Office that the discovery was based only on the inventor's insight after suggesting during prosecution that the discovery was based on results of clinical studies (438 F.3d at 1133). On appeal, the CAFC agreed with the trial court that Purdue's omission was material to the patentability of the invention and therefore, should have been disclosed to the Office. However, the omission was not as material as an affirmative misrepresentation to the Office (438 F.3d at 1133). When materiality is relatively low, the level of intent must be proportionately higher to support a finding of inequitable conduct (438 F.3d at 1134).

## PATENT TERM

A patent is awarded by individual government entities for a defined period of time. In most cases that period of time will run 20 years from the initial date of filing a nonprovisional application for patent. In some cases, term can be shortened, for example, by disclaimers of patent term in view of earlier issued patents, or lengthened, due to delays relating to appeals or regulatory approval. Provisional applications are useful for delaying the filing of a utility patent application, while simultaneously serving to establish priority over subject matter disclosed within the provisional application. However, provisional applications are not examined and will only result in a patent if a nonprovisional application is filed, which usually claims benefit of the earlier filed provisional application.

Under the revised U.S. patent law that was enacted as a result of GATT, the term of a patent issuing on a pre-GATT (i.e., filed before June 8, 1995) is seventeen years from the issue date or twenty years from the original date of filing or the filing date of the earlier nonprovisional application to which priority is claimed, whichever is greater; for patents issuing on applications filed post-GATT, only the 20-year term is applicable. The one year period between filing a provisional application and filing a nonprovisional patent application is not included in the term of the patent. Applicants therefore have more incentive to prosecute all claims related to a single invention in a single application in order to minimize costs for prosecuting and maintaining the patent and maximize available patent term. Under the law in effect prior to June 8, 1995, the patent term was seventeen years from the date of issue in the United States. Divisional and continuation applications were a commonly used method to extend patent protection to encompass different aspects of the technology over a period of time much greater than 17 years. For example, an application would be filed in 1990, and a single inventive concept (e.g., the composition) would be prosecuted in the first application. Three years later, when those claims were allowable and a patent was to issue, a divisional application would be filed with another set of the claims that had been restricted out of the original application. This divisional application would be prosecuted for another two to three years, the claims would be determined to be allowable, the second patent would issue with a 17-year term, and a third divisional application would be filed. The result is that patents on related technology would issue sequentially over several years, increasing the effective term of patent protection beyond twenty years. This is not possible under current law.

The GATT was signed into law in the United States on December 7, 1994, and the initial provisions affecting U.S. patent practice were implemented June 8, 1995. The most significant changes arising from enactment of that agreement, now called Uruguay Round Act, were changes in the patent term in the United States, the implementation of provisional patent applications, and the broadening of what constitutes infringement in the United States. The change in patent term has been discussed above. For those applications filed before June 8, 1995, the term of any issuing patent is seventeen years from the date of issue or twenty years from the filing date, whichever is longer. The term of any patent issued on an application filed June 8, 1995 or later is twenty years from the earliest claimed nonprovisional priority date. Extensions of terms are available upon delays in issuance arising from appeals or interferences. Additional extensions of terms are available for delays in obtaining regulatory approval by the Food & Drug Administration (FDA) for a device or a drug.

## Patent Term Extensions

Delays in examination, with many patents now not being examined for more than three years after filing and more stringent examination proceeding under 35 U.S.C. §112 (enablement and written description) in the bio-technology area and prior art in the pharmaceutical area, have led to many patents not issuing for at least as many as five to seven years from the original priority date. The result is that a high percentage of biotechnology and pharmaceutical patents have a substantially shortened term compared to preGATT patent terms. Because a patent extension can still be obtained for delays due to regulatory issues involving the FDA, as well as for appeals to the Board of Patent Appeals and Interferences, those in the United States who believe that their patent rights will be limited in term due to delays in prosecution should avail themselves of the Patent Extension Act, if at all possible. One must bear in mind, however, that an extension for regulatory delays can only be obtained on *one* patent for any particular product or process; thus, the inventor or licensee with multiple, related patents clearly should choose the most important patent or the patent subject to the greatest increase in patent term, when facing such a situation. The patent that is to be extended must be brought to the attention of the FDA, immediately following FDA approval of the product.

The right to a patent term extension based upon regulatory review is the result of the Drug Price Competition and Patent Term Restoration Act of 1984, Pub. L. No. 98-417, 98 Stat. 1585 (codified at 21 U.S.C. § 355(b), (j), (l); 35

U.S.C. § 156, 271, 282) (Hatch-Waxman Act). The act sought to eliminate two distortions to the normal "patent term produced by the requirement that certain products must receive premarket regulatory approval" (22). The first distortion was that the patent owner loses patent term during the early years of the patent because the product cannot be commercially marketed without approval from a regulatory agency. The second distortion occurred after the end of the patent term because competitors could not immediately enter the market upon expiration of the patent because they were not allowed to begin testing and other activities necessary to receive FDA approval before patent expiration.

The part of the act codified as 35 U.S.C. § 156 was designed to create new incentives for research and development of certain products subject to premarket government approval by a regulatory agency. The statute enables the owners of patents on certain human drugs, food or color additives, medical devices, animal drugs, and veterinary biological products to recover some of the patent term lost while obtaining premarket approval from a regulatory agency. The rights derived from extension of the patent term are limited to the approved product [as defined in 35 U.S.C. § 156(a)(4) and (a)(5); see also 35 U.S.C. § 156(b)]. Accordingly, if the patent claims other products in addition to the approved product, the exclusive patent rights to the additional products expire with the original expiration date of the patent.

This issue was addressed by the CAFC in *Pfizer v. Dr. Reddy's Laboratories*, which involved the drug amlodipine. Pfizer owned two patents with claims directed to amlodipine and pharmaceutically acceptable salts thereof. Amlodipine is marketed as Norvasc®. Pfizer obtained FDA approval to market and sell the besylate salt of amlodipine. During the approval process, Pfizer submitted clinical data for both the besylate salt of amlodipine as well as the maleate salt. Ultimately, Pfizer decided to market the besylate salt due to its greater ease of tableting. Pfizer's patent on amlodipine was to expire in 2003, but under the Act, the patent term was extended to 2006.

Dr. Reddy's Laboratories, a generic pharmaceutical manufacturer, filed an Abbreviated New Drug Application (ANDA) proposing to market the maleate salt of amlodipine. A New Drug Application (NDA) is required when approval is being sought for a new chemical entity. In contrast, an ANDA is filed when the applicant is seeking to market a generic version of a drug that has already been approved by the FDA. The filer of the ANDA is allowed to rely on the clinical data submitted in the NDA to show safety and efficacy, thus dramatically reducing the cost and time associated with approval. In the case of amlodipine, Dr. Reddy's based its application on the clinical data that Pfizer submitted in its NDA for amlodipine besylate.

The question before the Court was whether the extension applied to all forms of amlodipine, or only to the form that Pfizer actually marketed and sold (the besylate salt). Dr. Reddy's argued that the patent term extension applied only to the besylate salt of amlodipine and therefore, patent term for other salts of amlodipine, such as the maleate salt, expired in 2003. Pfizer disagreed and sued Dr. Reddy's for patent infringement, claiming that the patent term extension applied to all forms of amlodipine. The trial court agreed with Dr. Reddy's and dismissed Pfizer's lawsuit. The trial court's rationale was that the patent term extension was limited to amlodipine besylate because the act limits such extensions to "the product's first permitted commercial marketing or use."

Pfizer appealed to the CAFC. On appeal, Dr. Reddy's argued, in its request for an extension, Pfizer had identified the besylate salt as the approved product and therefore, the extension should apply to this product only. In contrast, Pfizer argued that the FDA's approval described the approved product as simply "amlodipine." Pfizer also argued that the commercial marketing and use are the same for the amlodipine maleate and that the choice of salt does not affect the activity of the active agent-amlodipine. It was Pfizer's position that if a change in the salt removes amlodipine from the Act's term extension benefit to the patent owner, it also removes it from the Act's counterpart benefits to the generic manufacturer. Thus, Dr. Reddy's could not rely on Pfizer's clinical data for FDA approval. The appellate court took notice of the fact that Dr. Reddy's ANDA relied on Pfizer's clinical data for both salts. The CAFC held that the active ingredient is amlodipine and therefore the drug is the same regardless of the salt. The CAFC said that the purpose of the Act is to strike a balance between preserving the innovation incentive by allowing for patent term extension and facilitating generic entry into the marketplace when that extended term expires. Thus, giving Dr. Reddy's the benefit of the Act, while denying the corresponding benefit to the patent owner, would defeat the intent of the Act. The Court reversed the dismissal of Pfizer's patent infringement claim.

35 U.S.C. § 271(e) provides that it shall not be an act of infringement to make and test a patented human or animal drug solely for the purpose of developing and submitting information for an ANDA. 35 U.S.C. § 271(e) (1). See Donald O. Beers, Generic and Innovator Drugs: A Guide to FDA Approval Requirements, Fifth Edition, Aspen Law & Business, 1999, 4.3[2] for a discussion of the Hatch-Waxman Act and infringement litigation. Congress provided that an ANDA cannot be filed until five years after the approval date of the product if the active ingredient or a salt or ester of the active ingredient had not been previously approved under section 505(b) of the Federal Food, Drug and Cosmetic Act. 21 U.S.C. 355(j) (4)(D)(ii) (23,24).

35 U.S.C. §156 also provides for interim extension of a patent where a product claimed by the patent was expected to be approved, but not until after the original expiration date of the patent. Public Law 103-179, Section 5.

An application for the extension of the term of a patent under 35 U.S.C. § 156 must be submitted by the owner of record of the patent or its agent within the 60-day period beginning on the date the product received permission for commercial marketing or use under the provision of law under which the applicable regulatory review period occurred for commercial marketing or use [see 35 U.S.C. § 156(d)(1)]. The USPTO initially determines whether the application is formally complete and whether the patent is eligible for extension. The statute requires the Director of the Patent and Trademark Office to notify the Secretary of Agriculture or the Secre-tary of Health and Human Services of the submission of an application for extension of patent term which complies with 35 U.S.C. § 156 within sixty days and to submit to the Secretary a copy of the application. Not later than thirty days after receipt of the application from the Direc-tor, the Secretary will determine the length of the applicable regula-tory review period and notify the Director of the determination. If the Director determines that the patent is eligible for extension, the Director calculates the length of extension for which the patent is eligible under the appropriate.

## INFRINGEMENT

In addition to changes in patent term and creation of provisional patent applications, passage of the GATT changed the definition of infringement in the United States. One who, without authority, makes, uses, offers to sell, or sells any patented invention, within the United States or imports into the United States any patented invention during the term of the patent therefore, infringes the patent (24). In the United States, a claim for infringement cannot be made until after issuance of the patent. In some other countries, including the European Patent Convention countries, translated claims can be filed prior to issuance of the patent and damages can be backdated to the date of filing the translated claim, once the patent issues.

A party who believes that an issued U.S. patent is not valid may file a request for re-examination, citing art that was not made of record during the prosecution of the patent. If the patent is asserted against the party, that party may go into federal district court and ask for a declaratory judgment that the patent claims are invalid or that they are not infringed. In Europe, and in many other countries, there is a postgrant opposition proceeding available. In the European Patent Office, there is also a process whereby one may file observations during the prosecution of an application, which is public, unlike in the United States. Third party observations can be used as a means to bring relevant prior art, mischaracterized prior art, or problems relating to enablement to the attention of the European patent examiner, and may result in revocation. In the United States, a party can file a request for re-examination to bring additional art to the attention of the Patent

Office. There is also a limited procedure available during prosecution for a third party to submit prior art.

As is now evident, intellectual property rights help increase the value of technology. This is easiest to place in perspective and understand in relation to patents. Patents give the patent owner the right to exclude competition. This is accomplished by asserting the patent against third parties who are marketing a product or service which falls within the scope of the claims. Referred to as "infringement," the criteria are totally different from the criteria for obtaining a patent, referred to as "patentability." In simple terms, a patent claim consists of "elements" in a defined relationship. Certain phrases expand or limit the scope of the claim. For example, the term "comprising" can be translated as "including at least," while "consisting" means "including only" If a claim reads

Composition comprising:

A,

B, and

C,

then the claim would cover any composition including A, B, C and any other component. Use of the term "consisting" would restrict the claim to a composition including *only* A, B and C. In determining infringement, one must look to the claims of the patent. Claims may be clear on their face, or require reference to the specification, or description, of the patent. Claims also may be limited by amendments or arguments made during prosecution, a doctrine referred to as "file wrapper estoppel." For example, if the prosecuting attorney argues that the claims distinguish over the prior art on the basis that the prior art does not disclose a particular feature that the attorney argues is essential to the claims in the patent, then the claims will be construed to require that limitation, even if not explicitly recited in the claims as issued.

## TRADE SECRETS, COPYRIGHTS, AND TRADEMARKS

Other types of intellectual property that may have applicability to drug delivery technology include trade secrets, and to a lesser degree copyrights and trademarks. Trade secret protection of an invention may be an appropriate alternative to patent protection for an invention or discovery, in certain competitive circumstances. Copyrights and trademarks, which do not protect ideas or inventions, may have value in protecting other facets of a business related to the drug delivery technology. These three types of intellectual property are only briefly described below.

### Trade Secrets

Trade secrets can be compositions or methods of manufacture or even uses that are maintained in secrecy. Most companies that have optimized methods for manufacture (e.g., methods for processing polymers to impart the most desirable physical and chemical properties) keep them secret. Trade secrets are unlimited in term but must be actively protected; they are lost if another party independently derives the same method or composition that is being maintained as a trade secret. Unlike patents, trade secrets are defined by and enforced pursuant to state laws. Trade secrets may be protected by asserting laws relating specifically to trade secrets, as well as unfair competition and business practices.

In order to maintain the process or product as a trade secret, one must (*i*) not disclose the process or product in public and (*ii*) must take affirmative steps to protect the information from public disclosure. This duty includes informing parties who may accidentally become aware of the technology, as well as those who are intentionally informed regarding the technology, that the material is a trade secret and is to be maintained in confidence. Laboratory notebooks describing processes or products that are considered proprietary should be maintained in designated areas labeled confidential or restricted access. Employees involved in the use of the trade secrets should be informed that the material is to be maintained as confidential and that breach of any agreement with the company by disclosing the trade secrets to a third party could result in irreparable harm and therefore be subject to injunctive relief. Trade secrets cease to be trade secrets upon public disclosure, as discussed above, or when they are independently developed by another party. If a third party independently develops the trade secret, the original holder of the trade secret has no recourse unless he can prove that the secret was acquired by theft, fraud, or other improper means. Unlike patents, which have a defined term during which the patentee can exclude others from competition, trade secrets are subject to no similar limitation. One of the most famous trade secrets is the formula for the original Coca-Cola® which has been kept in secret for decades and is enormously valuable, demonstrating that it is not just patents that have value as an asset to a company.

## Copyrights

Copyright protects original works of authorship fixed in any tangible medium of expression (25). Unlike patent and trade secret law however, copyrights do not protect an idea, rather only the expression of that idea. Copyright protection may extend, for example, to visual depictions of products, or to advertising material associated with the use and sale of products. Also, copyright may protect computer software programs, publications, protocols, or other materials. In many cases where the author is employed or engaged as a consultant, the copyrights will be owned by the party contracting with the author, the journal publishing the work, or the employer. Copyrights, which also can be extremely valuable, are transferable and enforceable under U.S. law and in many foreign jurisdictions, as a result of international agreements relating to copyrights.

## Trademarks

Trademarks typically are associated with the sale of goods or services and are used to denote the origin of the goods or services. Advantages of trademarks are that they are not limited in term and rights arise upon use in either intra- or interstate commerce. One very well-known trademark is Coca-Cola®, which has been in continuous use for over 100 years. The company has used the trademark in combination with retaining the formula as a trade secret to create enormous value for the company. A company name, as well as a product name, can be a trademark. A trademark can be a name design or combination thereof. The trademark cannot be generic or totally descriptive of the product, and it must be distinct enough from other trademarks in a similar field of use or similar good or service to avoid any likelihood of confusion as to the origin of the good or service among the consumers of the trademark good or service. Trademarks can be protected under either state or federal law. An applicant for a trademark registration must show that the trademark has been used in *intra*state commerce for a state registration and *inter*state commerce for a federal registration. A federal "intent to use" application can be used to preserve the right to use a trademark prior to actual use in commerce. This provides for an initial determination of the registerability of the trademark, i.e., that the mark is not already in use by another in a way that would be confusingly similar to the applicant's use, and that the mark is not generic or descriptive, and not contrary to the public interest.

## SUMMARY

Intellectual property rights provide a means for the owners of technology to recover their investment in the technology and, in some cases, to make a profit. More importantly, intellectual property rights provide a means for financing the incredibly expensive research and development and testing required for commercialization of new products and processes in the medical and biotechnology field. When the intellectual property rights have been lost or given away by publication, many times it is not possible to obtain the money required to see a product or process reach the clinic and benefit those for whom it is intended. It is only by protecting the technology that it can be used to help those who need it the most.

## ACKNOWLEDGMENTS

The author would like to thank Charles Vorndran, Ph.D and Michael J. Terapane, Ph.D for their contributions to this chapter.

## REFERENCES

1. 35 U.S.C. § 101(1988).
2. *Diamond v. Chakrabarty*, 447 U.S. 303, 206 U.S.P.Q. 193 (1980).
3. 35 U.S.C. § 102(1988).
4. *Philips Elec. & Pharmaceutical Indus. Corp. v. Thermal & Elec. Indus., Inc.*, 450 F.2d 1164, 1169–72, 171 U.S.P.Q. 641 (3d Cir. 1971); Gulliksen v. Halberg, 75 U.S.P.Q. 252 (Pat. Off. Bd. Int'f. 1937).
5. *Ciba-Geigy Corp. v. Alza Corp.*, 864 F. Supp. 429, 33 U.S.P.Q.2d 1018 (D.N.J. 1994).
6. See 35 U.S.C. § 103(1998).
7. *Graham v. John Deere Co.*, 383 U.S. 1, 148 U.S.P.Q. 459 (1966).
8. *KSR Int'l Co. v. Teleflex, Inc.*, 127 S. Ct. 1727, 82 U.S.P.Q.2d 1385 (2007).
9. *Univ. of Rochester v. G.D. Searle*, 358 F.3d 916, 921 (Fed. Cir. 2004).
10. *Reifflin v. Microsoft Corp.*, 214 F.3d 1342, 1345 (Fed. Cir. 2000).
11. *Enzo Biochem, Inc. v. Gen-Probe Inc.*, 323 F.3d 956, 963 (Fed. Cir. 2002).
12. *Hyatt v. Boone*, 146 F.3d 1348, 1353 (Fed. Cir. 1998).
13. 35 U.S.C. § 122(b).
14. *Pfizer, Inc. v. Ranbaxy Laboratories, Ltd.*, 405 F.Supp.2d 495 (D. Del. 2005).
15. *Pfizer, Inc. v. Ranbaxy Laboratories, Ltd.*, 79 U.S.P.Q.2d 1583 (Fed. Cir. 2006).
16. U.S. Const., art. 1, §8, cl. 8.
17. 35 U.S.C. § 111(1988).
18. 35 U.S.C. § 116(1988).
19. 35 U.S.C. § 256(1988).
20. 37 C.F.R. §§1.56, 1.97, 1.98 (1996).
21. *Purdue Pharma, L.P. v. Endo Pharmaceuticals, Inc.* 438 F.3d 1123, 77 USPQ2d 1767 (Fed. Cir. 2006).
22. *Eli Lilly & Co. v. Medtronic Inc.*, 496 U.S. 661, 669, 15 USPQ2d 1121, 1126 (1990).
23. *Lourie, Patent Term Restoration: History, Summary, and Appraisal, 40 Food, Drug and Cosmetic* L. J. 351, 353–60 (1985).
24. Lourie, Patent Term Restoration, 66 J. Pat. Off. Soc'y 526 (1984)
25. 35 U.S.C. § 271(1988).
26. 17 U.S.C. §§ 101–1101(1996 & Supp. 1997).

# 2

# Intellectual Property Developments and Issues in India

## B. Kombi

*Remfry & Sagar, New Delhi, India*

## INTRODUCTION

The present chapter deals generally with the intellectual property issues; especially pharmaceutical patent issues and more particularly, issues relating to "controlled drug delivery technology." The chapter will briefly deal with these issues giving a perspective to the reader about intellectual property in India, in particular pharmaceutical patents and the challenges arising out of them. The chapter will also provide the reader a bird's eye view of the law and practice governing these issues in the prevailing scenario.

## INTELLECTUAL PROPERTY ISSUES IN INDIA

A decade and a half ago, India's burgeoning population was deemed the villain impeding her developmental process. How the tables have turned! A leading daily recently ran the following headline—"Thank God We Failed at Population Control." Having neglected the value of abundant human and intellectual capital for so long, the process of coaxing the necessary fundamentals into place in various socioeconomic sectors, including the legal one, is now on at full steam.

India has a very strong and well-established administrative and judicial framework, which is extremely dynamic and constantly reforming to safeguard intellectual property rights in India covering all fields, namely, patents, trademarks, copyrights, and industrial designs. The Indian trademarks law, now also being extended to service marks, is strong, with more and more goods and service marks being registered and protected in the process.

The Copyright Act has been successfully used by many software and database companies to curtail piracy.

Protection of intellectual property rights continues to strengthen further with an appreciable dynamism and endeavor to be in harmony with the International law and practices and in compliance with India's obligation under Trade Related Aspects of Intellectual Property Rights (TRIPS). These include:

1. The Patents (Amendment) Act, 2005, amending the Patents Act, 1970, that provides for protection of product patents in all fields of technology, such as food, pharmaceuticals, and chemicals.
2. The Trade Mark Act, 1999, replacing the Trade and Merchandise Marks Act, 1958.
3. The Copyright (Amendment) Act, 1999, amending the Copyright Act of 1957.
4. The Designs Act, 2000, replacing the Designs Act, 1911.

The changes have been most pronounced in the field of patents. The inventions along with rights of the applicants have been safe guarded by the Indian Patents Act, enacted in the year 1970. In last ten years, Indian patent law has been amended from time to time in order to meet India's obligation under the TRIPS. It now also provides for the grant of a patent for a uniform term of twenty years from the filing of a patent application, which is in harmony with International norms.

## PHARMACEUTICAL PATENT ISSUES

As mentioned, the most visible and globally sought after changes have been in the field of our patent law. The recently amended Patents Act, which came into force with effect from January 1, 2005, has ushered in an era of a new-found milieu for foreign and national applicants to get their inventions protected under the new Act.

While the amendments have enlarged the scope of patentability in diverse fields of technology, the most pronounced and far reaching effects have been in the pharmaceutical sector.

Some of the highlights of the amendments directly affecting the patentability of pharmaceuticals are outlined below:

Inventions in the pharmaceuticals sector hitherto entitled to process patents have now become eligible for product patent protection. However, salts, esters, ethers, polymorphs, metabolites, pure form, particle size, isomers, mixtures of isomers, complexes, combinations, and other derivatives of a known substance have been excluded from patentability unless they differ significantly in properties with regard to efficacy. This forms part of the Section 3(d) of the amended Act. It is considered a major road block in the grant of a majority of pharmaceutical patent applications is under challenge in an Indian court.

Pre-grant opposition has been replaced with post-grant opposition procedure, the period for which would stretch for one year from the date of publication of grant of the patent. However, at the pending stage, there is now a provision for making a representation by way of opposition against the grant of a patent. This provision has been strengthened by making all eleven grounds of post-grant opposition applicable thereto as well as providing for a hearing at the pre-grant stage to a third party. The rules also provide for an opportunity to the applicant to file his statement and evidence in support of his application. The Indian pharmaceutical companies are particularly taking advantage of this provision and filing pre-grant representations in cases which conflict with their commercial interests. Sometimes, a single patent application faces rolling oppositions from different parties, which may also include nongovernmental organizations (NGOs) claiming to be saviors of the poor of this nation. This has a cascading effect on the grant of a patent. Thus, the new law that came into force amid a nationwide debate on the feasibility and consequences of the same still continues to stir emotions considering the rather complex sociopolitical situation existing in India.

A provision for enabling grant of compulsory licenses for export of medicines to countries that have insufficient or lack the manufacturing capacity for meeting public health emergencies has been introduced (in line with the Doha Declaration).

The law also enables a claim for damages in an infringement action retrospectively from the date of publication and not from the date of acceptance of the patent application as was provided earlier. However, in the case of mailbox applications covering pharmaceutical products filed prior to January 1, 2005, damages can be claimed only from the date of grant.

A patent holder in respect of a patent granted on a mailbox application is prohibited from instituting an infringement suit against enterprises which have made significant investment and were producing and marketing the concerned product prior to January 1, 2005 and which continue to manufacture the product covered by the patent on the date of grant of the patent. The patent holder shall only be entitled to receive reasonable royalty from such enterprises. The denial of injunctive relief to a patent holder is unprecedented and *ex-facie* violates the letter and spirit of the TRIPS Agreement as well as our Constitutional norms. We expect that sooner, rather than later, this amendment would be put to test in the highest instance.

## CONTROLLED-DRUG-RELEASE TECHNOLOGY PATENT ISSUES

It would be pertinent to understand a few important provisions of the new law, which directly or indirectly affect the patentability of the very specific "controlled-drug-release technology."

Under the Indian patent law, an invention is defined as a new product or process involving an inventive step and capable of industrial application; wherein the "inventive step" means a feature of an invention that involves a technical advance as compared to the existing knowledge or having economic significance or both and that makes the invention not obvious to a person skilled in the art.

A new invention is defined as "any invention or technology which has not been anticipated by publication in any document or used in the country or elsewhere in the world before the date of filing of the patent application with the complete specifications, i.e., the subject matter has not fallen in public domain or that it does not form a part of the state of the art."

In the context of the preceding paragraphs, it would thus mean that an invention relating to modified release drug delivery technology would be patentable under the Indian patents law if it is *novel, inventive*, and possesses *industrial applicability*.

A patent application for a drug delivery technology could be filed in India as an application directed towards a novel product or process obtained by employing the drug release technology.

For instance, in case of dry powder formulations, development may include powder recrystallization, formulation, dispersion, delivery, and deposition of the therapeutic agent in different regions of the target area.

In case the invention claims a process, Indian practice requires the main process claim to define all the starting materials, process steps and parameters viz. temperature, pressure, molar ratio of reactants, etc. that are critical to the novelty and inventiveness of the claimed process.

It must be noted here that dosage forms *per se* are not allowable under Indian Practice. However, such forms are generally allowable as either a product which is a result of a chemical reaction or a synergistic composition. In case what is being claimed is a modified drug release formulation with a single active component, the surprising properties of the product should also be indicated clearly in the description by way of data to overcome a rejection under Section 3(e) of the Act, if any which precludes from patentability mere admixtures of the known substances which results in aggregation of the properties of the components thereof or a process for producing such substance.

In other cases, as a practice, to overcome the objection under Section 3(e), it becomes necessary to incorporate specific ranges for the amount of individual components broadly expressed as molar ratios or percentage (w/w), in the main composition/formulation claim. It is generally understood that unless the specific amounts of the individual components is disclosed, the composition will not show synergism.

*Section 3(d)* of the Patents Act precludes patentability of the "mere discovery of a new form of a known substance which does not result in the enhancement of the known efficacy of that substance or the mere discovery of any new property or the new use for a known substance or of the mere use of a known process, machine or apparatus unless such known process results in a new product or employs at least one new reactant."

"For the purpose of this clause, salts, esters, ethers, polymorphs, metabolites, pure form, particle size, isomers, mixtures of isomers, complexes, combinations and other derivatives of known substance shall be considered to be the same substance, unless they differ significantly in the properties with regard to efficacy."

The above-mentioned provision is peculiar to the patent law and possesses a major challenge to the patent applications relating to derivatives.

A major aspect of Section 3(d) that has been left undefined in the Act is the definition of the term "enhanced efficacy."

The parameters that will assess the "enhanced efficacy" are not defined within the provisions of the said Section. 'Enhanced efficacy' as stated in the section 3(d) of the Patents Act could be interpreted as comparative assessment with respect to clinical parameters such as bioequivalence study, clinical trial data, or a comparative preclinical data. Section 3(d) as stated may also provide room for establishing enhanced efficacy by comparative evaluation with respect to non clinical parameters such as enhanced stability, better *in vitro* dissolution or a stability profile which directly or indirectly translates to enhanced availability of the active in the in vivo system. However, generally the Indian examiners give consideration to the clinical data supporting the efficacy over biophysical parameters.

The case law is still developing in this regard. Interestingly, in a recent case, the Indian patent office rejected an application under Section 3(d), even though the applicants provided data evidencing 30% enhanced bioavailability of the claimed polymorph. The case is under an appeal in the Indian Court of Law.

## SUMMARY

The Indian government, being fully aware of the implications of deviations, such as issues relating to Section 3(d) from being fully TRIPS compliant, had constituted a high-level technical committee, called Mashelkar Committee, to look into the various issues, particularly the one relating to the allowance of new forms of known substances. The report of this technical committee that was submitted to the government on December 29, 2006 and states that the amended law is ostensibly not in compliance with the TRIPS obligations, especially with respect to restriction of patentability on new forms of known substances. However, this report generated alot of controversy from several quarters including the left parties, non-governmental organizations, public health groups, and the Indian generic drug industry. Some sections even alleged plagiarism, stating that the report contains verbatum reproduction of passages from a published paper.

Following the large scale criticism of the report, in an upprecedente twist, the technical Expert Group on patent Law Issues withdrew its report on February 23, 2007. Thereafter, the chairman of this committee, Mr. R.A. Mashelkar resigned from this past. Till date, no substantial development has taken place in the regard.

# 3

# Parameter Claims at the European Patent Office

## Peter Klusmann

*Hoffmann-Eitle, Munich, Germany*

## INTRODUCTION

A good invention deserves good patent protection. There can be no doubt about this. Yet, this is easier said than done, and it is clearly one of the most frustrating experiences for an inventor when his good invention is denied protection for reasons unrelated to the invention as such. Unfair as it seems, this is not a rare event. In the pharmaceutical arts and especially in inventions relating to formulations, a frequent source for such frustrations are so-called parameter claims.

Parameter claims define the subject matter for which protection is sought in terms of one or more parameters reflecting physical characteristics or performance related characteristics of the invention. For example, steel compositions are normally defined in terms of their chemical compositions. An example of this might be a claim to steel characterized by containing 2% by weight of carbon, 3% by weight of chromium and a balance of iron. The description may show that such a steel has advantageous properties such as high melting point, high tensile strength and high hardness.

An ambitious Applicant could however seek to define this steel not by its composition but instead in terms of its properties, namely by reference to parameters such as high melting point, tensile strength and hardness. Such a claim might be directed to a steel having a melting point greater than $T\,^{\circ}C$, a tensile strength greater than $S\ N/m^2$ and a hardness greater than H Vickers units. As it is only based upon parameters, it would provide the Applicant with a much broader protective scope than the composition-type claim. It is not restricted to the composition being formed from any particular components, but it instead covers the steel whatever its composition as long as it has the (desirable) parameters, which are defined. While this makes a parameter claim attractive for an applicant, it also makes it very unattractive for an examiner. This is particularly true in the field of pharmaceutical formulations where many examples for parameter claims e.g., defining certain release profiles can be found. However, not everything that is popular is also a good and safe idea.

## BASIC CONSIDERATIONS

Parameter claims need to meet the same patentability requirements as any other type of claim, i.e., they must be novel and inventive. Furthermore, Art. 84 EPC (European Patent Convention) requires that the claims "shall be clear and concise and be supported by the description." The exact meaning of the term "clear" is open to interpretation, but this Article is normally taken to mean that a claim must provide a definite boundary between subject matter that is claimed and subject matter that is not so that there is no ambiguity as to whether a given activity falls within or outside the scope of the claim. As for the support requirement, this is understood to mean that the scope of a claim should not be so broad that it extends beyond the inventive subject matter, which is actually disclosed in the application.

Art. 83 EPC requires that the subject matter of the patent is disclosed "in a manner sufficiently clear and complete for it to be carried out by a person skilled in the art." The effect of this is that a skilled worker must be able to carry out the invention over the entire scope of the claims without undue burden using only the information contained in the specification and his general knowledge.

## TYPES OF PARAMETER CLAIMS

The simple case is a parameter claim wherein the parameter reflects the result to be achieved, but not the means to do so. Such claims are quaintly known as "free beer" claims. They, as a rule, find no mercy with the European Patent Office (EPO) examiners. One of the reasons claims of this type are considered objectionable is that it may well be that the prior art comprises a product that has the properties defined by the parameter without actually mentioning it. Although such prior art would anticipate the desideratum claim, the Search Examiner has little or no chance of finding it. Therefore, an adequate prior art search cannot be carried out. This puts the Examiner in a difficult situation. Not being able to search in a meaningful way does not mean that the invention is patentable. In an attempt to overcome this problem, the examiner will typically question the support of the claim by stating that the application does not contain enough information to meet the claimed parameter in all cases.

Once a case for lack of disclosure has been made by an EPO Examiner, the onus is on the Applicant to prove the contrary. As the Applicant typically is not in a position to do so, such claims typically do not go far in the EPO.

A second group of parameter claims that typically do not go far in the EPO are claims that are based on "creative parameters." "Creative parameters" are parameters that the Applicant devises to define the invention. Some applicants are more creative in imagining new parameters than they are in inventing new technology. Popular types of "creative parameters" are composite parameters, i.e., parameters that put unrelated properties into a mathematical relationship. Such parameters are generally viewed in a particularly unfavorable light by the EPO, because a comparison with the prior art is rendered impossible by virtue of the new parameter itself.

In their approach to such claims, the examiners are guided by the EPO examination Guidelines. Section C-III, 4.7a of the Guidelines states that: "… where the invention relates to a product it may be defined in a claim in various ways, viz. as a chemical product, by its chemical formula, as a product of a process (if no clearer definition is possible) or exceptionally by its parameters.

Parameters are characteristic values, which may be values of directly measurable properties (e.g., the melting point of a substance, the flexural strength of a steel, the resistance of an electrical conductor) or may be defined as more or less complicated mathematical combinations of several variables in the form of formulae.

Characterization of a product mainly by its parameters should only be allowed in those cases where the invention cannot be adequately defined in any other way, provided that those parameters can be clearly and reliably determined either by indications in the description or by objective procedures that are usual in the art (see T 94/82). The same applies to a process related feature that is defined by parameters. Cases in which unusual parameters are employed or a nonaccessible apparatus for measuring the parameter(s) is used are *prima facie* objectionable on grounds of lack of clarity, as no meaningful comparison with the prior art can be made. Such cases might also disguise a lack of novelty."

Such an approach was followed in the Decision T 12/81 where the Appeal Board stated that it is permissible to make the definition of a chemical substance more precise by additional product parameters such as melting point, hydrophilic properties, NMR coupling constant or product-by-process claims if the substance cannot be defined by a sufficiently accurate generic formula.

While one may say that "obvious desiderata" and "creative parameter" claims are extremes, they illustrate the general approach and difficulties with parameters of any kind. In addition, they also caused the EPO to apply stricter rules to all parameters, including those that are included in the claims for a good reason.

This rigorous policy is also reflected in the Examination Guidelines, Section C-IV, 7.5, which frequently provides the basis for novelty objections against parameter claims:

> In the case of a prior document, the lack of novelty may be apparent from what is explicitly stated in the document itself. Alternatively, it may be implicit in the sense that, in carrying out the teaching of the prior document, the skilled person would inevitably arrive at a result falling within the terms of the claim. An objection of lack of novelty of this kind should be raised by the Examiner only where there can be no reasonable doubt as to the practical effect of the prior teaching. Situations of this kind may also occur when the claims define the invention, or a feature thereof, by parameters. It may happen that in the relevant prior art a different parameter, or no parameter at all, is mentioned. If the known and the claimed products are identical in all other respects (which is to be expected if, for example, the starting products and the manufacturing processes are identical), then in the first place an objection of lack of novelty arises. If the Applicant is able to show, e.g., by appropriate comparison tests, that differences do exist with respect to the parameters, it is questionable whether the application discloses all the features essential to manufacture products having the parameters specified in the claims (Art. 83).

This approach actually puts the Applicant into an unfortunate squeeze. While a prior art document may not make it clear that a particular parameter requirement of the claim under consideration is fulfilled, the Examiner may decide that this is inevitably the case such that the claim is anticipated by a prior art teaching explicitly including all of the technical features of the claim apart from the parameter. In response to such prima facie novelty objection, the Applicant has little choice but to stress the importance of the parameter. This, however, then prompts an objection as to lack of sufficiency.

An example for this is the case underlying Decision T 666/89. Here the Board held that the term "made available to the public" clearly went beyond literal or diagrammatical description, and implied the communication, express or implicit, of technical information by other means as well.

One example of the available information content of a document extending beyond this literal descriptive or diagrammatical content was the case where the carrying out of the process, specifically or literally described in a prior art document, inevitably resulted in a product not described as such. In such a case, the Board stated that the prior art document would deprive a claim covering such a product of novelty. Faced with such an objection, the onus is on the Applicant to demonstrate that the parameter in question is in fact not fulfilled by the prior art teaching and that the parameter does provide a genuine technical distinction. This is normally proved by filing experimental evidence reproducing the prior art teaching and measuring the appropriate parameter.

However, even if such experimental material can be produced, the question of insufficiency remains. In order for a claim to be allowable, it must be reproducible by a person skilled in the art. Care must be taken in particular where unusual parameters are concerned to make sure that *all* the details of how the parameter is measured are fully explained, including complete experimental protocols. If it is not clear how one of the parameters is measured, or if the parameter can be measured in a variety of ways giving rise to different results, then the claim is insufficient. It is usually very difficult to rebut a technically well-founded insufficiency objection and so care must be taken to avoid this potential pitfall during drafting of the Application.

One example of this is the Decision T 225/93 where calcium carbonate particles were defined *inter alia* by means of their diameter, i.e., a parameter. However, the Opponent was able to show that there were different methods for measuring such a diameter and these did not always lead to the same result. As a consequence, the Appeal Board concluded that the disclosure was therefore insufficient. On the other hand, it was held in Decision T 492/ 92 that where it is obvious that a skilled person would select a particular analytical measuring method in the case that none is disclosed in the application in suit, the requirements of Article 83 EPC (sufficiency) are met.

A further objection often raised by Examiners when faced with parameter claims is that of lack of support and/or lack of disclosure. Such objections are based on Articles 83 and 84 EPC. These Articles can be considered to reflect the principle that the scope of a Patent claim should be justified by the inventor's contribution to the art. On this basis, an Examiner may object to a claim if he considers that the scope of the claim is so broad that it covers much more than the actual invention. This issue is addressed in the Guidelines, C-III, 6.1–6.2, which state that the extent of generalization permissible from particular examples is a matter for the Examiner to decide, and that a fair claim is one that is not so broad that it goes beyond the invention nor so narrow that it deprives the Applicant of a just reward for the disclosure of the invention.

At present, two contrasting lines of EPO case law exist regarding support and disclosure. According to a first approach, the full breadth of the claim must be supported and disclosed. This generally means that a reasonable number of Examples have to be included in the description spread out over the entire scope of the claim such that it is made credible that the technical advantages associated with the invention can in fact be achieved over the its entire scope. This approach is exemplified by T 409/91. In this particular case, the Applicant had invented a fuel additive that imparted very good, low temperature characteristics to fuel oil. The additive worked by preventing the formation of wax crystals, which were known to cause problems by blocking fuel filters. Rather than claiming the additive itself however, the claim was directed to a fuel oil having a very small wax crystal concentration at very low temperatures. The claim was refused because it was a desideratum claim that made no mention of the additive at all. The Examining Division argued that the claim was not supported over the whole of its breadth.

According to a second school of thought, the scope of a claim can be as broad as the prior art allows and should not be challenged on grounds of support unless tangible facts are produced that prove that the given scope is unreasonable. According to this doctrine, even a single Example may be sufficient to support a broad claim. This doctrine is typified by Decisions such as T 19/90 where a single disclosure of a genetically modified mouse was held to support a broad claim to "nonhuman mammals" that were genetically modified according to the invention.

Because of these two conflicting lines of case law, plausible arguments against a lack of support objection can be made by reference to the "one way" case law. However, if the Examiner is not receptive to such argumentation and maintains his objection that the scope of the claim is too broad, then it will be difficult to overcome such an objection given that the case law supports both approaches. Furthermore, the Examiner can also rely on C-III, 6.2 of the Guidelines, which states that the level of generalization allowable in claim drafting is a matter for the Examiner to decide.

As illustrated above, it is already rather hard to obtain a patent based on parameter claims. However, this is not the end of the difficulties as such claims are also rather vulnerable in post-grant proceedings such as opposition proceedings. This is the result of Article 123(3) EPC, which states that the claims of a Patent may not be amended during Opposition proceedings such that the scope of protection is extended. If, for example, an insufficiency objection is raised against a parameter claim during Opposition proceedings, this can cause the Proprietor to find himself in an inescapable trap whereby the parameter cannot be kept in the claim due to the insufficiency problem but on the other hand cannot be removed because the parameter constitutes a restriction and so its removal would broaden the claim. For this reason, it is particularly important when drafting claims to ensure that the experimental procedure underlying any parameter in a claim is fully described in order to avoid being caught in this trap.

## BENEFITS OF PARAMETER CLAIMS

The above shows that significant difficulties can arise when prosecuting parameter claims at the EPO because of the multiple types of objections that the Examiner can, and as a rule will, raise. Nonetheless, parameter claims are very popular among European Applicants as they provide broad protection and leave little room for design-arounds. This is understandable, but risky if the Applicant does not take utmost care and appreciates the potential pitfalls.

## HOW TO DRAFT PARAMETER-CLAIM APPLICATIONS

When drafting parameter claims one has to expect that the Examiner will raise at least one of the objections that have been discussed, and it is quite possible that the Examiner will maintain his objection regardless of any counter arguments that are filed. For this reason, it is generally not advisable to file these claims unless it really is the case that the invention cannot be adequately defined in any other way. In this case, great care must be taken to ensure that the parameters are well characterized in terms of their measurement and should not be directed to clearly obvious desiderata of the product in question. For instance, a claim to a conductive wire characterized by having a volume resistivity below a certain critical value may not be patentable regardless of the prior art and the actual value of the volume resistivity because the claim is clearly drawn to a desirable objective.

Well-founded insufficiency objections can be very bad news for any claim, particularly so during Opposition due to Article 123(3) EPC that means that it may not be possible to remove an insufficient feature from a claim post-grant if this removal extends the scope of protection. In order to avoid an insufficiency problem, it is important to ensure that all of the parameters used are repeatably measurable and unambiguously defined in the description before filing the application. In doing so, it is also very important to refer to measurements that are not dependent on a particular commercial apparatus as it is not guaranteed that this apparatus will be available over the entire lifetime of the patent.

Furthermore, it is important to have a backup plan in case the Examiner proves unwilling to allow the parameter claim. In such a situation, the description should be drafted to include an alternative definition of the invention in terms of more conventional features if possible that can be used to replace the parameter. The unfortunate flip side of the coin is that Section C-III-4.7a of the Examination Guidelines set out above states that parameters may only be used *where it is not possible* to define the invention conventionally. Having such a backup plan may cause the Examiner to object that it is possible to define the invention in a more conventional manner, and leaves the Applicant vulnerable to an objection based on this Section of the Guidelines. Nevertheless, having such a backup plan may save the application from refusal.

In the context of having a backup plan, it is of course also important to ensure that the relevant amendments can actually be carried out during the prosecution of the application without adding matter. For the parameter to be removable, it must not be mentioned as an essential feature of the invention throughout the description as then its removal would result in a new combination of technical features. Of course, when amending the claims during Opposition, also Art 123(3) EPC applies so that the scope of protection cannot be extended by amendment. Thus post-grant amendment at the EPO is often problematic.

When drafting the claim, it is also worthwhile to bear in mind that the presence of a parameter in a claim is more likely to lead to objection the more prominent it is in a claim. Thus the Examination Guidelines C-III-4.7a refers to situations where an invention is defined *mainly* in terms of parameters. In general, the more concrete technical features are included in the claim, the easier it is for the Examiner to compare its scope with the prior art, and so the more chance there is for the Examiner to be able to acknowledge the patentability of the claim based on some other (non-parameter) feature. Another important factor is how unusual the parameter is in the context in that it is used. Generally, Examiners are extremely reluctant to allow claims having complicated "homemade" parameters on the ground of lack of clarity. On the other hand, they are likely to be much more lenient if the parameter is a standard one such as melting point or density. It is not advisable to file claims at the EPO that include very unusual parameters unknown in the relevant technology as the Examiner will almost certainly not be very cooperative.

## EXAMPLE CASE—EP 0 819 258

This case concerns the European Phase of a PCT Patent Application filed in 1996 by Novartis relating to a contact lens capable of extended continuous wear with little or no discomfort for the user. The Application as filed contained 158 claims, 10 of these being independent claims. Claim 1 of the Application in essence read as follows:

> "*1. An ophthalmic lens* . . . *[that]* . . . allows oxygen permeation in an amount sufficient to maintain corneal health and wearer comfort during a period of extended, continuous contact with ocular tissue and ocular fluids, and
>     *wherein said lens allows ion or water permeation in an amount sufficient to enable the lens to move on the eye such that corneal health is not substantially harmed and wearer comfort is acceptable during a period of extended, continuous contact with ocular tissue and ocular fluids.*"

The International Preliminary Examination Report issued in 1997 by an EPO Examiner was not exactly promising insofar as all of the 158 claims were considered to lack novelty. Further, the Examiner stated that *inter alia* Claim 1 hardly imposed any limitation to the claimed lens and essentially defined a standard contact lens that was known at the priority date. With respect to the claims that define the invention in terms of conventional features such as the specific polymer materials used for making the lens, the Examiner reached the conclusion that these materials were all well-known in the art of making contact lenses, citing several prior art documents.

The next stage of the EPO prosecution of this case was the issuance of the first Official Action written by the same Examiner who authorized the IPER. Here, all of the 158 claims were objected to on the grounds of lack of clarity and lack of novelty with reference to his earlier reasoning expressed in the IPER. The response filed by Novartis simply added the following to claim 1:

> wherein said ophthalmic lens has an oxygen transmissibility of at least about 70 barrers/mm and an ion permeability characterized either by (1) an Ionoton Ion Permeability Coefficient of greater than about $0.2 \times 10^{-6}$ cm$^2$/sec, or (2) an Ionoflux Diffusion Coefficient of greater than about $1.5 \times 10^{-6}$ mm$^2$/min, wherein said ion permeability is measured with respect to sodium ions.

This claim further characterized by the inclusion of three parametric features that previously were to be found in three of the dependent claims. The main argument presented in the response was that the invention was in fact a major breakthrough in the field of contact lens manufacture. This bold statement was substantiated by the fact that the invention was the result of an extensive research program spanning several years and involving researchers from three continents. Further, it was explained that a contact lens that can be safely worn in the eye of a user during both day and night for several days had been sought after for a long time but so far not realized. Novartis submitted that their invention was based on the finding that the combination of high oxygen permeability and high ion permeability was what qualified materials as being suitable for forming such extended wear contact lenses, a fact that Novartis claimed had never been discussed previously in the literature. In their view, their discovery was a new fundamental concept and contact lenses that were invented on the basis of this discovery were therefore patentable. It was stated that the fundamentality and importance of this invention was reflected not only by the unusually high number of pages of the specification and many claims but also the unusually high number of inventors that had been named. As for the novelty objections that were raised, Novartis explained that none of the prior art references disclosed water and ion permeabilities falling within the parameters of the new Claim 1 and so this claim was novel. In fact none of the prior art discussed the parameters of oxygen transmissibility in terms of barrers/mm or ion permeability in terms of an Ionoton Ion Permeability Coefficient or an Ionoflux Diffusion Coefficient. These parameters were, and remain, "novel" in the sense that none of the prior art mentions them.

Accordingly, simple comparison between the claim and the prior art is precluded.

The main section of the claim corresponds exactly to original Claim 1 that the Examiner considered in the IPER to "define, in essence, merely an ophthalmic lens, e.g., a contact lens, made from oxygen and water permeable polymer material." As for the new features of this claim, these three parameters merely define extents of permeability.

The Examiner thus had a significant arsenal of objections available to him. He might have decided that the amended claim lacked novelty because the prior art disclosures, although not reciting these specific parameter values, would inevitably fulfill the requirements of the claim as it was known at the priority date of the patent to form contact lenses from a mixture of materials permeable to both oxygen and ions. Alternatively, the Examiner might have objected that the use of parameters in this case was not warranted in the light of Part C-III-4.7a given that it was clear from the dependent claims focusing on the chemistry of the lenses that the invention could be defined conventionally. The Examiner could also have argued that the scope of such a claim was not commensurate with the contribution to the art and that the description did not support such a claim over its entire scope.

The second Official Action was most surprising as the Examiner concluded that "the explanations in the Representative's letter have been read with interest and appear substantially convincing." He then listed a few relatively minor objections and concluded his letter by stating that if the specification were to be revised in order to meet these minor points then the Application could possibly proceed to grant as the next step. And this is what happened.

As one might expect, the consequences of the EPO Examiner allowing the application were significant for competitor companies. As a result the patent was opposed by both Bausch & Lomb and Johnson & Johnson in a case that came before the Opposition Division in September 2003. The result of the Hearing was the complete revocation of the patent for lack of novelty. In the end, the Opposition Division found that the Opponents had presented evidence that made it clear that the parameters were inevitably fulfilled in the prior art. Predictably, the decision was appealed by Novartis. The final outcome of this case is some way off.

## SUMMARY

When filing an application at the EPO, it is generally not generally advisable to include parameter features because the EPO are particularly suspicious about such applications. Parameter claims should be considered as an exception. This is because they fall under the category of Complex Applications, which are considered to cause problems during Examination. This is because parameter claims are often difficult to compare with the prior art, and so Examiners cannot carry out a proper assessment of their merits.

In spite of the problems associated with the prosecution of parameter claims, it must be recognized that claims of this form can be particularly valuable to Applicants. In some cases, defining an invention in terms of parameters makes it possible to get a claim having a relatively broad protective scope that extends beyond the actual invention. This may be particularly valuable in a technical area where development is rapid because such a claim is likely to encompass other solutions to the technical problem than that provided by the actual invention such that the patent obstructs competitors.

If parameter claims are filed, it is important to firstly ensure that a backup plan is available such that the parameter can be removed and replaced with more conventional technical features in the event that the Examiner cannot be persuaded to allow the parameter claim. Secondly, it is important to ensure that the parameter is sufficient by ensuring that all of the necessary measurement techniques are described in detail.

# 4

# Japan's Patent Issues Relating to Modified Drug Delivery Technology

### John A. Tessensohn
*Shusaku Yamamoto Patent Law Office, Osaka, Japan*

## INTRODUCTION

Japan's importance to the world's pharmaceutical drug marketplace is attributable to two simple facts. First, its irresistible size as the world's second largest pharmaceutical market (1). Second, Japanese pharmaceutical research and development (R&D) has a proven track record of success in the American pharmaceutical market (2,3). Therefore, it is important to understand Japanese patenting issues so that companies can make informed decisions when seeking to patent or commercialize their pharmaceutical and drug delivery inventions in Japan.

## INDUSTRIALLY APPLICABLE INVENTIONS: A MEDICAL METHOD NOT A STATUTORY MATTER

All patents must be industrially applicable under Japan's Patent Law (4). With regard to medicinal inventions, industrial applicability is very clear: anything that can be manufactured and sold is patentable subject matter in Japan, and thus compounds, compositions, and methods of making these products are patentable. Furthermore, methods of controlling the operation of medical devices are also patentable. However, medical activities normally practiced by a medical doctor such as methods for treatment of the human body by surgery or therapy and diagnostic methods practiced on the human body, are not industrially applicable and hence not statutory subject matter. However, compositions, devices, systems, or kits for use in the medical surgery, treatment or diagnosis to be practiced on the human body are industrially applicable and patentable subject matter.

## PHARMACEUTICAL COMPOSITIONS

First and second pharmaceutical uses are patentable in Japan, and although a novel product or composition is patentable *per se*, a pharmaceutical composition is generally required to be limited to a specific use or uses under Japanese practice. Thus, open-ended claims such as "A composition comprising X for use as a pharmaceutical" are usually not patentable, even if the application at hand provides the first disclosure of pharmaceutical effects.

Thus, regardless of whether it is a first or second medical use, under Japanese practice, pharmaceutical compositions are generally protected by claims of the format "A composition comprising X for treatment of Y." Claims of this sort are considered regular product claims. Unlike in the United States, the use limitation carries patentable weight and is read into the claim. Swiss-type claims are also patentable under Japanese practice, although composition claims offer a broader scope of coverage relative to Swiss-type claims under current Japanese practice.

## PATENTABILITY REQUIREMENTS

### Novelty

Japan requires absolute novelty for a pharmaceutical composition to be patented. As of January 1, 2000, inventions that were publicly known, publicly worked, or described in a publication distributed in Japan or elsewhere serve as novelty bars. Prior to this date, novelty was destroyed with regard to publicly known or worked inventions only if these acts were carried out in Japan.

### Section 29bis Novelty

Under Sections 29bis and 184terdecies of Japanese Patent Law, filed but not yet published national applications and Patent Cooperation Treaty (PCT) applications could serve as a novelty bar when the claims of an application (the junior case) have an effective filing date after a patent application (the senior case) which discloses or essentially discloses an identical invention, subject to certain conditions.

### Six-Month Novelty Grace Period

Japan has a six-month grace period against an inventor's own novelty destroying disclosures which include "experiment," "presentation in a printed or online publication," or "having made a presentation in writing at a study meeting held by a scientific body designated by the Commissioner of the

JPO" (5). The only two ways to legally claim the novelty grace period, is for the applicant to either file a patent application directly with the Japanese Patent Office (JPO), or an International PCT application designating Japan, within six months of the date of stipulated novelty destroying event.

## Selection Invention

Japan does recognize selection inventions where an invention with a generic concept is expressed in a cited reference, an invention with more specific concept selected from the generic concept is called "selection invention," if it is novel over the generic invention and pertains to a technical field in which an effect of a product is difficult to understand from its structure. A selection invention possesses inventive step, when it generates an advantageous effect, not disclosed in a cited reference, qualitatively different or qualitatively the same but quantitatively prominent in comparison with that of an invention with a generic concept in a cited invention, neither of the effect being foreseen by a person skilled in the art from the state of the art (6).

## OBVIOUSNESS

The obviousness standard in Japan is different from the U.S. structural nonobviousness *per se* is insufficient. Under Japanese patent practice the applicant must show that the claimed invention has significant effects that could not have been expected from the prior art or that there was undue difficulty encountered in obtaining the claimed invention, even using a well-known technique, or that one skilled in the art would not have reasonably expected to obtain the claimed invention.

Furthermore, even though a particular combination of elements may be structurally nonobvious, the JPO will still take the position that it would be obvious for one skilled in the art to conduct routine variation based on the prior art, and achieve the invention without any significant difficulty. Significant effects relied upon to establish nonobviousness of a claimed invention must be present in the application as originally filed. The Tokyo High Court held that if the specification as originally filed fails to specifically describe actual pharmacological effects of a claimed invention, such disclosure can not be used as a cited reference with regard to obviousness (7).

## SPECIFIC COMMENTARY ON DRUG DELIVERY SYSTEMS

For purposes of discussion, drug delivery systems are categorized into two general types: (1) novel delivery of a known pharmaceutical or (2) new delivery of a new pharmaceutical. As patentability of a new delivery system of a new pharmaceutical can be considered as described above for pharmaceutical compositions in general, the following comments are specifically directed to new delivery systems for known pharmaceutical products. Although technically patentable subject matter, the current JPO position on patentability of improved or new drug delivery systems is generally challenging, particularly with regard to obviousness.

## Novelty

Particular compositions for drug delivery can be patentably distinguishable if they are novel. The JPO allows a drug delivery system to be patented if the dosing interval, given dose, administration protocol, etc., is different from that known in the prior art, or in the following two situations:

1. In the case that one skilled in the art can clearly distinguish the target patent groups of the claimed invention from those of the prior art. In this instance, it becomes clear that the claimed invention is defined by being particularly effective to a particular patient (such as those of a specific genotype or the like).
2. In the case where one skilled in the art can clearly distinguish the desired target application area or treatment area from those disclosed in a prior publication.

If one skilled in the art can clearly distinguish the claimed drug delivery system in terms of its dosage or formulation alone and the disclosure of the prior art system, neither of the above scenarios are required (8).

## Obviousness

Despite the fact that the subject matter of drug delivery systems or administration protocols can be technically considered novel, it is generally more challenging to successfully assert that such inventions are nonobvious. Specifically, the JPO considers that the problems of increasing the medicinal effect of a drug, the reduction of side effects, and optimization of the mode or use of a medicine (by altering dosing interval, dose, or the like) are merely exercises in ordinary creativity for one skilled in the art.

Accordingly, in the case where a claimed drug delivery system demonstrates advantageous effects compared with the prior art, it is usually considered that such advantageous effects would be expected by one skilled in the art, as these would be obvious problems to be solved. As such, the JPO's "significant effect test" with regard to overcoming obviousness would not be fulfilled, and the inventive step of the claimed drug delivery system would likely be denied, even if the claimed drug delivery system is novel.

The Tokyo High Court has endorsed the JPO position when it ruled (8) that it is simply an exertion of ordinary creative ability for one skilled in the art to solve a well known problem involving the increase of medicinal effects, reduction of side effects, and/or optimization of the mode of the use of the known medicine (dosing interval, given dose, or the like). If these points are the only difference between the claimed invention and the cited invention, the non-obviousness of the claimed invention will ordinarily be denied. Thus, drug delivery systems which result in even dramatic improvements are generally considered obvious, as the JPO would consider that it would have been obvious for one skilled in the art to look for such improvements.

However, in the situation where there are other grounds for inferring the inventive step of a claimed drug delivery system such that the advantageous effects compared with the prior art are considered remarkable beyond the state of the art, the drug delivery system is considered to involve an inventive step. The JPO's examination guidelines (9) illustrate such a scenario is where a higher than usually tolerated dosage regime is found to be particularly effective in treating patients of a particular genotype. Thus, not only is the novel dose itself found to be more effective, it is surprisingly found to be effective in a subset of patients.

## ENABLEMENT, WRITTEN DESCRIPTION, AND COMPLETION

The enablement/written description requirement with regard to pharmaceutical compositions under Japanese patent law is rigorously strict, in that pharmacological data or its equivalent must be present in the specification as filed. A recent IP High Court decision (10) confirmed this hard line rule in that if the specification as originally filed fails to specifically describe actual pharmacological data relating to a claimed pharmaceutical composition, such a pharmaceutical composition is NOT recognized to be enabled and postfiling data showing such activity is not permissible.

Another enablement issue arises if the claims can be considered to encompass nonfunctional compounds within the composition, i.e., those which cannot be recognized to have utility or attain the effects of the claimed invention, the claimed invention will not be considered to fulfill the requirements of enablement (and likely written description). If only a small number of compounds are tested in pharmaceutical composition form, the JPO regularly assumes that nonfunctional compounds are encompassed by the claims. This position has been upheld at the Tokyo High Court where it was conclusively determined that: either usefulness in regard to all peptides included in the scope of the claims should be described in the specification, or such usefulness should be clear to a person skilled in the art from common general technical knowledge (11).

Drug-related inventions that do not have supporting pharmacological data in the specification as filed will also be rejected by the JPO on the basis that they do not satisfy the completion requirement under Section 29 of Japan's Patent Law (12).

It goes without saying that Japan's particularly strict enablement and written description requirements for pharmaceutical compositions in general are extended to drug delivery systems. Thus, the effects of a particular drug delivery system to be patented must be thoroughly described and extensively tested in the specification as filed to be considered patentable.

## PATENT TERM EXTENSION FOR REGULATORY APPROVAL DELAYS

Patent term extension is only available if the granted patent cannot be worked because regulatory delay in obtaining marketing approval from the Japanese Ministry of Health, Labor and Welfare. Japan does *not* have the U.S.-style patent term adjustment system to compensate for patent prosecution delays at the patent office.

## INVALIDATION

Effective January 1, 2004, Japan abolished its postgrant opposition system. Currently anyone (there is no standing or controversy requirement) seeking to invalidate a patent may file an Invalidation Appeal (IA) against a granted patent at any time at the Japanese Patent Office (13). An IA takes about 12 to 18 months to complete from filing to decision.

## INFRINGEMENT AND CLINICAL TRIAL IMMUNITY

Japan recognizes direct and indirect patent infringement. Doctrine of Equivalents (DOE) infringement is also recognized in Japan under applicable conditions (14). Clinical trials for regulatory approval are exempt from patent infringement (15). Section 69(1) Patent Law provides a research or experimental use exemption from patent infringement however this does not encompass economic or commercial research (conducted by any party including universities) (16).

## SUMMARY

Although pharmaceutical compositions and drug delivery systems are patentable subject matter under Japanese patent law, there are nuanced obviousness and enablement challenges under Japanese patent law that are very different from the United States and European position. In addition, routine attempts to improve pharmaceutical effects by developing improved drug delivery systems through dosing regimens or the like are very likely to be considered obvious, unless the effects achieved thereby are remarkably distinct.

Therefore, great care must be taken when drafting and prosecuting such patent applications in the world's second most important health-care market.

## ACKNOWLEDGMENT

I would like to especially thank my colleague Lisa M. Mandrusiak, a stellar biotechnology patent analyst, for her outstanding assistance in the preparation of this contribution. I, alas, retain full responsibility for any errors that remain.

## REFERENCES

1. Zaun T, *Japan Drug Maker to Buy a Rival for $7.7 Billion*, N.Y. Times, Feb. 26, 2005 at C3.
2. Landers P, *With Dry Pipelines, Big Drug Makers Stock Up in Japan*, Wall St J, Nov. 24, 2003 at A1.
3. Landers P, Singer J. Pharmaceutical Makers See Feast in Japan, Wall St J, Apr. 29, 2002 at C1.
4. Tokkyo Ho [Patent Law], Law No. 121 of 1959, as amended.
5. Tessensohn JA, Yamamoto S. *Japan's novelty grace period solves the problem of publish and perish.* Nature Biotechnol 2007; 25(1): 55.
6. *Allied Chemical Corp. v. Commissioner Japan Patent Office*, Showa 60 (gyo-ke) 51 dated Sep. 8, 1987 (Tokyo High Ct.).
7. *Glaxo Group Ltd. v. Commissioner Japan Patent Office*, Heisei 15 (gyo-ke) 104 dated Dec. 26, 2003 (Tokyo H. Ct.).
8. *Asta Medica AG. v. Commissioner Japan Patent Office*, Heisei 12 (Gyo Ke) 294 dated Mar. 28, 2001 (Tokyo H. Ct.).
9. Japan Patent Office. *Examination Guidelines for Patent and Utility Model in Japan* (2006).
10. *Astellas & Fujisawa v. Commissioner Japan Patent Office*, Heisei 17 (gyo-ke) 10312 dated Aug. 30, 2005 (Intellectual Property H. Ct.).
11. *Stanford University v. Commissioner Japan Patent Office* Heisei 10 (gyo-ke) 95 dated Feb. 22, 2000 (Tokyo H. Ct.).
12. *Scios v. Commissioner of Japan Patent Office*, Heisei 10 (gyo-ke) 393 dated Mar. 13, 2001 (Tokyo H. Ct.).
13. Tessensohn JA, Yamamoto S. *New invalidation appeal system.* Euro Intell Prop Rev 2003; 25(10):N-154.
14. *THK Co. v. Tsubakimoto Seiko Co.* 1630 Hanrei Jiho 32 (Sup. Ct., Feb. 24, 1998).
15. *Ono Pharmaceutical v. Kyoto Pharmaceutical* 1675 Hanrei Jiho 37 (Sup. Ct., Apr. 16, 1999).
16. *Monsanto Company v. Stauffer Japan KK* 1246 Hanrei Jiho 128 (Tokyo Dist Ct., July 10, 1987).

## Part II: Oral Mucosal Technologies

# 5

# Oral Transmucosal Drug Delivery

### S. Indiran Pather

*California Northstate College of Pharmacy, Rancho Cordova, California, U.S.A.*

### Michael J. Rathbone

*InterAg, Hamilton, New Zealand*

### Sevda Şenel

*Department of Pharmaceutical Technology,
Faculty of Pharmacy, Hacettepe University, Ankara, Turkey*

## INTRODUCTION

This chapter provides an introduction to the section dealing with oral transmucosal drug delivery. It starts with a historical perspective of the use of this route, and then some of the advantages and disadvantages are presented. Next, the structure of the oral mucosa and the pathways for drug absorption are briefly described. Some problems inherent in using isolated tissues for permeation experiments are mentioned and some common misconceptions are noted. A brief overview of some of the buccal/sublingual drugs on the U.S. market provides a snap shot of where we are today. The chapter also gives some insight into the difficulties encountered in developing these products. Lastly, it attempts to give an indication, in broad terms, of the progress that is likely to be made in this area of drug delivery and an assessment of the potential, in the authors' view, of the future of buccal and sublingual drugs.

There has been a great interest, for several years, in the delivery of drugs through the buccal and sublingual mucosae. There are many academic institutions performing basic research, often mechanistic in nature, dealing with drug permeation through the oral mucosa, permeation enhancers, mucoadhesion, etc. In addition, several pharmaceutical companies are actively involved with the development of oral transmucosal drugs; some of these companies have a stated aim of being solely involved with this route of drug administration.

A recently-published book (1) lists 93 companies involved with drugs delivered to the oral cavity, with many companies developing multiple drugs. The above list includes companies developing orally disintegrating tablets (ODT). Even if one were to exclude (for the reasons stated below) those companies involved solely with ODT, there would remain many companies intensely researching oral transmucosal drug delivery. Furthermore, the search term "buccal delivery" at the United States Patent and Trademark Office website (2) reveals 126 patents that were issued between 1976 and July 2007. While some of these patents make only an oblique reference to buccal delivery, many of the inventions are primarily related to this route of administration, indicating that novel formulations are being actively conceptualized and invented. The combination of academic and industrial research depicted above represents a significant investment of time and resources in this route of drug delivery.

In contrast to the fairly extensive research outlined above, a computer database search indicates that there are less than 50 registered products available for buccal/sublingual delivery in the United States at the time of writing (3). Many of these are multiple presentations of the same drug such as different flavors and strengths of nicotine chewing gum. Thus, only a handful of active pharmaceutical ingredients (APIs) have successfully reached the market place as drugs for oral transmucosal delivery. Some of these, such as nicotine and ergot alkaloids, have been used in buccal/sublingual delivery dosage forms for many years. This begs the question: why is there a disparity between the intense research activity over the last two decades and the drugs for oral transmucosal delivery actually reaching the market? We will return to this question after a discussion of some of the other topics mentioned in the introductory paragraph.

It is important to distinguish ODT from transmucosal dosage forms. The latter release the drug into the oral cavity for absorption through the oral mucosa. An absorption enhancer may, simultaneously, be released into the oral cavity to aid drug absorption. ODT, on the other hand, are generally not intended for oral cavity absorption. Instead, the drug-containing coated microcapsules (or other units) are released from the dosage form into the oral cavity, usually after rapid disintegration of the tablet. The microcapsules are then swallowed and the major portion of the drug is released distal to the oral cavity when the coating dissolves. The purpose of the coating is to prevent the patient experiencing the bad taste of the drug since the barrier coating retards the drug's dissolution. Since the major portion of the drug is not released in the oral cavity, ODT should not be considered buccal, or sublingual, delivery systems.

It may be worthwhile, at this point, to review some of the advantages and disadvantages of oral transmucosal delivery.

Advantages include:

1.  A drug administered through the mucosa of the oral cavity avoids the first-pass effect. Drugs in the oral cavity pass into the lingual, facial, and retromandibular veins, which open into the internal jugular vein (4). The latter eventually empties into the superior vena cava (via the subclavian vein) and thus into the general circulation, avoiding the hepatic first-pass effect.
2.  The oral cavity is generally considered to have a low enzyme content which, when considered together with its pH (5.8–7.4), presents a less hostile environment for labile drugs than the stomach (low pH and proteases) or the small intestines (bile salts and enzymes). As suggested by Jasti and Abraham (5), if peptides permeate via the paracellular route, it is the enzyme content in the paracellular channels (and not the content of mucosal homogenates) that is important, thus presenting an even lower enzymatic barrier to peptides.
3.  There is a much greater ease of administration with oral-cavity dosage forms than with many other dosage forms or devices for drug delivery.
4.  If side effects are seen, the dosage form may be easily removed. This advantage is, obviously, only relevant in the case of sustained release medication.
5.  Permeability enhancers may be more easily applied to the oral cavity, with less deleterious effects, than to other absorptive surfaces such as the gastrointestinal tract (GIT).
6.  The cellular turnaround time in the buccal region of the oral cavity is estimated to be from 4 to 14 days (6), which is in between the extremes of the skin (slow) and the GIT (fast). Thus a mucoadhesive device may be worn for many hours or even days without disturbing its adhesion due to rapid cell division. If slight tissue damage occurs from wearing a dosage form, fairly rapid recovery is possible.
7.  An often overlooked advantage is that the microenvironment of a dosage form placed in the oral cavity can directly and easily be modified. Thus, the physico-chemical conditions in a small volume of biological fluid can be changed, with minimal side effects, in contrast to altering the conditions in a large fluid compartment. Fentora, the fentanyl delivery system is an example of a dosage form which temporarily changes the pH of the saliva in the buccal cavity. The fact that the buffer capacity of saliva (unstimulated) is only 6 mmol/L/pH unit (7) facilitates easy pH modification.

Disadvantages include:

1. The oral cavity has a relatively small absorptive surface area of $0.01\,m^2$ (8) in comparison to the absorptive surface area of the small intestines of $100\,m^2$. The latter value does not take into account the additional surface area provided by the microvilli.
2. The mucosa of the oral cavity is less permeable than that of the small intestine.
3. Salivation and resulting swallowing effectively remove the drug from the preferred absorptive region. While salivary flow is slow (0.2–0.4 mL/min) when resting, it becomes considerably faster (2 mL/min) when stimulated (9). Placement of a dosage form in the oral cavity will provide some degree of stimulation, the extent depending on the nature of the dosage form. Thus, loss of drug due to faster salivation is to be expected.
4. The taste of the drug may present difficulties to patients and decrease compliance with the dosing regimen. This problem may be greater with certain patient populations such as the young, the elderly, and patients experiencing nausea either due to their illness or as a consequence of concomitant medications.
5. In the case of mucoadhesive systems, movements of the mouth or tongue may displace or otherwise affect the dosage form adversely.
6. Where a dosage form is to be held for any length of time in the oral cavity, with the instruction to avoid swallowing, the dosing instructions may not be accurately followed by some patient populations, e.g., the young, the elderly, and some physically or mentally impaired patients.

For rapid oral transmucosal delivery, the drug may be presented as lozenges, patches, sprays, or compressed tablets having a fairly rapid in-mouth disintegration time (15 minutes or less). Where prolonged action is required, the dosage form is usually mucoadhesive (patch or mucoadhesive tablet) and the drug is released slowly for slow absorption through the oral mucosa. Prochlorperazine (Buccastem®, Reckitt and Colman) is delivered in this manner for long-acting control of nausea. Some delivery systems are designed to deliver the drug unidirectionally (towards the mucosal surface only) with an impermeable surface exposed to the oral cavity (10).

There is no evidence that the thin films currently marketed (mostly for over the counter [OTC] products) deliver the drug through the oral mucosa but research is ongoing for such an application (11). In addition, ODT (with the exception of some freeze-dried products) do not allow significant oral transmucosal permeation, as mentioned previously. While bite capsules that release a drug solution have been described in the patent literature (12–14), the authors are not aware of a commercial product using this dosage form.

In contrast to what is commonly believed by the lay population, there is also no evidence that homeopathic products placed in the oral cavity deliver the active through the oral mucosa.

The first recorded use of transmucosal delivery appears to be an 1879 paper (15) describing the use of glyceryl trinitrate for treatment of angina. This drug penetrates the mucosa easily and does not require any enhancement. In spite of this early success, not much further development of this route occurred during the next 70 to 80 years. Then followed a period in which a few drugs were developed and, in the United States, a number of drugs were registered prior to 1982 (3). These include isosorbide dinitrate, Ergot alkaloids, nitroglycerine, nicotine, and testosterone and its derivatives. Isosorbide dinitrite and nitroglycerine are rapidly absorbed through the oral cavity membranes and provide rapid relief of anginal pain. Oral cavity transmucosal testosterone is useful to elevate male hormone levels, avoiding the degradation that occurs in the GIT and during first pass through the liver.

The most significant introduction of the "modern" era was the fentanyl lollipop (Actiq® by Anesta Corporation, now Cephalon Inc.) in 1998. This was the first product with a label claim for breakthrough cancer pain (other products had been used off label). The fentanyl effervescent dosage form, Fentora®, was introduced by CIMA LABS/Cephalon in September, 2006, as the second fentanyl oral transmucosal dosage form, also with an indication for breakthrough cancer pain. The tablet is placed in the buccal cavity (above a premolar, between the gum and the cheek) where it disintegrates over approximately 10 minutes releasing the drug. Cephalon is currently researching the use of this product for other pain indications such as breakthrough neuropathic pain (16).

In 2002, the FDA approved Subutex® (buprenorphine) for initiating treatment of addiction to drugs such heroin, and Suboxone® (buprenorphine plus naloxone) for continuing treatment of addicts. The naloxone is intended to be a safeguard against the extraction and intravenous injection, by drug abusers, of the active ingredient in this transmucosal dosage form. These drugs were introduced by Reckitt and Colman in an attempt to counter the wave of drugs of abuse. Reckitt and Colman also introduced Prochlorperazine buccal tablet (Buccastem®) in Europe for treatment of nausea and vomiting. The tablet is placed in the buccal area where it releases the drug over a few hours.

Noven Pharmaceuticals developed the Dentipatch®, a small ($2\,cm^2$) patch that is affixed to the gum line where it releases lidocaine for local anesthesia. The patch, which was approved by the FDA in 1996, produces sufficient desensitization for pain-free injection of a larger dose of local anesthetic for prolonged dental procedures. On its own, the patch may provide sufficient local anesthesia for short dental procedures (see Chapter 8 for further details on this technology).

The Periochip® is a thin film containing chlorhexidine for the adjunctive treatment of periodontal disease. A dentist inserts the chip into the periodontal sulcus where it releases chlorhexidine over a period of approximately 10 days. Repeat visits, at 3-month intervals, are required for the insertion of additional chips for long-term treatment. The currently marketed version of the Periochip was approved by the FDA in 2002 and has a shelf life of 2 years when stored at room temperature. The first version had to be stored at 4°C. The development of the Periochip is detailed in Chapter 11 of this book.

The above brief description, while not meant to be exhaustive, provides a flavor for the introduction of new products to the market. Let us now turn our attention to how drugs, after being released from pharmaceutical products placed in the oral cavity, cross the mucosa for penetration into blood capillaries. A familiarity with the structure of the oral mucosa is required to understand these mechanisms. Since this topic has been extensively described by several authors, only pertinent information to facilitate the discussion will be mentioned here. Short overviews of the structure of the oral mucosa are given in References 4 and 17 while a detailed account of the cellular structure and the molecular basis for the barrier function of the oral mucosa are given in Reference 18. The latter reference also provides a very good comparison of the barrier functions of the skin and the oral mucosa. The reader is referred to these documents for a more detailed account.

## STRUCTURE OF THE ORAL MUCOSA AND ROUTES OF ABSORPTION

Although there are regional differences in the structure of the mucosa from different parts of the mouth, the mucosa has similar general structure in all regions. It consists of an epithelium and connective tissue beneath this. The epithelium arises from a basal layer of cuboidal cells. From this actively dividing layer, cells are pushed upwards to the surface and become more flattened as they reach the uppermost layers which are described as squamous, stratified cells. The epithelium consists of 40 to 50 layers, only a few of which are shown in the diagrammatic representation depicted in Figure 1. The epithelium protects the underlying tissue from mechanical and chemical injury. The mechanical barrier enables us to chew on rough food while the chemical barrier prevents noxious chemicals from directly entering the systemic circulation (as previously mentioned, blood flowing from the oral cavity by-passes the liver). The efficiency of this chemical barrier is one of the major obstacles to the development of oral transmucosal delivery systems: the function of the epithelium is to keep out foreign chemicals whereas the aim of transmucosal delivery is to enable selected foreign chemicals (known as drugs) to permeate this tissue and reach the blood stream.

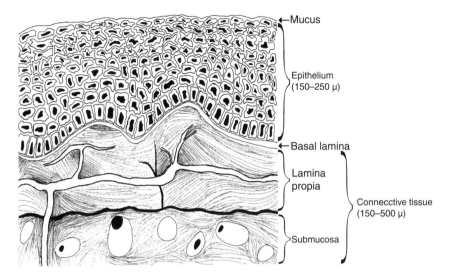

**Figure 1** Structure of the buccal mucosa. *Source*: Artwork by Jayd Pather.

The connective tissue supports the epithelium and consists of a lamina propria and sub mucosa as shown in Figure 1. The lamina propria contains a network of capillaries. It is difficult for drugs to permeate the tightly bound cell layers, especially the outermost layers, of the epithelium. However, once a drug has permeated through the layers of cells constituting the epithelium and the basement membrane, it can easily penetrate the capillaries and enter the general blood circulation. Hence, the epithelium is the barrier to drug permeation.

In general, drugs may permeate the mucosa through two routes: the paracellular route (through the spaces between the cells) or directly through the cell membranes. These routes are illustrated in Figure 2.

Depending on their physico-chemical properties (e.g., lipophilicity, molecular weight, etc.), some drugs may preferentially permeate the inter-cellular spaces, going around, and between, the cells rather than through the cells. This pathway, referred to as the paracellular route, is favored by hydrophilic drugs which dissolve more readily in the aqueous fluids filling the intercellular spaces. The transcellular pathway, on the other hand, involves drugs permeating the cell membrane and going through the cell to then penetrate the opposite cell membrane and into the next cell, and so on, as shown in Figure 2. An example of a drug known to penetrate via the transcellular pathway is fentanyl (19). It is feasible that some drugs may penetrate via both pathways and this may occur with drugs that have approximately balanced hydrophobic and hydrophilic properties, with a slight predominance of hydrophobicity. Such drugs will usually penetrate the fastest. Most often, however, one pathway predominates.

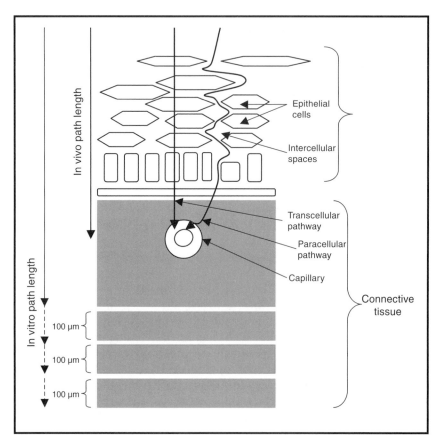

**Figure 2** Diagrammatic representation of pathways for drug delivery through the oral cavity mucosa showing (A) the direct transcellular and tortuous paracellular pathways, and (B) the in vivo and longer in vitro path lengths. Each 100 μm of additional connective tissue has a significant adverse effect on the permeation rate. *Source*: From Refs. 29 and 52.

It can readily be seen that the transcellular pathway is a more direct pathway, with drugs tending to move more directly across the cell layers with little lateral diffusion. For the paracellular pathway, the drug moves in a tortuous fashion around the cells, thus this is a longer pathway. It is important to make the following distinction: while the shortest pathway that the drug may take around the cells is longer than the transcellular pathway, there is also a greater tendency, in paracellular permeation, for the drug to diffuse laterally over a wider area of the mucosa. This may help to explain the longer lead time often observed with drugs that are known to be absorbed by the paracellular pathway. Caffeine is an example of a drug absorbed via the paracellular route and it is used as a marker of paracellular absorption (20).

While the transcellular route is more direct, the drug has to traverse the lipophilic cell membrane, then the hydrophilic interior of the cell before passing through two cell membranes to reach the cytoplasm of the next cell. Therefore, the predominantly hydrophobic drug should have some hydrophilicity, if absorption into the systemic circulation is required. If the drug is extremely hydrophobic, there would be a tendency for it to be retained in the more hydrophobic components of the mucosal tissue, such as the cell membranes of the superficial epithelial layers, and not reach the blood circulation in significant amounts. This, of course, would be a desirable feature for a topical effect (e.g., anti-inflammatory action) but not if a systemic effect is desired.

## IN VITRO EXPERIMENTS

In a landmark publication, Beckett and Triggs demonstrated that the loss of drug from a solution held in the mouth can be attributed to oral mucosal absorption (21). Swallowing and salivation can be accounted for by the changes in volume and concentration of a red dye in the original, and the expelled, solutions. A series of papers from Beckett's laboratory in the 1960s and 1970s demonstrated the buccal absorption of different drugs and the fact that the pH of the solution influences the absorption of many drugs. This work, an example of which is Reference 22, may have been the forerunner of the use of the in situ model to study drug absorption from the mouths of test animals. Specially designed cells containing drug solutions were affixed to the oral mucosae of a variety of test animals. In some instances, perfusion cells were used in human volunteers. These models have been comprehensively reviewed by Rathbone et al. (23). This type of experiment has largely been supplanted by the in vitro model in which a drug is allowed to pass from a donor cell through a piece of excised mucosa to the receiver cell. The concentration of the drug in the receiver cell is measured at fixed time intervals to determine the time course of permeation. The advantages of using excised tissue in an in vitro model are:

1. The experimental conditions can be tightly controlled in a contained environment.
2. Tissue from one animal can be used for a series of comparative experiments, thus minimizing the effect of biological variability.
3. It is cheaper.
4. Drug analysis in an aqueous medium is easier than analysis of the drug content of blood.

It is usual to use a surrogate for human oral mucosal tissue, such as porcine buccal tissue, in such experiments. The tissue may be excised from sacrificed animals or the local abattoir may provide a ready supply. Such experiments are commonly performed in the course of developing oral transmucosal dosage forms. However, the results of such experiments do not always lend themselves to unambiguous interpretation. Therefore, it may be useful to review the basic technique and some of the issues and common misconceptions.

In a typical experimental setup, the buccal epithelium from a sacrificed animal is placed between the donor and receiver cells with the mucosal surface of the tissue facing the donor compartment. A drug solution of known concentration is transferred to the donor cell and a physiologically compatible solution is added to the receiver cell. These chambers are of small volume and may be constructed to function side by side (Ussing chamber) or one below the other (Franz diffusion cells). The receiver chamber is sampled at fixed intervals and assayed for the drug that has been transferred through the membrane up to that point. The apparent permeability coefficient is determined from the slope of the linear portion of the permeation vs time plot, using equation 1.

$$P_{app} = (dC_r/dt) \times V_r/(A \times C_0) \tag{1}$$

where $P_{app}$ is the apparent permeability coefficient, $dC_r/dt$ is the slope of the cumulative concentration in the receiver compartment versus time plot, $V_r$ is the volume of the receiver compartment, $A$ is the surface area of buccal epithelium available for permeation, and $C_0$ is the initial concentration of the compound in the donor chamber.

It is extremely important to pay careful attention to the preparation of the tissue to be used in permeation experiments as the preparative method can lead to differences in the observed permeation rate. It is best to use fresh membranes, whenever possible. The storage of the membrane, if the permeation experiment cannot be conducted immediately after excision, is of utmost importance. For excised porcine buccal membrane, it was found that storage in Krebs' Ringer Lactate (pH = 7.4) at 4°C for 24 hours (but not 48 hours) was acceptable, as defined below (24). Storage of the membrane in phosphate buffered saline (pH = 7.4) at 4°C was acceptable up to 6 hours only whereas freezing was found to be unacceptable, presumably due to ice crystals damaging the membrane. Antipyrine and caffeine permeability values were used in the assessment of acceptability. A storage method was deemed acceptable if similar permeability values were seen for the stored membrane and the freshly excised tissues. The damage to the membranes due to freezing is worth noting as many authors have previously used frozen membranes for permeation studies. Examples of such studies are described in References 25 and 26.

The use of integrity markers and positive controls in the experiment is vital. Transepithelial electrical resistance (TEER) is a method of assessing the integrity of the membrane. If there are minute tears in the membrane, the electrical resistance between the donor and receiver cells is altered. This test should be conducted before and after the permeation experiment. The first test confirms that no damage to the membrane occurred during tissue preparation and experimental set up while the latter test confirms that the drug treatments did not compromise the integrity of a membrane that was acceptable to start with. It is good practice to include in the donor cells, together with the drug of interest, a compound known to have low permeability (such as Lucifer yellow) and a high permeability compound (such as caffeine) as markers of the level of membrane permeability. Caffeine is known to be rapidly, and completely, permeable through oral mucosa in vivo (20).

The addition of high- and low-permeability markers into the donor cells in every experiment enables a comparison of the permeation rates for that experiment with established values for these compounds. If the results for the permeability markers in an experiment (or in one replicate of an experiment) are very different from expected values, the results for the test compound should be regarded as suspect. Obviously, there should be no interaction between the permeability markers and the drug of interest either during permeation or in the analytical procedure.

The experimental design described above is very useful for certain purposes, such as the determination of whether buccal permeation does, or does not, occur to a useful extent with a particular drug. Also, one may discriminate between related drugs in a chemical series where the permeability difference is approximately 2 times or more. To attempt to discriminate between formulations or enhancers delivering small differences in permeability is often futile because of the variability associated with this experiment. This variability is evident even in well-conducted experiments.

Replicate experiments of the identical set up (same drug, concentration, enhancer and experimental conditions) may show a variability as high as 20–50%. With two sets of data, each with this extent of variability, it is often difficult to make a meaningful comparison where there is only a moderate difference in permeability. The sources of this variability are many and include, first, the animals themselves, which are subject to normal biological variation (a few experiments/replicates may be done with tissues from the same animal), their age and condition being important. Then there are the differences in the method of tissue excision and preparation, and method of storage, if the tissue is not used immediately.

Scientists new to the technique may be surprised that it takes longer for the drug to permeate the isolated tissue than it does in vivo. Thus, significant blood levels will be observed much faster than the in vitro experiment would indicate. This difference will be observed even when the absorption mechanism is known to be passive diffusion. The in vitro experiment merely provides the rank order of permeation rates of a series of compounds or the rank order of the efficacy of a series of enhancers, not an indication of the absolute permeation rates in vivo.

Part of the explanation for this phenomenon is the fact that, in a live animal, the blood flow through the capillaries, found in the connective tissue just below the basement membrane, provides perfect sink conditions. The absence of blood flow may make a significant difference to the rate of drug permeation through the excised mucosa. Related to this, is the fact that in a live animal the drug must penetrate only as far as the capillaries for absorption to occur, whereas in an isolated tissue experiment the drug must further traverse the connective tissue to reach the receiver cell. This longer pathway is depicted diagrammatically in Figure 2. The thickness of the connective tissue may vary between experiments, thus adding a variable additional path length for diffusion. This may have an impact on the results, as explained below.

While the epithelium has been correctly stated to be the major impediment to drug diffusion, the role of the connective tissue in *excised membranes* may have been under-rated since no specific mention is made of controlling its thickness in several publications, examples of which are References 27 and 28. In a recent study, the permeability of antipyrine and caffeine were shown to be inversely proportional to the tissue thickness (29). An increase of about 100 μm significantly decreased the permeability of these compounds ($p < 0.05$). It is imperative that each laboratory validates their tissue excision, preparation and handling methods in order to achieve the most consistent and reliable results.

The temperature at which the experiment is conducted and the analytical method are additional sources of error. The permeability of model compounds through excised porcine buccal mucosa was found to increase exponentially with temperature (30). Sensitive analytical methods are required, considering the small volumes of the receiver compartment and the analytical sample.

It may be possible to avoid some of the intricacies of the excision process, and the errors involved, by using cultured buccal tissue that is produced commercially. Non-keratized buccal cells (EpiOral™) plated in 6-well plates may be obtained from MatTek Corporation (31). The company also provides buffer solutions to be used as the donor and receiver solutions. The use of these tissue plates involves a cost greater than that associated with obtaining porcine buccal tissue from the local abattoir. There is a two-week lead time for growth and delivery of the plates and, if the cultured tissue does not meet QA criteria, a second batch would have to be produced, involving a further two-week delay. If a series of permeation studies is needed in the course of the development of a pharmaceutical product, careful planning will be required (taking into account these lead times) to ensure that the launch of the product is not delayed.

As an alternate model, human vaginal tissue has been used in permeation experiments as a surrogate for buccal tissue with apparent success (32). Human vaginal tissue is more easily available than human buccal tissue as some vaginal tissue may be excised during hysterectomies. Vaginal and buccal tissues share some structural similarities, making this a viable alternate tissue (33). Of course, legal and ethical considerations must be paramount in the decision to use human tissues for any experiment.

Reference was made initially to the research being undertaken by universities and to the transmucosal delivery systems development work of several companies. The basic work of universities sometimes feeds into the dosage form development work of companies. Some of the drugs currently in development in the United States will now be briefly discussed. Where this information has been made public, some of the problems encountered by the companies concerned will be mentioned. An overview of such issues provides a better understanding of the complexities of the development process.

## DRUGS IN DEVELOPMENT

The fact that the term "buccal delivery" appears in 126 patents issued between 1976 and July 2007 (2), indicates that this is a fairly active area of research and invention. Some of the products known to be in development are shown in Table 1. Which products can we expect to be approved by registering authorities and commercially launched in the medium term? The reader may want to draw his own conclusions after reviewing the following remarks and, perhaps, obtaining further information from the references cited.

Novadel specializes in sprays for oral transmucosal delivery; the droplets of fine mist adhere to the tissues and release their drug content for absorption through the mucosa. Nitroglycerine lingual spray (Nitromist™)

**Table 1** Some Oral Transmucosal Products in Development in the United States

| Company | Products |
| --- | --- |
| Generex | Insulin, "Ora-lyn" |
| | Low MW Heparin |
| | Fentanyl |
| | Morphine |
| Novadel | Sumatriptan |
| | Zolpidem |
| | Ondansetron |
| Biodelivery Sciences International | BEMA Fentanyl |
| | BEMA LA |
| | BEMA Zolpidem |
| | Prochlorperazine |
| Transcept Pharmaceuticals, Inc. | Zolpidem |

for the treatment of angina was approved by the FDA in November 2006 (34). This was the company's first marketing approval, which, they claim, validates both the technology and their ability to charter the 21 CFR 505(b) 2 course. Two studies comparing the effects of zolpidem spray and Ambien® tablets (healthy volunteers and elderly healthy volunteers) were completed in 2007 and the company expects to submit an New Drug Application (NDA) for zolpidem in 2007 (35). Novadel's licensee for the ondansetron buccal spray, Hana Biosciences, announced in February 2007 that there were issues with precipitation from the solution during stability studies of scaled up batches (36). Novadel stated that this necessitated a change in formulation and/or scale up, and that this issue would set the Ondansetron program back to some extent (37). In August 2007, Novadel announced a sublicense agreement with Par Pharmaceutical (38) in terms of which Novadel and Par would collaborate on the reformulation of the ondansetron spray, while Par was responsible for updates to the NDA and commercialization activities in North America. Par and Hana Biosciences entered into a separate licensing agreement.

Transoral Pharmaceuticals (now known as Transcept Pharmaceuticals) successfully completed a low dose zolpidem Phase 3 sleep laboratory study of a sublingual lozenge and is, at the time of writing, conducting a second Phase 3 study in outpatients (39). The company expects to submit an NDA in 2008 (39). Although Reckitt and Colman's Prochlorperazine has been on the European market for several years, the U.S. FDA asked for additional information in connection with a marketing application. Biodelivery Sciences International (BDSI) acquired the U.S. rights to this product and has submitted an NDA in the United States (see case study below).

Generex has done extensive work on oral mucosal delivery of insulin and the product is marketed in South America (40). The registration in 2005 in Ecuador is believed to be the first marketing approval in the world of a non-injectible insulin. It was approved for the treatment of type 1 and type 2 diabetes. The company's RapidMist device is used to supply a fine mist to the mouth. Insulin does not enter the lungs, it is claimed. A once-a-day long acting injection is still needed but the multiple injections associated with meals are avoided (41). A Phase 3 study is expected to be started by the end of 2007 with patient enrollment in the United States, Europe and Canada, and U.S. marketing approval is anticipated by 2009 (42). This product could represent a convenient method of administration of insulin. For diabetics who have to inject themselves daily (often multiple times), ease of administration is very important.

Oral transmucosal insulin could see comparable, if not better, patient acceptance because of even greater ease of use and, thus, this product could see good patient support. If this occurs, it would represent a significant improvement over the current, widely accepted therapy that involves multiple injections.

Having introduced several aspects of oral transmucosal drug delivery, it is appropriate to return to the question posed at the beginning of the chapter: Why is the development and approval of these dosage forms so slow? There may be several reasons which, when taken together, represent a fairly large challenge.

1. Often, these are low dose drugs with special characteristics which may present formulation difficulties such as content uniformity issues, difficulty in attaining very fast dissolution or, conversely, attaining steady, sustained release over a predetermined time. The achievement of the optimal formulation may be difficult for the drug in question. (The dosage form is often either very rapidly releasing, or it may have a combination of sustained release and mucoadhesive properties.)

2. There needs to be a good understanding of the underlying biology and permeability issues and the complexity of these questions may be underestimated.

3. There is often a need to have a special mechanism to enhance the absorption of the drug without causing undue side effects.

4. The taste of the drug and patient acceptability may be a problem.

5. While an increase in the absorption rate and an enhancement of bio-availability are both desirable attributes, the extent of improvement may have been underestimated during early development. Dose titration for in vivo studies may prove to be difficult.

6. With a novel route of administration, it may be somewhat more difficult convincing regulatory agencies of the acceptability of a new product. The agency may display greater circumspection, in keeping with their aim of protecting the public.

7. Oral transmucosal delivery research and dosage form development are often undertaken by smaller companies who do not have the resources of the larger pharmaceutical companies. This may become a significant issue, noting the other difficulties mentioned in this section.

8. The 505(b)2 regulatory path is often followed for a known drug delivered by a new route of administration and companies may not be fully cognizant of the difficulties associated with this type of submission. While the 21 CFR 505(b)2 path is certainly less onerous than the NDA path with its requirements for toxicity studies etc., it is not as straightforward as the Abbreviated New Drug Application (ANDA) path. The requirements for the latter are very clearly spelled out in regulations and FDA guidances. The requirements for approval of a 21 CFR 505(b)2 application are often the subject of negotiation and agreement with the agency. It may require a higher level of expertise and sophistication on the part of the applicant company to successfully charter the regulatory course.

Some of these points are illustrated in the following regulatory case study.

## Regulatory Case Study: Prochlorperazine

BDSI acquired the rights to develop prochlorperazine buccal tablets in the United States from Reckitt Benckiser (previously Reckitt and Colman) via their acquisition of Arius Pharmaceuticals (43). Reckitt Benckiser retained the right to sell the product in Europe (as "Buccastem") and in certain other countries such as Japan. In view of the fact that this product had been on sale in Europe for several years before the U.S. regulatory submission, it may reasonably have been expected to have a relatively straightforward regulatory passage. In addition, the company had the cooperation and experience of Reckitt Benckiser to support them in their application.

On 2 May 2005, BDSI announced that it had submitted a 21 CFR 505 (b)2 NDA for prochlorperazine (44) and that, they believed, they adhered to the requirements agreed upon with the FDA in the pre-NDA meeting. This submission occurred less than 3 months after the announcement, on February 9, 2005, of completion of clinical studies required for the NDA (46) and was BDSI's first NDA (44) and the first product for buccal delivery of an anti-nausea drug in the United States (45). On July 20, 2005, BDSI announced that the drug had been accepted for review by the FDA (46). However, on March 1, 2006, the company announced that it was "extremely surprised and disappointed" to have received a letter from the FDA on 28 February stating that the application was nonapprovable and that additional information was required (47).

BDSI met with the FDA's Division of Gastroenterology Products on May 17, 2006 and agreed in principle on the approach for BDSI to potentially achieve regulatory approval of the prochlorperazine product, Emezine® buccal tablets (48). BDSI believes two small pharmacokinetic (PK) studies are appropriate, one of which will be in older patients. The tolerance in the oral cavity and the metabolic profile after delivery through the buccal mucosa must also be assessed in any future PK studies. The slower absorption in the first 1–2 hours (compared to the oral swallowed tablet) observed in the PK studies submitted with the NDA caused the FDA to be concerned about onset of action. The higher $C_{max}$ values seen in these studies led the FDA to question the drug's impact on older patients, hence the request for a study in this population group.

A reading of the company's statement (48) leads one to believe that the FDA had four major concerns: (*i*) low initial blood levels and onset of action; (*ii*) high $C_{max}$ and its effect on elderly patients; (*iii*) local tolerance; (*iv*) differences in metabolism via the buccal route. The metabolism question may not have been expected. Could the other questions have been anticipated?

## FUTURE

What can we expect in the future? The ongoing research and development are expected to yield at least a few successes in the form of products approved for marketing. This success may encourage research by new entrants into the field and stimulate more vigorous development by existing players. There may also be some consolidation, mergers, or acquisitions by the companies involved in this field. This has already happened to some extent with the acquisition by Cephalon of both Anesta Corporation and CIMA LABS, Inc. The acquisition by BDSI of Arius Pharmaceuticals, Inc. in 2004 (43) is another example. Arius had, itself, acquired an exclusive world wide license to the BEMA technology of Atrix Laboratories, Inc. also in 2004 (49). In terms of the agreement, Atrix retained the right to co promote BEMA fentanyl. Apart from acquisitions, other forms of cooperative agreements between the small companies engaged in this field may continue to occur in order to leverage the strengths of each other.

Initial successes are likely to lead to some opportunistic entrants into this field. However, it must be borne in mind that careful selection of drugs is needed for successful transmucosal delivery. In the first place, buccal/sublingual delivery must offer a definite therapeutic advantage for it to be useful. Examples of a therapeutic advantage are: reducing the first-pass effect, or the faster attainment of clinically relevant blood levels. Where buccal delivery allows the avoidance of more intrusive delivery mechanisms, such as injections, it would also be useful. It is ideal for drugs that are not absorbed in the GIT or those that are largely destroyed in the GIT. The delivery of peptides by this route would be a major advantage since it avoids injections.

Only 22 new chemical entities (NCEs) and biologics were the subject of new drug approvals in the United States in 2006 while 53 were approved in 1996 (50). The tremendous reduction in the number of new approvals comes with a doubling of the total research budget. This is a very strong indication that it is increasingly more difficult to register drug products containing NCEs. A greater reliance should be placed on improving the delivery of currently-marketed drugs, in the future, in view of the fact that it is so expensive and time consuming to develop an NCE. As previously mentioned, such enhanced delivery must offer a definite therapeutic improvement (51). With such an approach, the twin objectives of enhanced therapy as well as improving the bottom line of companies may be achieved. In this light, oral transmucosal delivery may be one of the delivery mechanisms that becomes important in the future.

## REFERENCES

1.  Ghosh TK, Pfister WR, eds. Drug Delivery to the Oral Cavity: Molecules to Market. Boca Raton, FL: CRC Press, 2005; Appendix 1:357–83.
2.  The United States Patent and Trademark Office website. http://www.uspto.gov/patft/index.html
3.  Food and Drug Administration. The Electronic Orange Book: Approved Drugs Products with Therapeutic Equivalence Evaluations, 2007. http://www.fda.gov/cder/ob/default.htm
4.  Squier CA, Wertz PW. Structure and function of the oral mucosa and implications for drug delivery. In: Rathbone MJ, ed. Oral Mucosal Delivery. New York: Marcel Dekker, 1996.
5.  Jasti BR, Abraham W. Oral transmucosal delivery of protein and peptide therapeutics. In: Ghosh TK, Pfister WR, eds. Drug Delivery to the Oral Cavity: Molecules to Market. Boca Raton, FL: CRC Press, 2005.
6.  Hill MW. Cell renewal in oral epithelia. In: Meyer J, Squier CA, Gerson SJ, eds. The Structure and Function of Oral Mucosa, New York: Pergamon, 1984.
7.  Bardow A, Moe D, Nyvad B, Nauntofte B. The buffer capacity and buffer systems of human whole saliva measured without loss of $CO_2$. Arch Oral Biol 2000; 45(1):1–12.
8.  DeFelippis, MR. Overcoming the challenges of noninvasive protein and peptide delivery. Am Pharm Review 2003; 6(4):21–30.
9.  Li B, Robinson JR, Preclinical assessment of oral mucosal drug delivery systems. In: Ghosh TK, Pfister WR, eds. Drug Delivery to the Oral Cavity: Molecules to Market. Boca Raton, FL: CRC Press, 2005.
10. Alur HH, Beal JD, Pather SI, Mitra AK, Johnston TP. Evaluation of a novel, natural oligosaccharide gum as a sustained-release and mucoadhesive component of calcitonin buccal tablets. J Pharm Sci 1999; 88:1313–9.
11. MonoSol Rx website. http://www.monosolrx.com/index.html
12. Dugger, HA III. Buccal, polar and non-polar spray or capsule. United States Patent 6,998,110. Issued 14 February 2006.
13. Dugger HA III. Buccal, polar and non-polar spray or capsule containing drugs for treating disorders of the central nervous system. United States Patent 6,977,070. Issued 20 December 2005.
14. Dugger HA III. Buccal, polar and non-polar spray or capsule containing drugs for treating pain. United States Patent 6,969,508. Issued 29 November 2005.
15. Murrell W. Nitroglycerin as a remedy for angina pectoris, Lancet 1879; 151: 225–7.
16. Simpson DM, Messina J, Xie F, Hale M. Fentanyl buccal tablet for the relief of breakthrough pain in opioid-tolerant adult patients with chronic neuropathic pain: a multicenter, randomized, double-blind, placebo-controlled study. Clin Ther 2007; 29(4):588–601.
17. Harris D, Robinson JR. Drug delivery via the mucous membranes of the oral cavity. J Pharm Sci 1992; 81(1):1–10.
18. Wertz PW, Squier CA. Cellular and molecular basis of barrier function in oral epithelium. Crit Rev Ther Drug Carrier Syst 1991; 8:237–69.

19. Zhang J, Streisand J, Niu S, et al. Estimation of bucccal fentanyl absorption bioavailability by measuring drug depletion from vehicle solutions: validation of the method in dogs. Pharm Res 1992; 9:S177.

20. Kamimori GH, Karyekar CS, Otterstetter R, Cox DS, Belenky GL, Eddington ND. The rate of absorption and relative bioavailability of caffeine administered in chewing gum versus capsules to normal healthy volunteers. Int J Pharm 2002; 234:159–67.

21. Beckett AH, Triggs EJ. Buccal absorption of basic drugs and its application as an in vivo model of passive drug transfer through lipid membranes. J Pharm Pharmacol 1967; 19:31S.

22. Beckett AH, Moffat AC. The influence of substitution in phenylacetic acids on their performance in the buccal absorption test. J Pharm Pharmacol 1969; 21: 139S.

23. Rathbone MJ, Purves R, Ghazali FA, Ho PC. In vivo techniques for studying the oral mucosal absorption characteristics of drugs in animals and humans. In: Rathbone MJ, ed. Oral Mucosal Delivery. New York: Marcel Dekker, 1996.

24. Jasti B, Mahalingam R, Li X, Kulkarni U, Pather I. Influence of biological and experimental variables on the in vitro transbuccal permeation of antipyrine and caffeine. AAPS Journal, Vol. 8(S2): Abstract T2134 (2006).

25. Manganaro AM, Wertz PW. The effects of permeabilizers on the in vitro penetration of propranolol through porcine buccal epithelium. Mil Med 1996; 161(11):669–72.

26. Işcan YY, Çapan Y, Şenel S, Şahin MF, Kes S, Duchêne D, Hıncal AA. Formulation and in vitro/in vivo evaluation of buccal bioadhesive captopril tablets. STP Pharma Sci 1998; 8(6):357–63.

27. Lee Y, Chien YW. Oral mucosa controlled delivery of LHRH by bilayer mucoadhesive polymer systems. J Contr Rel 1995; 37(3):251–61.

28. Shojaei AH, Zhuo S-L, Li X. Transbuccal delivery of acyclovir (II): feasibility, system design, and in vitro permeation studies. J Pharm Pharmaceut Sci 1998; 1(2):66–73.

29. Jasti B, Mahalingam R, Li X, Kulkarni U, Pather I. Influence of the thickness of buccal mucosa and effect of heat separation on the in vitro transbuccal permeation of antipyrine and caffeine. AAPS Journal, Vol. 8(S2): Abstract T2133 (2006).

30. Kulkarni U, Mahalingam R, Pather SI, Li X, Jasti B. Effect of temperature on the in vitro transbuccal permeation. 34th Annual Meeting and Exposition of the Controlled Release Society, 7–11 July 2007.

31. Mattek Corporation, Ashland, MA. http://www.mattek.com

32. van der Bijl P, Penkler L, van Eyk AD. Permeation of sumatriptan through human vaginal and buccal mucosa. Headache 2000; 40(2):137–41.

33. Thompson IOC, van der Bijl P, van Wyk CW, van Eyk AD. A comparative light-microscopic, electron-microscopic and chemical study of human vaginal and buccal epithelium. Archives of oral biology 2001; 46(12):1091–8.

34. Novadel press release, 3 November 2006. NovaDel Pharma receives FDA approval of NitroMist™. http://www.integratir.com/newsrelease.asp?news= 2130980802&ticker = NVD&lang = EN

35.  Novadel press release, 5 June 2007. NovaDel announces positive data from two studies comparing zolpidem oral spray to Ambien® Tablets. http://www.integratir.com/newsrelease.asp?news = 2130983049&ticker = NVD&lang = EN

36.  Hana Biosciences press release, 20 February 2007. Hana Biosciences reports likely delay in launch of Zensana™. http://ir.hanabiosciences.com/phoenix.zhtml?c = 183701&p = irol-newsArticle&ID = 965237&highlight =

37.  Novadel press release, 20 February 2007. Novadel comments on delay in Zensana™ Launch, as announced by Hana BioSciences. http://www.integratir.com/newsrelease.asp?news = 2130981877&ticker = NVD&lang = EN

38.  Novadel press release, 1 August 2007 NovaDel announces sublicense agreement for Zensana™. http://www.integratir.com/newsrelease.asp?news = 2130983541&ticker = NVD&lang = EN

39.  Transcept Pharmaceuticals press release, 13 June 2007. TransOral Pharmaceuticals, Inc. reports positive Phase 3 trial results with Intermezzo™ (low dose sublingual zolpidem tartrate) in treating insomnia patients with middle of the night awakenings. http://www.transcept.com/index.php?option = com_content&task = view&id = 21&Itemid = 31

40.  Medical News Today, 11 May 2005. First regulatory approval of non-injectible insulin, Generex Biotechnology announces. http://www.medicalnewstoday.com/articles/24174.php

41.  Medical News Today, 14 March 2005. Generex Biotechnology's Oral-lyn™ matches fast-acting insulin in phase IIb study. http://www.medicalnewstoday.com/articles/21213.php

42.  Reuters, 25 June 2007. UPDATE 1-Generex to start phase 3 trials for insulin spray. http://www.reuters.com/article/comktnews/idUSN2539964020070625?rpc = 77

43.  Biodelivery Sciences International press release, 24 August 2004. BioDelivery Sciences International, Inc. announces the closing of the Arius Pharmaceuticals acquisition. http://www.biodeliverysciences.com/news/webpr/pdf/8-24-2004%20Arius%20Acquisition.pdf

44.  Biodelivery Sciences International press release, 2 May 2005. BDSI Announces submission of NDA for Emezine. http://www.biodeliverysciences.com/news/documents/5-2-2005NDA.pdf

45.  Biodelivery Sciences International press release, 9 February 2005. BDSI completes clinical trials for its formulation of Emezine. http://www.biodeliverysciences.com/news/documents/2-9-2005ClinicalTrialsforEmezineComplete.pdf

46.  Biodelivery Sciences International press release, 20 July 2005. BDSI announces acceptance of Emezine® NDA for review by FDA. http://www.biodeliverysciences.com/news/documents/07-20-05EmezineNDAReview.pdf

47.  Biodelivery Sciences International press release, 1 March 2006. BioDelivery Sciences receives non-approvable notification from FDA on Emezine®. http://www.biodeliverysciences.com/news/documents/03-01-06EmezineNotApprovable.pdf

48.  Biodelivery Sciences International press release, 9 June 2006. BioDelivery Sciences announces promising results of meeting with FDA on Emezine®. http://www.biodeliverysciences.com/news/documents/06-09-06BDSIReleaseFDAMeeting.pdf

49.  Biotech Patent News, 1 July 2004. Atrix licenses BEMA technology to Arius. Reported in Allbusiness. http://www.allbusiness.com/technology/206530-2.html

50. PricewaterhouseCooper Report. Pharma 2020: The vision (2007). http://www. pwc.com/gx/eng/about/ind/pharma/pharma2020final.pdf

51. Senel S, Hıncal AA. Drug permeation enhancement via buccal route: possibilities and limitations. J Control Release 2001; 72(1–3):133–44.

# 6

# Pilocarpine Buccal Insert

Janet A. Halliday and Steve Robertson
*Controlled Therapeutics (Scotland) Limited, East Kilbride, Scotland, U.K.*

## INTRODUCTION

The Pilobuc™ pilocarpine buccal insert is a treatment for xerostomia. Xerostomia, or dry mouth, may be a result of Sjögren's syndrome, an autoimmune disease, or of certain treatments (e.g., head and neck radiotherapy), or medications. The condition distorts the patient's senses of taste and smell and can lead to recurrent mouth infections and dental caries, causing severe discomfort and malnutrition in extreme cases (1).

The market for xerostomia treatments is currently relatively small, in large part because it is underserved. Sialogogues, such as pilocarpine (Salagen®) and cevimeline (Evoxac®), when taken by mouth, are generally effective in stimulating residual salivary function, but may cause uncomfortable systemic side effects that outweigh perceived therapeutic benefits. As a result, patients frequently do not comply with these treatments or stop taking them after their initial prescription.

The Pilobuc insert is a controlled-release form of pilocarpine delivered via a buccal insert. The insert achieves therapeutic effect by delivering the drug to the salivary gland target tissues. The controlled release sustained method of administering pilocarpine reduces systemic side effects associated with oral bolus doses of the drug. Reducing side effects should lead to better patient compliance and improved therapeutic outcomes.

The delivery of pilocarpine and other sialogogues is covered by a U.S. patent (2).

## DEVELOPMENT HISTORY

The hydrogel polymer technology was invented by Professor Neil Graham at the University of Strathclyde in the early 1980s. The technology was patented by the British Technology Group plc and rights to certain applications licensed to Controlled Therapeutics. The first product to be developed using this technology was a vaginal insert containing dinoprostone. This product, sold under the trademarks Cervidil® and Propess® around the world, is currently licensed for cervical ripening and has been marketed since 1995. The buccal insert uses the same polymer. Development for use as a buccal insert has been carried out with advice from experts on oral medicine.

## DESCRIPTION OF TECHNOLOGY

Pilobuc is a controlled-release polymer chip impregnated with pilocarpine, a muscarinic agonist known to be effective in the treatment of xerostomia. The chip is placed in the upper or lower sulcus (the cavity between the upper or lower gum and the cheek), where it adheres due to its mildly mucoadhesive property. While in place, the chip releases pilocarpine, which is absorbed through the mucosa and, to a lesser degree, by swallowing. The chip is designed to remain in place for two to three hours, during which time it releases drug in a controlled fashion. Clinical studies are required to determine whether two or three applications will be needed to improve mouth comfort scores over 24 hour. The chip is not biodegradable and is removed and discarded after use. The Pilobuc controlled-release polymer chip is shown in Figure 1.

The hydrogel technology is based on a polyurethane polymer composed of polyethylene glycol, chain extended with an isocyanate and cross-linked with a triol described in standard texts (3). By adjusting the crystallinity and solvent uptake properties the polymer controls the release of drug over a period of many hours. When placed in an aqueous environment the polymer absorbs the solvent and any compounds dissolved therein. By drying off the solvent the drug then remains trapped in the matrix. Placing the drug loaded polymer matrix in body fluids rehydrates the polymer, the drug dissolves and is then released.

The properties of the hydrogel also make it suitable for use in buccal delivery. As with the vaginal formulations the polymer is removed at the end of the dosage period and drug delivery can be stopped simply by removing the insert from the site of application.

## CLINICAL RESULTS

Early clinical trials confirm that Pilobuc is equivalent to other xerostomia treatments in augmenting saliva production, yet it is able to achieve this

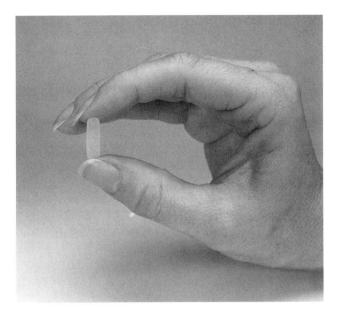

**Figure 1**  Pilobuc pilocarpine buccal insert.

beneficial effect with fewer systemic side effects. The reduction in side effects is due both to the local administration of the drug and to its controlled release. The latter avoids the pharmacokinetic "peaks and valleys" associated with serial oral administration of bolus doses in tablet form. It is believed that Pilobuc will have a lower dosing frequency than oral tablets, thereby making its use more convenient for patients.

Trials with Pilobuc show a reduction in side effects compared to Salagen® oral tablets and an improvement in both oral and eye comfort accompanied by increased saliva flow. The results of two, 8-patient, Phase I trials showed safety and tolerability of 5 mg and 10 mg Pilobuc inserts of various thicknesses. Acceptable mouth comfort scores were observed and are shown in Figure 2, and side effects were observed to be minimal and of the type anticipated with pilocarpine (4).

A further study was conducted in healthy volunteers to determine the pharmacokinetics of a 10 mg Pilobuc insert in the upper and the lower sulcus compared with two 5 mg tablets of Salagen taken orally. Results showed similar saliva flow for Pilobuc, with lower systemic exposure and fewer side effects.

Another study comprised a four-center, Phase II study conducted in the United Kingdom. This double blind, crossover study in 24 Sjögren's patients tested three Pilobuc doses versus placebo. The results showed an unequivocal dose response and clear efficacy in the higher doses for a

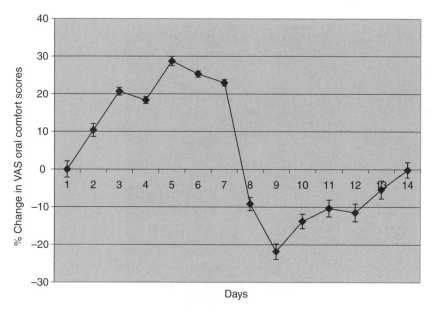

**Figure 2**  Change in oral comfort score with time.

number of endpoints. Saliva flow observed as a result of treatment in this trial is shown in Table 1.

The study also showed that safety was acceptable with few significant adverse events. The next step in Pilobuc development will be a Phase 2, placebo-controlled clinical trial to select the appropriate dose and frequency of usage in patients with Sjögren's syndrome and head and neck cancer.

## REGULATORY PLAN

The 505(b) (2) route, in the United States, would seem to be conventional and applicable filing strategy for this product. This approach is appropriate

**Table 1**  Saliva Flow After Four Days Treatment with Placebo, 2.5-, 5-, and 10-mg Reservoir

| | Treatment | Median saliva flow (mL/min) | | | |
|---|---|---|---|---|---|
| | Dose | Placebo | 2.5 mg | 5 mg | 10 mg |
| Day | Number of patients | 25 | 24 | 25 | 26 |
| 1 | Pretreatment | 0.05 | 0.05 | 0.03 | 0.05 |
| 1 | Posttreatment | 0.07 | 0.08 | 0.05 | 0.14[a] |
| 4 | Pretreatment | 0.05 | 0.05 | 0.06 | 0.06 |
| 4 | Posttreatment | 0.05 | 0.07 | 0.08 | 0.13[a] |

[a]Statistically significant.

when changing the route of administration of an approved drug; the case with pilocarpine, as it is already marketed in oral form. The polymer used in the buccal insert is well known to regulatory authorities as it is the same as that approved around the world in CTS' Cervidil and Propess vaginal inserts. The use of pilocarpine is already approved in xerostomia associated with Sjögren's syndrome and radiation therapy, and is supported by a large body of medical literature.

## CLINICAL NEED

The prevalence of Sjögren's syndrome is estimated at two to four million in the United States. The wide range is attributed to differences in age groups studied, the classification criteria used, and the methods for objectively evaluating lachrymal and salivary gland hypo-function. The prevalence of Sjögren's syndrome is expected to grow as awareness of the condition increases and the benefits of earlier diagnosis and treatment are appreciated.

More than 55,000 Americans are diagnosed with head and neck cancer each year. Most are treated with radiation, and virtually all will develop xerostomia. Provided some salivary function remains, the patient may benefit from a treatment such as Pilobuc.

Certain medications, particularly antidepressants, antipsychotics, chemotherapeutic agents, sedatives and hypnotics, can also cause xerostomia. This is a particular problem in the elderly, where thin oral tissues make them more susceptible to the sequelae of xerostomia, such as rampant caries and oral infections. This group represents a growing but untapped market for xerostomia treatments.

Finally, aging itself can lead to a decline in salivary function. An aging Western population suggests that this problem and market will only increase.

## COMPETITIVE ADVANTAGE

U.S. sales of Salagen (pilocarpine) and Evoxac (cevimiline) total less than $50 million (5). This market size is viewed as under-representing the true market and can be attributed to the combination of bothersome side effects with moderate benefit from these oral tablets. Dentists prescribe a variety of artificial saliva and dental caries protection products in the attempt to counteract the lack of protective saliva. Sales of caries preventative products such as PreviDent® are estimated at $40 million (6).

In Europe, oral pilocarpine sales revenues are lower than in the United States, principally due to pricing. The market for the rest of the world is difficult to estimate, both because of problems with existing products and because these markets have not been developed. Moreover, all markets face the challenges of under diagnosis and under treatment. Moreover, anecdotal reports from physicians working in this field indicate that a dentist or oral surgeon is as likely to initiate the diagnosis as a rheumatologist or other physician due to the sudden occurrence of dental caries, rather than to complaints of dry mouth by the patient.

The case of radiotherapy-induced xerostomia is different from autoimmune-induced disease, probably because the immediate radiation damage to the salivary tissues leads to an accelerated onset of symptoms. This rapid onset leaves the patient extremely uncomfortable and in need of urgent treatment to avoid recurrent mouth infections and tooth damage. The same may be true of certain medications that immediately diminish salivary flow.

## MARKET POTENTIAL

The challenge of the xerostomia market is to identify the health care professionals to whom to promote the product. Analysis reveals that rheumatologists and radiation oncologists are the most frequent prescribers of Salagen and Evoxac prescriptions in the United States. Perhaps xerostomia is an area where direct-to-consumer advertising might be particularly useful. Restasis®, a dry eye treatment from Allergan, where such direct-to-consumer advertising has succeeded, is a case in point (6). The product has achieved substantial sales since its launch in 2003 and is promoted extensively on TV and in print.

Artificial tears and saliva provide short-term symptomatic relief, but have the inconvenience of requiring administration many times daily. However, they are the principal symptomatic treatment for dry eye and mouth and are used by most patients with Sjögren's syndrome. Only 10–20% of patients in the United Kingdom currently use oral pilocarpine and, based upon pilocarpine sales, the percentage is probably even smaller in the United States.

The major disadvantages of pilocarpine, cevimeline, and other oral muscarinic agonists are the adverse effects associated with exaggerated parasympathetic stimulation. In clinical trials with oral pilocarpine, very commonly reported adverse effects (> 10% patients) were flu-like symptoms, sweating, headache, and urinary frequency. Other reported adverse effects (1–10%) included asthenia, chills, rhinitis, skin rashes, pruritus, dizziness, gastro-intestinal symptoms, salivation, flushing (vasodilatation), hypertension, palpitations, blurred vision, and lachrymation.

Some patients with Sjögren's syndrome tolerate these adverse effects because of the improvement in dry mouth symptoms. Taking pilocarpine after food and titrating the dose up over several weeks can improve tolerability. However, many patients are still unable to tolerate oral pilocarpine, so there is a need for a product that reduces side effects while maintaining effectiveness.

Perhaps the greatest market opportunity involves an eventual shift to consumer product sales. While Sjögren's syndrome and head and neck radiotherapy patients will generally be under the care of a physician, there is considerable scope for a dental OTC product that will stimulate saliva production for consumers suffering from mild or transient dry mouth due to medication or aging.

## FUTURE DIRECTIONS

The novel nature of the product creates manufacturing challenges. A scaled up process for polymer manufacture is under development. The volume of the product will be dictated by the nature of the consumer.

## REFERENCES

1. Manthorpe R, et al. Epidemiology of Sjögren's syndrome. Annales de Medecine Interne 1998; 149:7–11.
2. Halliday JA, Robertson S. US 6,488,953. Granted 2002.
3. Graham NB. Poly(ethylene oxide) and related hydrogels. In: Peppas NA, ed. Hydrogels in Medicine and Pharmacy, Vol. 2. Boca Raton, FL: CRC Press, 1987:95–113.
4. Gibson J, Halliday JA, Ewert K, Robertson S. Brit Dent J 2007; 202:E17.
5. IMS 2004.
6. Allergan's 10Q report quarter ending March 25, 2005. Restasis sold $37.5 million.

# 7

# OraVescent® Drug Delivery System: A Novel Technology for the Transmucosal Delivery of Drugs

**Ehab Hamed**

*Formulation Development, CIMA LABS INC., Brooklyn Park, Minnesota, U.S.A.*

**Steve L. Durfee**

*Drug Delivery Research, Cephalon Inc., Salt Lake City, Utah, U.S.A.*

## INTRODUCTION

The OraVescent® sublingual and buccal drug delivery systems have been designed to promote drug absorption through the oral mucosa. This may enable more rapid absorption of drugs that have a long $T_{max}$. In other instances, this route of administration may be desirable in order to avoid the first pass effect and as a result improve the bioavailability of the drug. Some drugs are not absorbed to a significant extent when administered orally, and delivery through the oral cavity mucosa may represent a convenient method of administration. The formulation of drugs of this type into tablets for transmucosal absorption may replace injection as the route of administration. In some instances, the pathological condition of the patient detracts from efficient absorption of a drug that would otherwise be well absorbed. An obvious example is the patient who is vomiting frequently. In addition, gastrointestinal (GI) transit may be so severely compromised during a migraine attack as to render efficient drug absorption unlikely. Under these circumstances, a transmucosal system may be advantageous. The technology is patent-protected as described in the technical section; additional patents are pending.

## HISTORICAL DEVELOPMENT

The $CO_2$-liberating reaction has been known and utilized in pharmaceutical dosage forms for a long time; the first patent was issued in 1872 (1). $CO_2$ is released as a result of the interaction of an acid with a carbonate or a bicarbonate salt. More recently, Eichman and Robinson explored the potential for $CO_2$ to promote the transport of a drug across a biological membrane (2). The mechanisms by which $CO_2$ acts as an absorption promoter are summarized as follows:

1. Solvent drag effect
2. Opening of tight junctions
3. Increase in the hydrophobicity of the cell membrane, thus promoting the absorption of hydrophobic drugs

The research described above illustrates the principle that $CO_2$-liberating reaction can enhance drug absorption. However, these authors did not set out to develop a practical system that could be utilized in drug delivery, nor was such a system described. Cima Labs scientists sought to utilize this principle to develop practical dosage forms. Systems that utilize the $CO_2$-liberating reaction for delivery of drugs through the oral mucosa (buccal and sublingual delivery) will be described in this monograph. Additional drug delivery systems based on the same principles and intended for administration via other routes are detailed in additional patents, but will not be described here.

Absorption enhancement illustrated by Robinson and Eichman may be improved by several additional effects, among them mucoadhesives, penetration enhancers and, in particular, pH effects. The latter will be examined in more detail.

## DESCRIPTION OF THE TECHNOLOGY

The relationship between solubility, $pK_a$, partitioning into a lipid phase, and pH in the GI tract has been described in the pharmaceutical literature as the "pH partition" hypothesis (3). This hypothesis states that for two aqueous environments separated by a lipid phase, permeability of a drug is most favored when it is in its unionized form. For drugs that are bases, this occurs when the pH is near to, or higher than, $pK_a$.

Besides the GI tract, the pH partition hypothesis has also been supported by certain drugs in percutaneous delivery, which show the expected dependence on pH relative to $pK_a$ (4,5). For other drugs, percutaneous penetration has been shown to have concentration dependence in a pH range in which the drug is largely ionized (6,7). These results have been interpreted to imply that there are multiple transdermal pathways. There is a large body of literature describing models for various pathways through the skin.

The existence of multiple pathways has been less clearly demonstrated in transmucosal permeability, which has generally been found to follow the pH partition hypothesis (8) because the chief barrier to permeability is an intercellular lipid layer (9), although there appear to be exceptions (10,11). As further evidence of a lipid barrier, many penetration enhancers operate by surfactant or solvent properties to decrease the lipid characteristics of the mucosa, allowing greater penetration of polar or ionized drugs.

The chief mechanism by which OraVescent technology promotes permeability by the nonpolar route was described by Pather et al. (12). Because it increases both solubility and concentration of unionized drug, OraVescent technology promotes both polar and nonpolar routes of penetration for drugs with a $pK_a$ within the approximate range of 4–10. The relative concentrations of citric acid, sodium carbonate and sodium bicarbonate may be adjusted to obtain the desired pH range. When a tablet formulated from these three ingredients first dissolves, citric acid ($H_3Ct$) dissolves causing the pH to decrease.

$$H_2O + H_3Ct \underset{\leftarrow}{\longrightarrow} H_3O^+ + H_2Ct^- \tag{1}$$

As the citric acid is dissolving the sodium bicarbonate also dissolves, leaving bicarbonate in solution

$$NaHCO_3(s) \underset{\leftarrow}{\longrightarrow} Na^+ + HCO_3^- \tag{2}$$

The decreasing pH facilitates rapid dissolution of the drug (D) by shifting equilibrium toward the ionized form.

$$D(s) + H_3O^+ \underset{\leftarrow}{\longrightarrow} D(aq) + H_3O^+ \underset{\leftarrow}{\longrightarrow} HD^+(aq) + H_2O(l) \tag{3}$$

As reactions (1) and (2) progress and the acidity of the solution increases, the bicarbonate neutralizes the acid and then effervesces.

$$H_3O^+ + HCO_3^- \underset{\leftarrow}{\longrightarrow} 2H_2O + CO_2(aq) \tag{4}$$

$$CO_2(aq) \underset{\leftarrow}{\longrightarrow} CO_2(g) \tag{5}$$

As the pH increases because of the loss of $CO_2$, protonated drug becomes increasingly unionized,

$$HD^+(aq) + OH^- \underset{\leftarrow}{\longrightarrow} D(aq) + H_2O(l) \tag{6}$$

Because recrystallization is a relatively slow process, the solution may ultimately become supersaturated with unionized drug, thus creating a driving force for the drug to partition into the lipid barrier of the mucosa.

Figure 1 shows the calculated apparent solubility and apparent partition coefficient for fentanyl (13–15), a basic drug with a $pK_a$ near 7.3. From Figure 1, it can be seen that OraVescent technology can promote both nonpolar and polar routes of absorption. When the tablet initially dissolves, the concentration of dissolved, ionized drug may be as much as 10 times higher than it would be at neutral pH, which promotes permeability by the polar route. Then, as the pH increases and the drug become predominantly unionized (and may be supersaturated as well), the nonpolar route is favored.

## RESEARCH AND DEVELOPMENT

The hypothesis that the above reactions and the resulting pH transition can be utilized to enhance the delivery of poorly soluble weak bases was tested

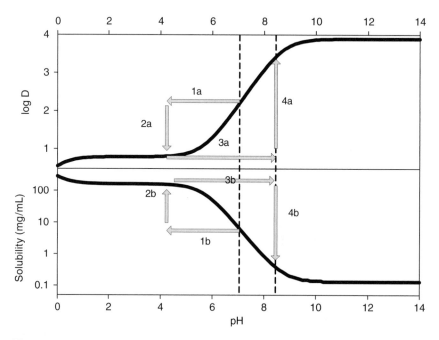

**Figure 1**   Log D and solubility curves for fentanyl. This figure shows both the log D and solubility curves for fentanyl. Arrows show the changes in pH and the corresponding changes in physical characteristics that occur in an OraVescent tablet as it dissolves. When the tablet first dissolves the pH decreases to about pH 4 (1a,1b). As it does so, the solubility increases by about one log(2b) and the apparent partition coefficient decreases by about one log(2a). As the solution effervesces, the pH increases (3a,3b). At a pH a little above 8, there is about a two-log increase in the partition coefficient (4a) and the solubility has decreased to about 1% of what it was (4b).

using fentanyl as the model compound. Fentanyl has been used for more than 40 years as an anesthetic and analgesic. It was chosen as a candidate for transmucosal delivery since its absorption via the GI tract is slow with significant gut wall and extensive hepatic metabolism. The $pK_a$ values of fentanyl are 7.3 and 8.4, and its unionized form is highly lipophilic, making it an ideal drug to test the hypothesis outlined above.

## Pharmacokinetics of OraVescent Buccal Tablets Containing Fentanyl

In one study, twelve healthy volunteers were given one of three dosing regimens according to a randomization schedule:

A.  An OraVescent buccal tablet containing fentanyl citrate
B.  A tablet that was similar to A in size, shape, and drug content but which contained lactose in place of the absorption-enhancing components; and
C.  An Actiq® oral transmucosal fentanyl citrate lozenge.

Subjects receiving treatments A and B were asked to place the tablet between the upper gum and inside of the cheek, above a premolar tooth. The tablets were left in place for 10 minutes. If, at this time, a subject felt that a portion of the tablet remained undissolved, he was told to gently massage the area of the outer cheek, corresponding to the tablet's placement, for a maximum of 5 minutes. A member of the clinic staff checked the subjects' mouths at 15 minutes to see if any portion of the tablet remained. The residue, if any, was allowed to dissolve on its own without further manipulation.

Administration of treatment C was according to the directions on the package insert of the product. After removal from the wrapper, the lozenge-on-a-stick delivery system was placed between the lower gum and cheek with the handle protruding from the subject's mouth. From time to time, the unit was moved to the other side of his mouth. Subjects were instructed to suck and not to chew the unit. The results of the study are shown in Figure 2 and Table 1.

The OraVescent enhanced delivery system displayed superior pharmacokinetics when compared to either the nonenhanced tablet (B) or the commercial dosage form (C). The OraVescent tablets had higher peak serum levels (~0.6 ng/mL compared to ~0.4 ng/mL for Actiq lozenges) and higher systemic fentanyl bioavailability (the AUC is approximately 1.47 times as high). Also, fentanyl was more rapidly absorbed from the OraVescent tablets ($T_{max}$ is 0.5 hr compared to 2 hr). A comparison of the enhanced and nonenhanced formulations (A *vs.* B) indicates that the improved pharmacokinetics of fentanyl is attributed to the OraVescent absorption enhancement components. In Figure 3, the serum levels obtained during the first 30 minutes are plotted on an expanded scale. These graphs clearly reveal the

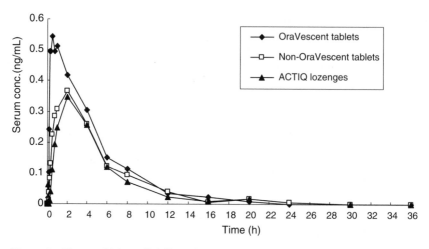

**Figure 2**  Fentanyl bioavailability after buccal administration.

faster absorption of fentanyl from the OraVescent formulation during the initial stages.

Similar superior pharmacokinetics of OraVescent buccal tablets containing fentanyl citrate were shown in other studies in healthy volunteers (16,17). In one study, 400 μg fentanyl in OraVescent tablets containing fentanyl citrate were administered transmucosally (FEBT$_{TrM}$) as described above and compared against:

1. 800 μg fentanyl in Actiq oral transmucosal fentanyl citrate lozenges administered transmucosally (OTFC$_{TrM}$);
2. 800 μg fentanyl in OraVescent tablets administered orally (FEBT$_{ORAL}$);
3. 400 μg fentanyl administered intravenously (Fentanyl$_{IV}$).

FEBT$_{TrM}$ had the highest absolute bioavailability (0.65) compared to OTFC$_{TrM}$ (0.47) and FEBT$_{ORAL}$ (0.31). $T_{max}$ was also fastest with FEBT$_{TrM}$ (47 minutes) when compared to either OTFC$_{TrM}$ (91 min) and

**Table 1**  Summary of Fentanyl Pharmacokinetics

|  | OraVescent® buccal tablets (A) | Nonenhanced buccal (B) | Actiq lozenges (C) |
|---|---|---|---|
| $C_{max}$ (ng/mL) | 0.64 (± 0.28) | 0.40 (± 0.07) | 0.41 (± 0.1537) |
| AUC (0–$t$) (ng*hr/mL) | 2.66 (± 0.6729) | 2.04 (± 0.87) | 1.81 (± 0.94) |
| Median $T_{max}$ (hr) | 0.5 | 2.0 | 2.0 |

*Note*: All values for OraVescent tablets are significantly different compared to corresponding values for the nonenhanced tablet and Actiq lozenges.

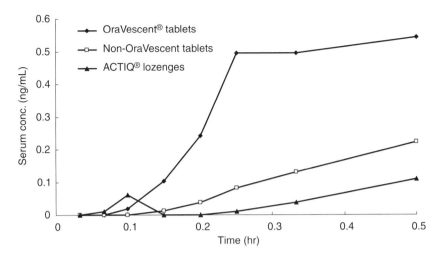

**Figure 3** Early phase fentanyl serum levels.

FEBT$_{ORAL}$ (90 minutes). It was concluded that approximately 30% smaller fentanyl doses in OraVescent buccal tablets would achieve equivalent systemic exposure to Actiq oral transmucosal fentanyl citrate lozenges. Similar short fentanyl $T_{max}$ values were also obtained after multiple dose administration of OraVescent buccal tablets (18), as well as in dose proportionality studies irrespective of the doses administered (19).

As it is the case with any new delivery system or administration route for a known compound, the question of absorption saturation and dose proportionality must be addressed. When OraVescent tablets containing fentanyl were tested for dose proportionality (200–1080 µg) in healthy subjects (19), the AUC$_\infty$ was linear over the full range of the study, while the increase in $C_{max}$ was linear between 200 and 810 µg. The increase in $C_{max}$ was 20% less than proportional at the 1080 µg dose. Dose proportionality after administration of 100–800 µg fentanyl in OraVescent buccal tablets was also confirmed in other studies (20–22). This linear fentanyl dose range has been shown to be safe and effective in treating pain in cancer patients.

## OraVescent Fentanyl Citrate Buccal Tablets and Breakthrough Pain

The fact that the OraVescent delivery system provides rapid initial rise in fentanyl serum levels indicates this delivery system has the potential to provide early onset of pain relief which is much needed in cancer patients with breakthrough pain (BTP). BTP is a transitory exacerbation of pain of severe-to-excruciating intensity that occurs on a background of otherwise controlled persistence pain. BTP is reported in 24–95% of cancer patients (23) and 70–80% of patients with chronic noncancer pain (24,25). An episode of BTP can reach maximum intensity within a median time of 10 minutes and last an average of 60 minutes (25). The onset of analgesic action of short-acting oral opioids used to alleviate BTP is approximately 30 minutes or more. OraVescent buccal tablets with faster absorption and significantly earlier $T_{max}$ can clearly offer a better alternative to patients with BTP.

To test whether OraVescent technology can provide early onset of analgesia in patients with BTP, OraVescent buccal tablets containing fentanyl were administered to opioid-treated patients with chronic pain associated with cancer who also suffer BTP (23,26). Pain intensity and pain relief were reported at 15, 30, 45, and 60 minutes and patient ratings of global medication performance were recorded at 30 and 60 minutes. The analgesic effect of fentanyl in OraVescent buccal tablets was apparent at 15 minutes, and the duration of relief was found through 60 minutes. Similar results were also reported in a well-designed phase III trial in opioid-tolerant patients with cancer (27). A single dose administration of OraVescent tablets containing 100–800 μg fentanyl provided clinically significant improvements in pain intensity from 15 to 60 minutes after the dose (27).

In all of the studies conducted, fentanyl delivery using OraVescent technology was well tolerated in patients (26,28–30) even after long-term usage (1 year) at a dose range of 100–800 μg (28). Of the 129 patients receiving OraVescent tablets therapy, only two patients discontinued the study because of oral mucosal adverse events (28).

## FUTURE DIRECTIONS

Other molecules that could potentially benefit from the OraVescent technology are presently being investigated.

## Note

Trademark OraVescent® is owned by CIMA LABS INC. Trademark Actiq® is owned by Anesta Corporation, a subsidiary of Cephalon, Inc.

## REFERENCES

1. Cooper. Improvements in preparing or making up medicated and other effervescing mixtures. British patent 3160.
2. Eichman JD, Robinson JR. Mechanistic studies on effervescent-induced permeability enhancement. Pharm Res 1998; 15:925–30.
3. Shore PA, Brodie BB, Hogben CA. The gastric secretion of drugs: a pH partition hypothesis. J Pharmacol Exp Ther 1957; 119:361–9.
4. Leveque N, Makki S, Hadgraft J, Humbert P. Comparison of Franz cells and microdialysis for assessing salicylic acid penetration through human skin. Int J Pharm 2004; 269:323–8.

5. Smith JC, Irwin WJ. Ionisation and the effect of absorption enhancers on transport of salicylic acid through silastic rubber and human skin. Int J Pharm 2000; 210:69–82.

6. Francoeur ML, Golden GM, Potts RO. Oleic acid: its effects on stratum corneum in relation to (trans)dermal drug delivery. Pharm Res 1990; 7:621–7.

7. Hadgraft J, Valenta C. pH, pK(a) and dermal delivery. Int J Pharm 2000; 200: 243–7.

8. Rathbone MJ, Tucker IG. Mechanisms, barriers and pathways of oral mucosal drug permeation. Adv Drug Delivery Rev 1993; 12:41–60.

9. Nicolazzo JA, Reed BL, Finnin BC. Buccal penetration enhancers—how do they really work? J Control Release 2005; 105:1–15.

10. Birudaraj R, Berner B, Shen S, Li X. Buccal permeation of buspirone: mechanistic studies on transport pathways. J Pharm Sci 2005; 94:70–8.

11. McElnay JC, Al-Furaih TA, Hughes CM, Scott MG, Elborn JS, Nicholls DP. Buccal absorption of enalapril and lisinopril. Eur J Clin Pharmacol 1998; 54: 609–14.

12. Pather SI, Khankari R, Siebert J. OraVescent: A Novel Technology for the Transmucosal Delivery of Drugs. In: Modified-Release Drug Delivery Technology. Rathbone MJ, Hadgraft J, Roberts MS, eds. New York: Marcel Dekker, 2003: pp. 463–216.

13. ACD/Labs, Version 10.0. Advanced Chemistry Development, Inc. Toronto, Ontario, Canada.

14. ACD/LogD, Version 10.0. Advanced Chemistry Development, Inc. Toronto, Ontario, Canada.

15. ACD/Solubility DB, Version 10.0. Advanced Chemistry Development, Inc. Toronto, Ontario, Canada.

16. Darwish M, Kirby M, Robertson P, Tracewell W, Jiang JG. Absolute and relative bioavailability of fentanyl buccal tablet and oral transmucosal fentanyl citrate. J Clin Pharmacol 2007; 47(3):343–50.

17. Darwish M, Kirby M, Robertson P, Tracewell W, Jiang JG. Comparative bioavailability of the novel fentanyl effervescent buccal tablet formulation: an open-label crossover study. Poster Presentation at the American Pain Society Annual Meeting, May 3–6, San Antonio, TX, 2006.

18. Darwish M, Kirby M, Robertson P, Hellriegel E, Jiang JG. Single-dose and steady-state pharmacokinetics of fentanyl buccal tablet in healthy volunteers. J Clin Pharmacol 2007; 47(1):56–63.

19. Darwish M, Tempro K, Kirby M, Thompson J. Pharmacokinetics and dose proportionality of fentanyl effervescent Buccal tablets in healthy volunteers. Clin Pharmacokinet 2005; 44(12):1279–86.

20. Darwish M, Kirby M, Robertson P, Tracewell W, Jiang JG. Pharmacokinetic properties of fentanyl effervescent buccal tablets: an open-label, crossover study in healthy adults. Poster Presentation at the American Academy of Pain Medicine Annual Meeting, February 22–25, San Diego, CA, 2006.

21. Darwish M, Kirby M, Robertson P, Tracewell W, Jiang JG. Pharmacokinetic properties of fentanyl effervescent buccal tablets: a phase I, open-label, crossover study of single-dose 100, 200, 400, and 800 microg in healthy adult volunteers. Clin Ther 2006; 28(5):707–14.

22. Darwish M, Messina J, Tempro K. Relative bioavailability and dose proportionality of a novel effervescent form of fentanyl in healthy volunteers. Poster Presentation at the American Society of Anesthesiologists Annual Meeting, October 24, Atlanta, GA, 2005.

23. Portenoy R, Taylor D, Messina J, Tremmel L. Fentanyl effervescent buccal tablets for relief of breakthrough pain in opioid-treated patients with cancer: a randomized, placebo-controlled study. Poster Presentation at the American Pain Society Annual Meeting, May 3–6, San Antonio, TX, 2006.

24. Webster L, Taylor D, Peppin J, Niebler G. Open-label study of fentanyl effervescent buccal tablets in patients with chronic noncancer pain and breakthrough pain: patient preference assessment. Poster Presentation at the American Pain Society Annual Meeting, May 3–6, San Antonio, TX, 2006.

25. Portenoy RK, Bennett DS, Rauck R, Simon S, Taylor D, Brennan M, Shoemaker S. Prevalence and characteristics of breakthrough pain in opioid-treated patients with chronic noncancer pain. J Pain 2006; 7(8): 583–91.

26. Portenoy R, Taylor D, Messina J, Tremmel L. A randomized, placebo-controlled study of fentanyl buccal tablet for breakthrough pain in opioid-treated patients with cancer. Clin J Pain 2006; 22(9):805–11.

27. Blick SK, Wagstaff AJ. Fentanyl buccal tablet: in breakthrough pain in opioid-tolerant patients with cancer. Drugs 2006; 66(18):2387–93; discussion 2394–5.

28. Segal T, Jhangiani H, Niebler G. Patients experience with fentanyl effervescent buccal tablets: interim analysis of a long-term, multicenter, open label study in cancer-related breakthrough pain. Poster Presentation at the American Pain Society Annual Meeting, May 3–6, San Antonio, TX, 2006.

29. Hale M, Webster L, Peppin J, Messina J. Open-label study with fentanyl effervescent buccal tablets in patients with chronic pain and breakthrough pain: interim safety and tolerability results. Poster Presentation at the American Academy of Pain Medicine Annual Meeting, February 22–25, San Diego, CA, 2006.

30. Portenoy RK, Messina J, Xie F, Peppin J. Fentanyl buccal tablet (FBT) for relief of breakthrough pain in opioid-treated patients with chronic low back pain: a randomized, placebo-controlled study. Curr Med Res Opin 2007; 23(1): 223–33.

# 8

# DentiPatch® Development

### Juan A. Mantelle

*Noven Pharmaceuticals, Inc., Miami, Florida, U.S.A.*

## BACKGROUND

Dental procedures, whether simple or complex, are typically associated with pain. The patient anticipates this pain, fears it, and postpones the visit to the dentist until such time as the discomfort or pain is such that he or she has to go. The dentist, on the other hand, knows that the patient is fearful and tries to make the visit as painless as possible so the patient will return on a more regular basis and thus minimize the need for the more painful procedures. Usually the mode used by the dentist to ameliorate the pain of the procedure is an injection of a local anesthetic, typically in combination with a vaso-constrictor, so as to extend the duration of the anesthesia. The problem is that the injection itself is painful, and the patient remembers the pain of the needle, the post procedure pain, as well as the uncomfortable feeling of the anesthetic "wearing off" for an hour or two after the visit.

Beginning in 1990, Noven Pharmaceuticals, historically a developer and manufacturer of transdermal products, set out to develop a transmucosal delivery system (TMDS) for pre-injection numbing that would address the shared desire of patients and dentists for a better, less painful approach. The target product profile (TPP) called for a system that would provide pain relief "to the bone," with rapid onset (less than 15 minutes after patch application) and a moderate duration (less than 30 minutes after removal). Ideally, the product would block the pain of injection and, in the case of less invasive procedures, actually eliminate the need for an injection altogether. The result was DentiPatch®, a small ($2\,cm^2$) patch that adheres to the gum line, delivering lidocaine locally and numbing the area to the bone. DentiPatch was approved by the FDA in 1996 and has been used successfully throughout the United States to ease the pain of injections and to permit certain procedures without the use of needles.

When the idea for DentiPatch was conceived, there were no commercially available examples of transmucosal patches. The path leading to the approval of DentiPatch (Fig. 1) included extensive research and intellectual property (IP) analysis in the areas of anesthetics, mucosal/gingival tissue composition/permeation properties, and mucoadhesives, as well as visual analog scales (VAS) for pain, and current dental practices, including allotted "chair times" for the various procedures and other practical considerations for the dentist.

This chapter will focus on the evaluation of relevant IP, the selection of the appropriate anesthetic, the development of the first-of-its-kind mucoadhesive platform, and the clinical trials leading to FDA approval of the DentiPatch system.

## INTELLECTUAL PROPERTY

During the development of DentiPatch, hundreds of patents were evaluated in order to understand what was the "state of the art" in anesthetics, specifically with respect to their use in dentistry and in TMDS. Table 1 shows the patents that were determined to be the most relevant given the TPP established for the product.

By experimenting with some of the compositions described in the above IP, the Noven formulators determined that mucoadhesion, although adequate, would not meet standards set forth by the DentiPatch TPP with respect to the onset and duration of anesthesia. This led to the development of the composition described by Mantelle in U.S. Patent 5,234,957, issued August 10, 1993, and subsequent patents assigned to Noven describing the DentiPatch system. The specific composition and its attributes will be discussed later in this chapter.

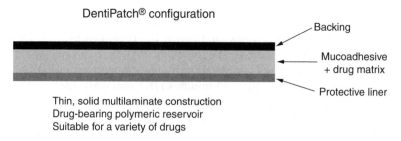

DentiPatch® configuration

Backing

Mucoadhesive + drug matrix

Protective liner

Thin, solid multilaminate construction
Drug-bearing polymeric reservoir
Suitable for a variety of drugs

**Figure 1**   The path leading to the approval of DentiPatch.

**Table 1** Key Patents Most Relevant to the Concept of the DentiPatch Target Product Profile

| Most relevant claim of patent | Reference |
| --- | --- |
| Incorporation of aminobenzoates in ointments that can be applied to mucosal tissues without irritation | (1) |
| The use of pH adjustments used on anesthetic mixtures for mucosal applications | (2) |
| The development of microadhesive systems with a focus on adherence evaluation as a function of compositional variables | (3) |
| The use of a lidocaine-saturated film capable of producing local anesthesia | (4) |
| The delivery of oxytocin to the oral mucosa using an adhesive patch | (5) |
| The use of a reservoir patch for delivering anesthetics | (6) |
| The use of eutectic compositions comprising etidocaine, lidocaine, prilocaine, tetracaine, or bupivacaine bases | (7) |
| The concept of a "soft patch" which consisted of embedded anesthetic agents in an ethylene (vinyl) acetate copolymer on a soft backing. Adhesion was achieved via the use of an oleaginous substance with polyhydric alcohol and a tactifier | (8) |
| The use of a single or multilayered bioadhesive film that could be utilized with a wide range of active agents. Extended or sustained release was contemplated from these films | (9) |

## ANESTHETIC SELECTION

Local anesthetics act by inhibiting depolarization and ion conduction of nerve fibers which, in turn, result in the blockage of pain perception. To achieve this blockage, the anesthetic must first permeate the target tissue, which in this case would be the gingival mucosa proximate to the intended site of the injection or procedure. Like transdermal systems (TDDS), a transmucosal system could use the base form of the active compound and benefit from the fact that the base is generally lipophilic. The salt form, although somewhat permeable through the gingiva, would be more hydrophilic and accordingly would take longer to permeate and require the buffering capacity of the mucosa in order to permeate the nerve membrane. DentiPatch, it was decided, would use the base form of the active compound.

With that decision made, the next decision was selection of the appropriate anesthetic. As per the TPP, the selected base would offer rapid onset, significant localized anesthesia to allow for minor procedures without injection, and moderate duration of action so that the anesthetic effects would wear off shortly after the patch is removed and the patient leaves the dentist's chair.

Table 2 shows a compilation of properties for the more commonly used anesthetic agents. The first criterion used to narrow the list of candidates was frequency of use in dental practices by injection. This eliminated benzocaine (not injected), dibucaine, procaine, cocaine, and pramoxine. Mepivacaine was eliminated due to its short duration of action. (Although catacholamines are used to extend the duration of anesthesia in injections, they are ineffective topically, so an extended duration of action of topical mepivacaine could not be achieved in this manner.) Tetracaine, although extremely effective in the DentiPatch platform and capable of providing up to one hour of localized anesthesia with a 15-minute wear time, was eliminated due to the potential for allergic reactions to "ester-based" anesthetics.

Noven developed formulations for four of the remaining anesthetics: lidocaine, bupivacaine, prilocaine, and dyclonine. Etidocaine was not formulated because the raw material could not be sourced at the time. These formulations were studied to assess depth of anesthesia, onset, duration and irritation of the mucosal tissue. Dyclonine was eliminated due to irritation potential, and prilocaine was eliminated because the depth of anesthesia that is offered was significantly less than lidocaine and bupivacaine.

With only two compounds remaining, it was time to decide between lidocaine and bupivacaine. The latter provided good depth of anesthesia and onset time and a longer duration of action, but the regulatory pathway to the approval of lidocaine appeared to be much shorter due to the long history of lidocaine use in dentistry. (Bupivacaine is used much less frequently in dentistry.) The formulators decided to proceed with lidocaine as a first generation product, and to follow with bupivacaine in the second generation.

## MUCOADHESIVE SELECTION

Noven's expertise was in transdermal systems that used pressure sensitive adhesives (PSAs), but PSAs were not suited to the moist environment of the mouth. The shift from PSAs to adhesives capable of adhering to moist mucosal tissues was challenging. In reviewing the existing literature and IP, it became apparent that, from among many possible approaches, the most expeditious route would use natural products such as gums, gelatins, and starches to create a gentle, removable adhesive capable of absorbing moisture and using it as a plasticizer (or tackifier) for the mucoadhesive.

This mucoadhesive would need to be swellable yet substantially insoluble so as to retain its shape while in use. In Addition, the mucoadhesive properties would have to be retained even when loaded over 60% with a combination of drug, co-solvents, sweeteners, and flavoring agents.

Formulators evaluated xanthan, tragacanth, and karaya gums alone and in combination with each other, as well as with polyacrylic acid, polyvinyl pyrrolidones, polisiloxanes, and ethylene oxide polymers. Several of these combinations yielded acceptable adhesives, but karaya gum stood out

**Table 2** Properties of the More Commonly Used Anesthetic Agents

| Local anesthetic[a] | Onset of anesthesia | Duration of effect | $pK_a$ (at 25°C) | Molecular weight | Chemical classification |
|---|---|---|---|---|---|
| 1. Benzocaine[a] | 1 | Short | 2.5 | 165.19 | Ester |
| 2. Lidocaine[b] | 2–5 | Medium | 7.9 | 234.33 | Amide |
| 3. Mepivacaine[b] | 1.5–4 | Short | 7.6 | 246.34 | Amide |
| 4. Bupivacaine[b] | 4–8 | Long | 8.1 | 288.43 | Amide |
| 5. Etidocaine[b] | 2–5 | Long | 7.7 | 276.42 | Amide |
| 6. Dibucaine | 3–10 | Long | N/A | 343.92 | Amide |
| 7. Tetracaine[b] | 3–8 | Long | 8.5 | 264.83 | Ester |
| 8. Prilocaine[b] | 2–5 | Medium | 7.9 | 220.31 | Amide |
| 9. Procaine | 5–10 | Short | 8.9 | 236.30 | Ester |
| 10. Dyclonine[b] | <10 | Medium | N/A | 289.43 | Ketone |
| 11. Cocaine | 2–5 | Long | 5.6 | 303.35 | Ester |
| 12. Pramoxine | 3–5 | Short | N/A | 293.39 | Ester |

[a]Commonly used topical local anesthetics for oral mucosal applications.
[b]Used as injectable agents in specific dental procedures.
*Source:* Compiled from Refs. 10–12.

as the most rugged in terms of processing and chemical stability and came the closest to achieving the properties set forth in the TPP.

The Noven team developed a co-solvent system comprised of lecithin, propylene glycol, and dipropylene glycol as solvation aids for what would be a 20% lidocaine base. Glycerine was utilized to impart gel properties to the karaya gum. Sweeteners and flavoring agents were added to mask the taste of the excipients.

The formulators currently contemplate a second generation of this transmucosal platform that uses polyacrylic acid and/or polyvinyl pyrrolidone as tackifiers to enhance mucoadhesion. This platform is viewed as a suitable vehicle for the delivery of bupivacaine, providing deeper anesthesia with prolonged duration and enhanced wear properties for up to several hours. However, the efficacy of this advanced platform has not been tested in humans as of the date of this writing.

## PIVOTAL CLINICAL TRIALS

The pivotal clinical trials supporting the FDA's approval of the DentiPatch product consisted of two randomized, placebo-controlled, double blind studies in healthy adults between the ages of 18 and 65 with no known contraindications to lidocaine or other local anesthetics. Subjects were trained in the use of the VAS and a verbal pain rating.

During the first screening visit, subjects received a single blind placebo applied to the buccal mucosa for 10 minutes at a site 2 mm above the mucogingival junction over the maxillary and mandibular premolars. Pain intensity was assessed via the use of a 25-gauge needle, which was inserted at a 45° angle to a depth of 2 mm apical to the mucogingival junction where the tip of the needle contacted the bone. The needle was removed immediately. A score of at least 2 on the five-point verbal scale was required for inclusion in further studies.

A total of 122 subjects were randomized to the double blind portion of the study. Over two visits, subjects received either a placebo or an active patch. Active patches contained either 10% or 20% lidocaine. A baseline 25-gauge needle stick was conducted as per the above procedure prior to patch application, and the VAS and verbal scores were recorded. This needle stick was then repeated at 5, 10, and 15 minutes post-patch application (with the patch in place) and the VAS and verbal scores recorded for each needle stick. Local irritation was rated using a 4-point scale as follows: $0 =$ no irritation, $1 =$ minimal, $2 =$ moderate, and $3 =$ severe.

Figure 2 shows the results of this clinical study (116 participants completed). These data show that both the 10% and 20% formulations significantly reduced needle stick pains ($p < 0.001$) compared with placebo at all of the measured time points. Onset of anesthesia was within 5 minutes

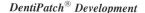

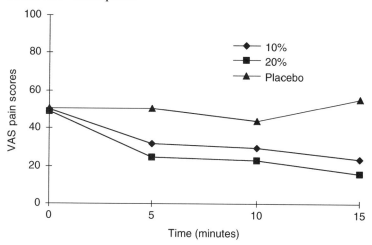

**Figure 2**    Mean change in VAS pain scores from 116 subjects receiving either a placebo or an active patch. *Abbreviation*: VAS, visual analog scales.

and peak anesthetic effect occurred at the 15-minute evaluation point. Overall, the mean reduction in pain was 49% and 65% for the 10% and 20% lidocaine formulations, respectively. Minimal irritation was noted in 15% of the placebo patients, 10% of the 10% lidocaine group and 8% of the 20% lidocaine group. No scores greater than 1 were noted for irritation on any of the three groups.

## CONCLUSION

DentiPatch was launched in 1996 and still remains the only product of its kind—a transmucosal patch for localized administration of therapeutic agents, in this case, lidocaine. The mucoadhesive platform upon which it was developed constitutes a very versatile vehicle for delivery of various therapeutic agents, either locally or systemically.

Subsequent generations of this platform have been formulated, and IP has been applied for and granted for technologies with enhanced adhesion over prolonged periods of time—multiple hours in some cases. Attesting to the versatility of the platform, these subsequent generations have been tested utilizing a range of therapeutic agents, including other anesthetics, non-steroidal anti-inflammatory drugs, steroids, antifungals, anti-migraine products, pain killers, breath fresheners, and insulin. Noven Pharmaceuticals holds the IP and know-how for this delivery platform, and intends to make this technology available for licensing and further development on a case-by-case basis.

## REFERENCES

1.  Tisza ET. US Patent 2,142,537. 1939. Anesthetic ointment.
2.  Curtis D. US Patent 2,277,038. 1942. Anesthetic preparation.
3.  Shrontz, DC. US Patent 2,501,544.1950. Therapeutic product.
4.  Davis SG, Mass, Swedish Publication 17747/70. 1972. Manufactured films containing anesthetics.
5.  Zaffaroni A. US Patent 3,699,963. 1972. Therapeutic adhesive patch.
6.  Zaffaroni A. US Patent 3,948,262. 1976. Novel drug delivery device.
7.  Broberg BFJ, Hans ECA. US Patent 4,562,060. 1985. Local anesthetic mixture for topical application, process for its preparation, as well as, method for obtaining local anesthesia.
8.  Kigasawa K, Ohtani H, Tanska M. European Patent Application 0,159,168. 1985. Soft patch drug preparation.
9.  Schiraldi MT, Rubin H, Perl MM. US Patent 4,713,243. 1987. Bioadhesive extruded film for intra-oral drug delivery and process.
10. Drugs Facts and Comparisons, 1990 Edition, J.B. Lippincort Company, St. Louis, MO, p. 601.
11. Merck Index, 1989-11th Edition, Merck & Co., Rahway, NJ.
12. Tucker GT, Mather LE, Clinical Pharmacokinetics of Local Anesthetics. ADIS Press Australasia Pty Ltd., 1979 Edition, pp. 242–78.

# 9

# Medicated Chewing Gum

Jette Jacobsen

*Department of Pharmaceutics and Analytical Chemistry, Faculty of Pharmaceutical Sciences, University of Copenhagen, Copenhagen, Denmark*

Margrethe Rømer Rassing

*Copenhagen, Denmark*

## INTRODUCTION

Chewing gum has been used worldwide since ancient times when man experienced the pleasure of chewing a variety of substances. Now, chewing gum is also used as a convenient modified-release drug delivery system. Commercially available medicated chewing gums are used for pain relief, smoking cessation, motion sickness, and freshening of the breath. In addition, a large number of chewing gums intended for caries prevention, xerostomia alleviation, tooth whitening, and vitamin/mineral supplementation are also on the market.

Medicated chewing gum offers advantages in comparison to conventional oromucosal and oral dosage forms for both (*i*) local treatment of mouth diseases and (*ii*) systemic effect after absorption through the buccal and sublingual mucosa or from the gastrointestinal tract. First, chewing gum can be retained in the oral cavity for long periods. Second, if the drug is readily absorbed across the oral mucosa, chewing gum can provide a fast on-set time for a systemic effect and the potential for avoidance of gastrointestinal and hepatic first-pass metabolism of susceptible drugs. Finally, chewing gum can be formulated to deliver drugs to the gastrointestinal tract to provide less irritation to the stomach owing to the drug already being dissolved or suspended in saliva when reaching the stomach. Generally, medicated chewing gum has good stability, the medicine can be taken easily and discretely without the prerequisite of water, and if required, prompt discontinuation of medication is possible.

Several factors affect release of drug from chewing gum including the physicochemical properties of the drug (i.e., aqueous solubility, lipid solubility, $pK_a$ value, distribution between gum-saliva), product properties (i.e., composition, mass, texture, manufacturing process), and the process of chewing (i.e., chewing time, chewing rate). The many possibilities for varying the formulations and the manufacturing process make chewing gum a drug delivery system of current interest when rate-controlled drug delivery for an extended period of time is required.

This chapter reviews the fundamentals of medicated chewing gum, historical development, regulatory issues, technologies, in vitro and in vivo evaluation of drug release, safety aspects, and future developments.

## HISTORICAL DEVELOPMENT

Gum-like substances, e.g., tree resins, leaves, waxes, and animal skins, have been chewed for many centuries. For a comprehensive review of the history of chewing gum, the reader is referred to Hendrickson (1) and Cloys and coworkers (2).

The first commercial chewing gum, "State of Maine pure spruce gum" was marketed in 1848 in the United States. The first patent on chewing gum was filed in 1869. This gum was intended as a dentifrice but it was never marketed (1,3). In 1927, the first medicated chewing gum, Caroxin® containing hydrogen peroxide, was marketed (4). In 1928, the second medicated chewing gum, Aspergum®, was commercially introduced. It contained acetylsalicylic acid (5).

The manufacturing processes and components of gums have been developed and improved over the years. Synthetic gum bases were developed during World War II due to shortage of natural gum bases (1). In the early 1950s artificially sweetened formulations became available (2).

Today, chewing gum as a drug delivery system is commercially available for several drugs, including acetylsalicylic acid, ascorbic acid, calcium carbonate, carbamide, chlorhexidine diacetate, dimenhydrinate, nicotine, sodium fluoride, and zinc salts.

## REGULATORY ISSUES

The first monograph on the dosage form, "Medicated Chewing Gum," was published in the *European Pharmacopoeia* in 1998. It describes the use of a solid tasteless masticatory gum base and coating, if necessary, to protect from humidity and light. Being a single-dose preparation, medicated chewing gum has to comply with tests ensuring the consistency of dosage units. In addition, the microbial quality has to be ensured.

Release testing is prescribed, e.g., a dissolution test. A monograph on a principle horizontal chewing apparatus and a procedure for the determination of drug release from medicated chewing gum is published in the *European Pharmacopoeia* (6).

A monograph for Nicotine Polacrilex Gum is published in the United States Pharmacopoeia (7).

Chewing gum must be chewed in order to release the drug(s) and it is accepted that residual drug(s) may be left in the chewing gum after chewing. Generally, a reproducible amount of residual lipophilic drug will remain after chewing a gum at a constant rate for a predetermined period of time. In some cases, e.g., smoking cessation, one only chews the gum until the desired effect is obtained, hence the expelled gum will have inter-individual variations in the amount of residual drug.

## COMPONENTS OF MEDICATED CHEWING GUM

### Main Components

Medicated chewing gum has a core consisting of the components given in Table 1.

The core normally weighs approximately 1 g. It may be provided with a coating either as a film of polymer, wax, or sugar/sugar alcohol or as a thicker layer of the latter.

The gum base consists of elastomers, resins, fats, emulsifiers, fillers, and possibly antioxidants. There are a number of different commercially available gum bases, each with different characteristics. All gum bases are insoluble in saliva and it is the gum base that determines the basic characteristics of the product. The characteristics that will be influenced by the choice of gum base include texture, drug release, stability, and the processing method. It is possible to manufacture chewing gum with either a larger or a smaller amount of gum base as described in Table 1. As an example, nicotine chewing gums contain approximately 70% gum base to adjust the release rate of nicotine from the product.

**Table 1**  Components of Conventional Chewing Gum

| Components | Concentration (%) |
|---|---|
| Active ingredient(s) | Max. approximately 50 |
| Gum base | 20–40 |
| Sugars/sugar alcohols | 30–75 |
| Softeners | 0–10 |
| Flavoring agents | 1–5 |
| Coloring agents | <1 |

## Taste and Mouthfeel

In contrast to most oromucosal formulations, chewing gum has a relatively long duration time within the oral cavity. Consequently, sensory parameters are important.

Unpleasant tastes of drugs can vary, e.g., they can be bitter, astringent, or metallic. There is no general, systematic description of methods for taste masking of chewing gum components and it is therefore necessary to rely on experience and consultation with flavor suppliers.

To obtain reliable statistical data on the sensory parameters of chewing gum, descriptive sensory analysis parameters are utilized in practice. A few relevant parameters are listed in Figure 1, which shows a quantitative descriptive analysis of two competitive products (8). In general, the parameters are assessed over time, relevant to the treatment period. Fundamental aspects are discussed by Meilgaard and (9), who describe concepts such as "*first bite*," "*first chew*," "*chew down*," and "*residual*" as important periods in the product's lifetime in the mouth.

## MANUFACTURING PROCESS

### Methods

#### Conventional Method

Chewing gum can be manufactured in different ways. The most common method includes the following steps:

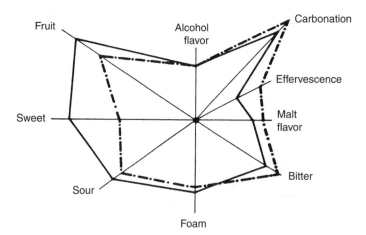

**Figure 1**   Quantitative descriptive analysis of two competitive chewing gum products; the distance from the center is the mean value for that attribute, and the angels between the outer lines are derived from the correlation coefficients. Solid line, product 1; dashed line, product 2. *Source*: From Ref. 8.

1. Mixing the gum base with excipients and active ingredient(s) in a Z-blade mixer (Fig. 2A)
2. Transferring the mixture to a cooling tunnel or storing it for 20–120 minutes in a separate container to cool the product
3. Rolling out and scoring of the chewing gum into pieces (Fig. 2B)
4. Storing for further cooling of the chewing gum pieces
5. Coating
6. Packaging

The gum base can either be added in a solid form and softened through heating from the jacket of the mixer or from the frictional heat generated during the mixing process, or it can be added in a melted form. The fact that the texture of the chewing gum is semifluid or dough-like during the mixing process and is hardened to a solid unchangeable form after the manufacturing process, makes it easy to obtain good homogeneity, and there are no segregation problems.

Another manufacturing method comprises a continuous extrusion process where the components are added at a fixed rate and place in an extruder (10).

### Compression Method

Chewing gum can also be manufactured by compression of gum powders or granulates on a conventional tablet machine. A particulate form of a gum base can be obtained by different patented techniques such as grinding the gum base under reduced temperature, or using underwater pelletizing (11).

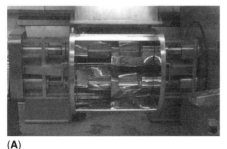 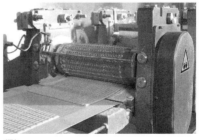

(A)  (B)

Figure 2  (A) Chewing gum mixer with Z-blades. The working volume of the mixer chamber is 800 L corresponding to approximately 650 kg chewing gum. (B) Scoring of chewing gum on a rolling and scoring machine. Capacity is 1–2 million pieces of gum/hour.

The compression method provides a number of advantages and disadvantages compared to conventional manufactured chewing gum.

Advantages:

- Different components can be separated and thereby any potential unwanted chemical interactions avoided.
- The process operates at lower temperature, which is suitable for heat sensitive active ingredients.
- Products look more like a pharmaceutical tablet.
- Multiple-layer chewing gum (two or more layers) is possible (Fig. 3). In multiple-layer chewing gum a combined fast and slow release of one or more active ingredients can be obtained. For different release profiles, each layer may have a different concentration of gum base.

Disadvantages:

- Poor chewability of the gum, but new developments have reduced this problem.
- Special requirements for the particle properties of the ingredients especially the gum base components.
- Controlled temperature and humidity conditions during handling and storage of the gum base, and during processing.
- As compressed chewing gums become more accepted and thereby more widespread as confectionary products, they are also likely to be increasingly used for medicated products.

## Scale-Up Issues

By using the conventional method, the majority of scale-up issues are related to the achievement of a proper texture as this is critical to obtain the proper mass and dimensions of the cores. These problems may be solved by choosing the right type and size of mixer and roller.

Using the compression method, the problem is that chewing gum softens at temperatures above 30°C and thereby deforms. Therefore, it is necessary to use equipment which operates at a lower temperature.

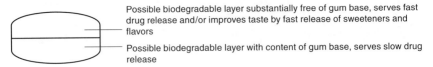

Possible biodegradable layer substantially free of gum base, serves fast drug release and/or improves taste by fast release of sweeteners and flavors

Possible biodegradable layer with content of gum base, serves slow drug release

**Figure 3** Cross section of a compressed two layer chewing gum. At least one layer contains one or more active ingredients. The concave shape gives a pleasant initial mouthfeel. The gum preferably has a diameter in the range of 8–20 mm and a thickness in the range of 4–10 mm. *Source*: From Ref. 33.

## STABILITY

The stability of chewing gum is comparable to that of most other solid delivery systems. Chewing gum normally contains little water (2–5%) and the water can be bound to other components in the product and is therefore not very reactive. The water activity ($a_w$) in chewing gum is normally below 0.6 and typically 0.4–0.5. If the water content is very critical for the stability of an active ingredient, the chewing gum can be manufactured without water (less than 0.2%). This will, however, often make the product hygroscopic and affect the texture. The low water activity also prevents microbial growth in the chewing gum during storage.

Special attention should be focused on the quality of the gum base and the flavors used in the formulation to avoid oxidation of the active ingredient. Normally, antioxidants are added with the gum base. Furthermore, the product can be protected against oxidation by a sealed coat and by an appropriate packaging.

For very temperature labile components, e.g., enzymes, a process temperature of 50–60°C while mixing can cause stability problems. It is, however, possible to operate the process at a lower temperature to avoid this issue (12).

## RELEASE OF DRUGS, SWEETENERS, AND FLAVORS

### Factors Affecting Release

For products intended for treating disorders in the oral cavity and in the throat as well as for systemic effect, it is often necessary to establish a constant concentration of the active ingredient in the saliva over a longer period of time. From a practical point of view, a realistic release period over which this can be achieved is 0.5–1 hour. To obtain a fast systemic effect a release period of 10–15 minutes is desirable.

The release rate of a drug is determined by a number of factors related to the chewer, the drug, and the chewing gum.

#### The Chewer

Release from chewing gum can be compared to an extraction process and the chewer-related factors are chewing-time, chewing-frequency, chewing-intensity and the volume of saliva (13).

#### The Drug

The release rate of a drug is first and foremost dependent on the solubility of the active ingredient in water/saliva. Very water-soluble active ingredients will be nearly completely released from chewing gum in 10–15 minutes. Active ingredients with a water solubility of less than 1 g/100 g will exhibit a slow and possibly incomplete release.

Lipid-soluble active ingredients are dissolved in the lipophilic components of the gum base and thereby slowly and incompletely released. An increase of the gum base percentage decreases the release rate and may increase the residual amount of active ingredient in the gum after chewing.

To obtain an optimal formulation that produces the desired release profile it is nearly always necessary to adjust the release rate of the active ingredient from the gum, either to obtain a slower release of readily water-soluble component or to obtain a faster or more complete release of a water-insoluble component.

The Chewing Gum

Several methods are available to modify the release of active ingredients from chewing gum by modification of the gum base and use of solubilizing excipients.

Nicotine has been formulated as a complex bound to a cation exchange resin, e.g., divinylbenzenemethacrylic acid or styrene-divinylbenzene. A higher percentage of ion exchange gives a slower release rate (14). The ion exchange principle could also be used for other ionic active ingredients.

An alternative method to increase the release of a lipophilic active ingredient is to produce a hydrophilic cyclodextrin complex (15,16).

It has been shown that the release rate from chewing gum can also be influenced by encapsulation of the active ingredient. A general description of encapsulation techniques for modified release from chewing gum is given in the patent literature (e.g., Reference 17). One method comprises a hydrophilic or a hydrophobic coating of particles of the active ingredient, normally by spray coating. To reduce the release rate a coating with ethyl cellulose can be used (18).

Other methods to modify release of active ingredients from chewing gum comprise granulation of the active ingredient with hydrophilic components/melted lipids or by mixing the active ingredient with a melted polymer (19). In addition, flavor oils can be adsorbed to organic or inorganic carriers, e.g., polymer gum base (20) components or silica (21,22), and thereby prolong the release.

Solubilization can be used as a method to increase the release of sparingly water-soluble active ingredients by adding emulsifying components. However, a problem with this technique is that it has a softening or dissolving effect on the gum base which requires a special gum base (23).

For further examples of principles for affecting drug release from chewing gum see the reviews by Rømer Rassing (13,24).

## Release Methods and Requirements

In vitro release methods mimicking the in vivo release are a desirable prerequisite for development of chewing gum formulations as drug delivery systems.

Previous in vitro methodologies and apparatuses for assessing drug release from medicated chewing gum have been reviewed by Rassing (13,24). Further, a vertical chewing apparatus has been reported (25). Requirements of appropriate release of active ingredient(s) are determined for each individual product according to the therapeutic needs on a case-by-case basis.

## In Vitro/In Vivo Correlation

A few studies have been reported concerning in vitro/in vivo release correlations. In one study, chewing gums containing 30 mg of urea were chewed for different periods of time up to 30 minutes. A chewing method similar to the method described in the *European Pharmacopoeia* was used for the in vitro release experiment. Volunteers chewed the gums and the residual amount of urea in the gum was analyzed to determine the in vivo release profile. A linear in vitro/in vivo correlation was obtained, $r = 0.9992$ (26).

In another study, using the same in vitro and in vivo release methods described above, four different chewing gum formulations containing water-soluble ascorbic acid were evaluated. The correlation between the in vitro and in vivo release profiles was linear within the first 5 minutes and between 5 and 15 minutes (27).

Adequate in vitro in vivo release profiles of chewing gum were reported applying suitable settings of the release equipment developed by Kvist and coworkers (25). In one study chewing gum containing 2 mg nicotine was tested (25). Another study tested a decapeptide in artificial saliva and an in vitro/in vivo correlation coefficient greater than 0.99 was obtained (28).

The in vitro and the in vivo release of the poorly water-soluble active ingredient, miconazole, from four different chewing gums has also been reported (29). The in vitro release method was according to the *European Pharmacopoeia*. However, for the in vivo study the gums were chewed for 30 minutes, and saliva samples collected at regular time intervals (29). The in vitro release profiles correlated well with the in vivo release profiles. The in vivo release resulted in therapeutically active concentrations of miconazole in saliva.

## SAFETY ASPECTS

Generally, today it is perfectly safe to chew a gum. Previously, hard chewing gums have caused broken teeth. Extensive chewing for a long period of time may cause painful jaw muscles, and extensive use of sugar alcohol-containing chewing gum may cause diarrhea. Long-term frequent chewing on gums has been reported to cause increased release of mercury vapor from dental amalgam fillings (30,31). However, medicated chewing gum does not normally require extensive chewing, or consumption to a great extent.

Flavors, colors etc., may cause allergic reactions.

Overdosing by use of chewing gum is unlikely because a large amount of gum has to be chewed in a short period of time to achieve this. Swallowing pieces of medicated chewing gum is likely to cause only minor release of the active ingredient due to difficulties of drug release from a gum base.

As a general rule, medicated chewing gum has (like other medicines) to be kept out of reach of children. In addition, if required, drug delivery may be promptly terminated by removal of the gum.


## FUTURE DEVELOPMENTS

Development of environmentally friendly chewing gums has been an issue for many years. That is, a biodegradable gum which will disappear by means of natures own remedies, i.e., water, light, and bacteria when left in nature or a gum that can easily be removed from indoor and outdoor surfaces by conventional cleaning methods and technologies (32).

Many efforts have been made by the chewing gum industry to develop chewing gum with these properties, which is illustrated by an increased number of issued patents on this topic. However no successful commercial products have so far been introduced on the market.

Chewing gum with a center filled with either liquid or powder is essentially based on a well-known technique for confectionary products and might also be used for medicated chewing gum. The production process takes place at a lower temperature as the gum is being produced by extrusion. Furthermore, the active ingredient is placed in the center which may result in better stability and a faster release.

In the future chewing gum as a drug delivery system will likely be forthcoming for the treatment of mouth and throat diseases, both of which require a long period of local drug release to the oral cavity.

By using optimal release systems and a better utilization of flavors, more active ingredients will be successfully formulated in chewing gum in the future.


## REFERENCES

1.  Hendrickson R. The Great American Chewing Gum Book. 1st Edn. Radnor, Pennsylvania: Clinton Book Company, 1976.
2.  Cloys LA, Christensen AG, Christensen JA. The development and history of chewing gum. Bull Hist Dent 1992; 40:57–65.
3.  Anonymous. A concise history of chewing gum. Dent Stud Mag 1969; 47: 626–44.
4.  Lützen CE. Solid oral anticariogenic composition. 1995, US 5,470,566.
5.  Growth through research: A history of Schering–Plough Corporation. Corporation brochure. 1992. pp. 3, 6.

6. Council of Europe. *European Pharmacopoeia*, 3rd ed. Strasbourg: European Directorate for the quality of medicines. 2001. pp. 129–30.
7. The United States Pharmacopeial Convention. Nicotine Polacrilex gum. In: USP 30–NF 18, Suppl. May 2007: 2751.
8. Stone H, Sidel J, Oliver S, Woolsey A, Singleton RC. Sensory evaluation by quantitative descriptive analysis. Food Tech 1974; 28:24–32.
9. Meilgaard M, Civille GV, Carr BT. Sensory Evaluation Techniques. 2nd ed. Boca Raton, FL: CRC Press, 1991: 162–9.
10. Broderick KB, Townsend DJ, Record DW, Song JH, Schnell PG, Sundstrom CE. 1995. Continuous chewing gum manufacturing process yielding gum with improved flavor perception. EP 0763330.
11. Mikkelsen R, Nielsen KH, Schmidt NR. A method for producing chewing gum granules and compressed gum products, and a chewing gum granulating system. 2004, WO 2004/098306 A1.
12. US Angel. 1994. Chewing gum and process for manufacture thereof. EP 2078186.
13. Rassing MR. Specialized oral mucosal drug delivery systems: chewing gum. In: Rathbone MJ, ed. Oral Mucosal Drug Delivery. New York: Marcel Dekker, 1996: 319–57.
14. Lichtneckert S, Lundgren C, Ferno O. 1974. Chewable smoking substitute composition. US patent 3,901,248.
15. Jacobsen J, Bjerregaard S, Pedersen M. Cyclodextrin inclusion complexes of antimycotics intended to act in the oral cavity—drug supersaturation, toxicity on TR146 cells and release from a delivery system. Eur J Pharm Biopharm 1999; 48:217–24.
16. Szejtli J, Pütter S. 1993. Chewing gum compositions. EP 0575 977.
17. McGrew GN, Barkalow DG, Johnson SS, et al. 1999. Chewing gum containing medicament active agents. WO 00/35298A1.
18. Morella AM, Lukas S. 1992. Microcapsule composition and process. CA 2068366.
19. Yang RK. 1987. Encapsulation composition for use with chewing gum and edible products. US patent 4,740,376.
20. D'Amelia RP, Cea TR, Beam JE, White RA, Agro SC. 1994. Chewing gum containing flavorant adsorbed in cross-linked elastomeric polymer. US patent 5,458,891.
21. Song JH, Courtright SB. 1990. Flavor releasing structures for chewing gum. US patent 5,128,155.
22. Bell W, Carroll TJ. 1993. Chewing gum or confection containing flavorant adsorbed on silica. US patent 5,338,809.
23. Andersen C, Pedersen M. 1990. Chewing gum composition with accelerated, controlled release of active agents. EP 486563.
24. Rassing MR. Chewing gum as a drug delivery system. Adv Drug Del Rev 1994; 13:89–121.
25. Kvist C, Andersson SB, Fors S, Wennergren B, Berglund J. Apparatus for studying in vitro drug release from medicated chewing gums. Int J Pharm 1999; 189:57–65.
26. Martinsen P. Ureas enhancereffekt på permeation over cellekulturen TR146 og release fra V6® tyggegummi samt β-lupeols permeation over cellekulturen. Masters thesis, The Royal Danish School of Pharmacy, Copenhagen, 1998.

27. Christrup LL, Møller N. Chewing gum as a drug delivery system. Arch Pharm Chem Sci Ed 1986; 14:30–6.

28. Na DH, Faraj J, Capan Y. Chewing gum of antimicrobial decapeptide (KSL) as a sustained antiplaque agent: preformulation study. J Control Release 2005; 107:122–30.

29. Pedersen M, Rassing MR. Miconazole chewing gum as a drug delivery system. Application of solid dispersion technique and lecithin. Drug Dev Ind Pharm 1990; 16:2015–30.

30. Sallstan G, Thoren J, Barrefard L, Schutz A, Skarping G. Long-term use of nicotine chewing gum and mercury exposure from dental amalgam fillings. J Dent Res 1996; 75:594–98.

31. Mackert JR, Berglund A. Mercury exposure from dental amalgam fillings: Absorbed dose and the potential for adverse health effects. Crit Rev Oral Biol Med 1997; 8:410–36.

32. Nissen V, Wittorff H, Andersen L. Compressed chewing gum tablet. 2004, WO 2004/068965.

33. Schmidt NR. Layered chewing gum tablet. 2005, EP 1 554 935 A1.

# 10

# The Oral PowderJect Device for Mucosal Drug Delivery

George Costigan and Brian J. Bellhouse
*Medical Engineering Unit, University of Oxford, Oxford, U.K.*

## INTRODUCTION

Oral PowderJect (OPJ) has been designed to deliver powdered drug to mucosal tissue in the mouth. Worldwide patents for the devices described below have been granted to PowderJect Pharmaceuticals plc.

There are several methods of accelerating powdered drug or vaccine particles to velocities high enough to penetrate skin or mucosal tissues. A shock tube forms the basis of the dermal PowderJect delivery device: it is capable of achieving high particle velocities in a jet of gas directed towards the target. However, the sudden release of this gas into the oral cavity was not considered desirable.

One alternative is the light gas gun in which a free piston is accelerated along a barrel by an expanding gas. Powder, placed on the upper surface of the piston, is thrown off at high velocity when the piston is brought to rest at the end of the barrel by a stopper ring. This device works well, but the possibility of piston escape or break up at high velocity did not commend it for use in the mouth.

The OPJ device uses the energy of a shock wave, traveling through a gas, to invert a flexible dome, on which the drug powder is placed. The powder is thrown off the dome with sufficient velocity to allow the particles to penetrate mucosal tissue. Gas is not released into the mouth, the dome is retained intact and the device is relatively quiet in operation.

A clinical study on 14 adult volunteers (1) concluded that an early design of inverting dome device could safely deliver powdered lidocaine hydrochloride to the oral mucosa, without causing tissue damage. This significantly reduced the pain of a needle probe at 1-minute post delivery. In this trial there was no means of retaining the drug on the dome; therefore it could fall off if the device was not held vertically. Consequently a number of different dome designs and manufacturing methods were investigated. Development and testing of the device to date have been focused on the delivery of lidocaine powder to the gum to produce an anesthetic effect. It is appreciated that it may be desirable to deliver other therapeutic agents by the mucosal route; the results and understanding gained from the lidocaine development program are making the achievement of this objective easier.

## DESCRIPTION OF THE ORAL POWDERJECT

OPJ is essentially a shock tube with a closed end, which can move (the inverting dome). The theory underlying shock tube operation has been described by Glass and Patterson (2), and Anderson (3). The performance of shock tubes with moveable end walls was considered by Nabulsi et al. (4).

Figure 1 shows a cross-section of an assembled prototype OPJ device. The functions of the labeled components are described below.

### Driver Gas Reservoir

The driver gas reservoir contains high-pressure gas which is released into the rupture chamber when the plunger is depressed. The rupture chamber and shock tube normally contain air at atmospheric pressure. The driver gas in the reservoir is usually helium, since this gives the greatest shock strength when the bursting diaphragm ruptures. The pressure and volume of the driver gas are selected so that, when released into the rupture chamber, a pressure high enough to burst the diaphragm is achieved.

### Bursting Diaphram

The diaphragm is required to burst rapidly, at a predetermined pressure, to set up the shock wave. The diaphragm burst pressure depends upon its diameter, the material used and its thickness. Burst pressure is also influenced by the strain rate applied, with low strain rates resulting in lower burst pressures.

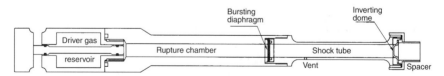

**Figure 1** Components of the prototype Oral PowderJect.

## Rupture Chamber

The longer the rupture chamber is, the more time will elapse before an expansion wave, reflected from the reservoir end of the rupture chamber, catches up with—and reduces the strength of—the initial shock wave. It is desirable to ensure that this interaction occurs well after the dome has inverted.

## Shock Tube

The shock tube diameter is fixed by the diameter of the dome. A minimum shock tube length of order five or six diameters is usually recommended, to allow a normal shock wave to form.

## Vent

The shock tube is vented to atmosphere in the OPJ device, to allow a controlled decay of pressure and minimize the possibility of dome rupture.

## Inverting Dome

The dome must be light and flexible to enable it to invert rapidly. It must also be resistant to rupture. It should retain drug particles under normal handling conditions, and release them uniformly when it inverts.

A photograph of the OPJ is shown in Figure 2.

## DOME DESIGN

Dome design is crucial to the satisfactory performance of the OPJ and considerable effort was expended to arrive at the current design, which is still subject to refinement as our studies of dome behavior progress. The domes used to produce the results described herein were all molded from

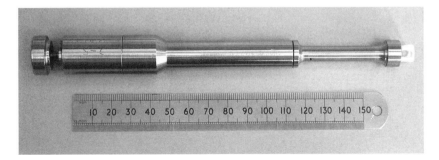

**Figure 2** A prototype Oral PowderJect.

Hytrel® (Du Pont) polyester elastomer. A cross section of a typical dome is shown in Figure 3, with a photograph below it.

The domes are shaped like soup plates, with a flat base and a ridge around the outer edge, which forms a retaining seal. A total of 81 short fibers are molded into the dome base to retain the lidocaine powder. Shaking tests demonstrated that this arrangement retains 100% of a payload of 3 mg of mannitol powder (size fraction 38–53 µm) at an acceleration of 2 g and 90% at an acceleration of 6 g. Lidocaine hydrochloride powder is much less "free running" than mannitol, so that the drug loaded domes can be manipulated easily without loss of powder.

In vitro testing of these domes confirmed that their performance did not deteriorate after degreasing and sterilization with chemicals or by gamma irradiation.

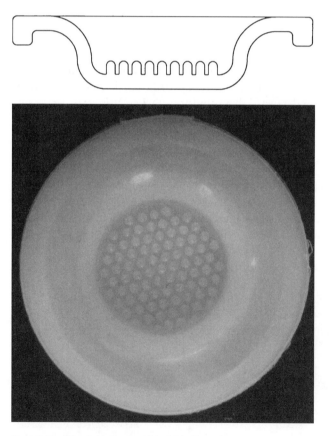

**Figure 3**   The injection molded 81 fiber dome.

## IN VITRO DEVICE TESTS

An instrumented version of the straight shock tube OPJ (Fig. 1) was used to collect performance data for a wide range of operating conditions. Driver cylinder pressure, rupture chamber, and shock tube pressures were recorded. The pressure measurements indicated shock strengths and velocities.

Powder velocities were deduced by cross correlating the obscuration signals from two photo diodes. The photo diodes were illuminated by two light emitting diodes placed 4 mm apart, with the lower beam located 10 mm above the dome clamping plane. The domes were loaded with $1.5 \pm 0.5$ mg of mannitol powder (size 53–75 μm) for these tests. The velocities obtained relate to the leading edge of the powder cloud as it passed through the beams. By varying the driver conditions velocities between 150 and 250 m/sec were achieved. The measured velocities were used as a criterion of performance of the device.

Results using particle sizes up to 800 μm (all particles with densities around $1 \text{ g/cm}^3$) showed that their velocities were independent of particle size for fixed driver conditions (driver gas pressure, diaphragm material, thickness, etc.). Since particle penetration depth depends upon particle size, density, and velocity, larger particles might be expected to penetrate further than small ones. This was confirmed by penetration measurements.

Oral devices were also tested by discharging them, loaded with a known payload (up to 3 mg) of model particles (usually polystyrene beads of known diameter), above a 3% agar gel target. The vented spacer fitted to the exit plane of each device kept it at a fixed distance from the target surface and at right angles to it. The gel surface was then photographed to record the delivery footprint. Then the gel target was sliced across a diameter and thin sections were photographed through a microscope, to establish the depth of penetration of the individual particles.

In general the device footprint was a 6 mm diameter circle and particles were distributed on the target in a pattern which reflected the positions of the fibers on the dome (Fig. 4).

No significant penetration was observed using 48 μm diameter polystyrene spheres, but 99 μm diameter particles penetrated the agar gel target to a maximum depth of 200 μm (Fig. 5).

Measurements of the penetration of similar model particles into excised mucosal tissue from pigs and dogs have also been made.

## IN VIVO TESTS (ANIMALS)

A study of the tolerability, efficacy and pharmacokinetic performance of the OPJ, when used to administer drugs to the oral mucosa of dogs has been started, but results were not available at the time of writing.

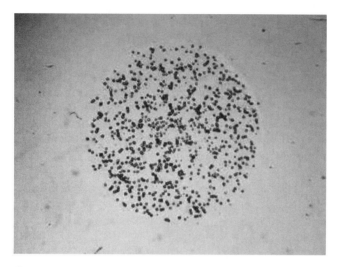

**Figure 4**   The Oral PowderJect device footprint on agar gel target.

## IN VIVO TESTS (HUMANS)

A number of small scale, in-house clinical trials of the device were conducted in a local dental surgery. A small number of volunteers received administrations of $1.5 \pm 0.1$ mg of powdered lidocaine from the OPJ device and the tolerability and efficacy of these doses were assessed. For all tests a 5 mL 24 bar cylinder of helium was used.

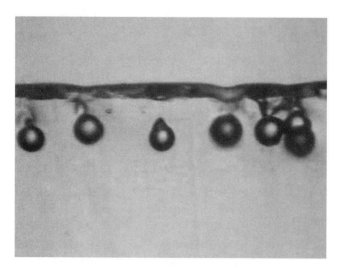

**Figure 5**   Penetration of 99 μm diameter polystyrene spheres into 3% agar gel.

## Tolerability Tests

For tolerability testing two aluminium diaphragm of thickness 20 and 30 μm were used. Four particle size ranges were tested ranging from 53 to 250 μm.

All particles were tolerated well, but the 180–250 μm size fraction left a number of small micro bleeds in the mucosal tissue.

## Efficacy Tests

### Experimental Methods

**Response to a hypodermic needle probe:** Two administrations of lidocaine (size fraction of 75–106 μm) were made to the buccal mucosa of each volunteer, a third administration of the device contained no powder. Operator and subject were unaware of which of the three administrations was the sham. Each site was probed at 30 and 60 seconds after administration using a 27 g needle inserted to a depth of 1.5 mm. Pain on administration and after probing was recorded on a 100 mm VAS scale.

For the purpose of comparison 5 mg of pure lidocaine and 5 mg of sugar were placed on two sites on the buccal sulcus. Both sites were probed with a needle after 60 seconds. In a similar way the effect of applying a commercially available topical anesthetic gel was compared with the application of a placebo gel. Again two sites on the buccal sulcus were probed with a hypodermic needle.

**Response to a dental injection:** Two sites on the buccal sulcus (one active, one sham) were used to test the pain of a dental injection. Lidocaine particles with diameters between 125 and 180 μm were used. After 60 seconds an injection of local anesthetic was administered to each site.

### Summary of Results

The above tests have been documented by Duckworth (5) who summarized his findings as follows:

- There is no pain on administration.
- There is no visible tissue damage.
- Anesthesia is very impressive.
- Reduces the pain of a needle probe to the gum in 30 seconds: median VAS scores 3.3 active versus 43.2 sham.
- Reduces the pain of a dental injection into the gum in 60 seconds: medium VAS scores 4.3 active versus 35.2 sham.
- Lidocaine powder applied topically is no more effective than a placebo after 60 seconds.
- Commercial anesthetic gel is no more effective than a placebo after 60 seconds.

## CONCLUSIONS

A typical operating condition for the existing design of OPJ uses a 5 mL cylinder of helium at 25 bar and a 30 μm aluminium bursting diaphragm to achieve powder velocities of 236 m/sec. At this condition particles of 100 μm in diameter with densities around 1 g/cm$^3$, penetrate mucosal tissue. In-house clinical trials have demonstrated the effectiveness and speed of the OPJ in producing anesthesia in the gum.

Higher particle velocities will enable the device to deliver smaller particles into the oral mucosa. In the future a device will be designed to deliver lidocaine, which is simpler and cheaper than the prototypes descri-bed here.

## REFERENCES

1. Duckworth GM, Millward HR, Potter CDO, Hewson G, Burkoth TL, Bellhouse BJ. Oral PowderJect: a novel system for administering local anaes-thetic to the oral mucosa. Brit Dent J 1998; 185:536–9.
2. Glass II and , Patterson GN. A theoretical and experimental study of shock-tube flows. J Aeronautic Sci 1955; 22:73–100.
3. Anderson JD Jr. Modern Compressible Flow. New York: McGraw-Hill, 1990.
4. Nabulsi SM, Millward HR, Bellhouse BJ. The use of a shock tube for the delivery of powdered drugs into the oral mucosa. 22nd Int. Symp. on Shock Waves, Imperial College, London. Paper #170, 1999.
5. Duckworth GM. Trial reports PJP-OPJ-BUCCAL-001 to 004. 2000.

# 11

# The PerioChip™: A Biodegradable Device for the Controlled Delivery of Chlorhexidine in the Subgingival Environment

**Wilfred Aubrey Soskolne**

*Department of Periodontology, Hebrew University-Hadassah Faculty of Dentistry, Jerusalem, Israel*

## INTRODUCTION

### Historical Background

In the 1970s it became clear that the subgingival environment was not accessible to antibacterial agents delivered to the oral cavity in the form of tooth pastes and mouth washes due to their limited ability to penetrate into the subgingival environment (1,2). The irrigation of the pockets with antibacterial agents was found to be clinically ineffective probably due to the rapid washout of the drugs to ineffective levels (3,4). This led to the development of devices that could be introduced into periodontal pockets to deliver their active antibacterial ingredients over an extended period of time (5–10).

   At the beginning of our studies we made the strategic decision to develop a fixed dimension delivery platform in the form of a film/slab that contained a fixed unit dose of the active agent. Based on previous studies (9,11), a prototype device was developed to establish the proof of concept. This device was an ethyl cellulose film, cast from ethanol or chloroform solutions of the polymer, with a plasticizing agent and the appropriate drug incorporated into the solution (10). A number of antibacterial agents including chlorhexidine (CHX) (10,12), minocycline (13), and tetracycline

(14,15) were tested in this platform and their degree of effectiveness in altering the subgingival microflora established. Based on our studies (10,12,16) CHX was chosen as the drug of choice for a number of reasons including the long history of safety and efficacy for its use in the oral cavity, its broad spectrum of antibacterial activity, no reported development of bacterial resistance and its safety for long term repeated multiple use.

After establishing the principle that controlled subgingival CHX release was effective in treating periodontal disease (10,12,16) and before scaling up to a good manufacturing practices (GMP) production line for clinical trials, a further strategic decision was made to develop a biodegradable platform. Maintaining the same physical form for ease of use a biodegradable platform would reduce the number of patient treatment visits needed and improve patient compliance compared to a non-degradable platform such as ethyl cellulose. A biodegradable platform, based on a cross-linked hydrolyzed gelatin matrix, was developed (17). The final formulation was then taken through all the required regulatory steps, in the individual countries, before marketing it as the PerioChip.

### Description of PerioChip

The device is in the form of a film consisting of a degradable matrix of cross-linked hydrolyzed gelatin 350 μm thick and measuring 4 mm in width and 5 mm in length. The one end is rounded for ease of insertion. It weighs 7.4 mg and contains 2.5 mg of chlorhexidine digluconate (Fig. 1). Although it initially had to be stored at about 4°C, FDA approval was obtained in February 2002 for a stabilized formulation that now allows storage at room temperature. It has a shelf life of 2 years.

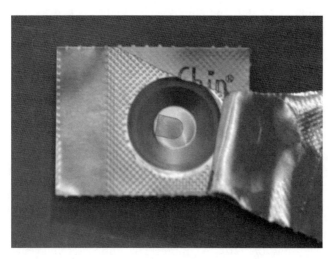

**Figure 1** A single PerioChip™ is seen in an opened blister package.

The PerioChip has a number of unique features when compared to other available technologies for the controlled subgingival delivery of drugs:

1. It is marketed as a fixed unit dosage for individual subgingival sites.
2. The placement of the device is extremely simple taking only a few seconds.
3. It is the only subgingival delivery platform whose active ingredient is an antiseptic (CHX) eradicating the possible adverse effects associated with the use of antibiotics.
4. It is degradable.

## Research and Development

Toxicology (Perio Products Ltd.—In-House Data)

A number of studies were carried out to establish the toxicity and safety of the PerioChip in cell cultures and animal models. A study was carried out to assess the toxicity of PerioChip powder administered via gastric intubation to rats. Dosages of 7.5, 37.5, and 125 mg PerioChip powder/kg/day were administered for 30 days to groups of 24 animals. Controls received the same dosages of vehicle (PEG 400). There was no effect of the treatments on body weight, food and water consumption, hematology or clinical chemistry parameters during the 30 days. Six animals receiving the high-dose treatment with PerioChip powder died during the study and except for pulmonary edema noted in these 6 animals, gross and microscopic findings occurred with equal frequency in control and experimental animals. Therefore the "no effect" level for 30 days oral administration of PerioChip powder was considered to be 37.5 mg/kg/day.

The effect of the CHX containing chip on the hamster cheek pouch mucosa, isolated from the oral cavity by a purse-string suture, was compared to the effect of a placebo chip, a polyvinyl chloride (PVC) chip (positive control) and sham suturing without a chip. The results indicated that 7 and 14 days of exposure to the CHX chip resulted in significantly more mucosal edema than in either the sham sutured or placebo chip treated groups. The PVC chip treated pouches resulted in significantly greater edema than did the CHX chip. The measure of erythema was similar in all three chip treated groups and after 14 days of exposure was significantly greater than in the sham sutured group. Histology indicated that there was slightly more inflammation in the CHX chip and PVC chip groups than in the placebo chip and sham sutured groups. This difference reached significance after 14 days of exposure. All clinical and histological changes had disappeared after a 7 day recovery period. These results indicated that the active CHX chip had some irritative effect on the mucosa. However, recovery was complete in 7 days.

The mice micronucleus test was carried out to establish the effect on chromosome structure in bone marrow cells following acute oral administration of different doses of PerioChip. The results indicated that, under the conditions of the test, there was no evidence of induced chromosomal or other damage leading to micronucleus formation in immature erythrocytes of treated mice 24, 48, or 72 hours after oral administration of PerioChip.

A study was carried out to determine the toxicity of PerioChip powder and PerioChip matrix to Chinese hamster lung cells (V79) in the presence and absence of a rat liver derived metabolic activation system (S-9 mix). The PerioChip powder alone showed marked toxicity with an $LC_{50}$ value of $17\,\mu g/mL$. The addition of S-9 mix had a detoxifying effect, giving a $LC_{50}$ value of $57\,\mu g/mL$. PerioChip matrix was considerably less toxic with $LC_{50}$ values of $300\,\mu g/mL$ alone and $600-1000\,\mu g/mL$ when S-9 mix was included. Chlorhexidine digluconate alone was extremely toxic giving an $LC_{50}$ of $1.5\,\mu g/mL$ which increased to $12.2\,\mu g/mL$ in the presence of S-9mix.

These data indicated that, at the dosages used for the treatment of human periodontitis, the PerioChip could be considered safe for use as a therapeutic agent.

## Pharmacokinetics

To establish the pharmacokinetics of CHX release from the chip into the subgingival environment and its systemic distribution, an open label, single center, 10-day pharmacokinetic study was conducted on 19 volunteers with chronic adult periodontitis (18). Each volunteer had a single chip (refrigerated version) inserted at time 0 into each of four selected pockets, with probing pocket depths (PPDs) of between 5 and 8 mm. Gingival crevicular fluid (GCF) samples were collected using filter paper strips prior to chip placement and at 2, 4, 24 hours and 2, 3, 4, 5, 6, 8, and 9 days post chip placement. The GCF volume was measured using a calibrated Periotron 6000. Blood samples were collected at times 0, 1, 4, 8, 12 hours and 5 days post dosing. Urine was collected as a total 24-hour specimen, immediately post dosing and two single samples at time 0 and 5 days. The CHX was then eluted from the paper strips and the CHX levels in GCF, blood and urine quantified using HPLC. The results (Fig. 2) indicate an initial peak concentration of CHX in the GCF at 2 hours post chip insertion ($2007\,\mu g/mL$) with slightly lower concentrations of between 1300 and $1900\,\mu g/mL$ being maintained over the next 96 hours. The CHX concentration then progressively decreased until the conclusion of the study. CHX concentrations ($57\,\mu g/mL$) were still detectable at day 10. CHX was not detectable in any of the plasma or urine sample at any time point during the study.

## Efficacy and Safety Studies

**As an adjunct to scaling and root planing:**   The efficacy and safety of the chip as an adjunct to the treatment of periodontitis was established in

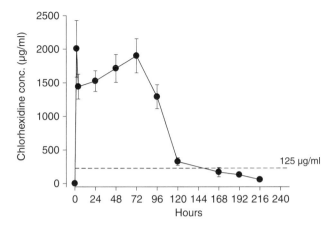

**Figure 2** The mean chlorhexidine concentration in the gingival crevicular fluid from periodontal pockets treated with a single PerioChip™. The vertical bars represent the standard error of the means.

three multicenter studies. The first was a 6-month, randomized, blinded, multicenter study of 118 patients with moderate periodontitis, carried out at three different centers in Europe (19). A split-mouth design was used to compare the treatment outcomes of scaling and root planing (SRP) alone with the combined use of SRP and the chip in pockets with probing depths of 5–8 mm. The two maxillary quadrants were used for the two treatment arms of the study. SRP was performed at baseline only, while the chip was inserted both at baseline and at three months. Clinical and safety measurements including PPD, probing attachment level (PAL), bleeding on probing (BOP) as well as gingivitis, plaque, and staining indices were recorded at baseline, 1, 3, and 6 months.

The average PPD reduction in the chip treated sites was significantly greater than in the sites receiving SRP alone at both 3 and 6 months with a mean difference of 0.42 mm ($p \leq 0.01$) at 6 months. The reduction in PAL at the chip treated sites was greater than at the sites receiving SRP alone. The difference was statistically significant at the 6 month visit only. An analysis of patients with initial PPDs of 7–8 mm ($n = 47$) revealed a significantly greater reduction in PPD and PAL in those pockets treated with the chip compared to SRP alone at both 3 and 6 months. The mean differences between test and control sites at 6 months were 0.71 and 0.56 mm for PPD and PAL respectively.

The two other double blind, randomized, placebo controlled multicenter clinical trials of 9-month duration were conducted in the United States. Their results were pooled and reported as a single study from 10 centers (20). At baseline, patients free of supra-gingival calculus, were provided with 1 hour of SRP. Sites targeted for treatment were sites that bled on probing with PPD of 5–8 mm. Study sites in the active chip subjects received, either CHX chip plus SRP or SRP alone (to maintain study blind). Sites in placebo chip subjects received, either a placebo chip plus SRP or SRP alone. Chip placement was repeated at 3 and/or 6 months if PPD remained ≥ 5mm. Examinations were performed at baseline; 7 days; 6 weeks; and 3, 6, and 9 months. At 9 months the CHX chip showed significantly greater reductions in both PPD (CHX chip plus SRP, $0.95 \pm 0.05$ mm; SRP alone $0.65 \pm 0.05$ mm, $p < 0.001$: placebo chip plus SRP, $0.69 \pm 0.05$mm, $p < 0.001$) and PAL (CHX chip plus SRP $0.75 \pm 0.06$ mm; SRP alone, $0.58 \pm 0.06$ mm, $p < 0.05$; placebo chip plus SRP, $0.55 \pm 0.06$ mm, $p < 0.05$) compared to the controls. The percentage of patients who had a PPD reduction from baseline of 2 mm or more at 9 months (19.1%) in the CHX chip group compared with (8%) in the SRP controls. Adverse effects were minor and transient. Toothache was the most common complaint occurring more often in the CHX chip group than in the placebo chip group ($p = 0.042$).

In a subset of 45 patients from the above U.S. multicenter study quantitative digital subtraction radiography on standardized radiographs taken at baseline and 9 months was used to measure changes in bone height at the targeted sites (21). Although the results showed that 15% of the sites receiving SRP alone, and 11% of those receiving a placebo chip + SRP lost bone height over the 9 month study period, none of the sites treated with the CHX chip lost bone ($p < 0.01$). Bone height gain was seen at 25% of the sites treated with the CHX chip but in only 0% and 5% of sites receiving SRP only and the placebo chip respectively.

In two additional studies, on limited patient numbers, mixed results have been shown. In a recent study based on 34 patients (22), a significant clinical advantage was shown for the adjunctive use of the chip whereas in a study of 19 patients (23) the authors were unable to demonstrate a significant adjunctive clinical effect of the chip.

These data demonstrate that the adjunctive use of the CHX chip results in a significant reduction of PPD when compared with both SRP alone and the adjunctive use of a placebo chip. In addition the CHX chip significantly reduces loss of alveolar bone.

**In supportive periodontal therapy:** Having established that the subgingival controlled release of CHX is a safe and effective adjunctive chemotherapy for the treatment of periodontitis, the use of the CHX chip for the long-term management of adult periodontitis patients needed to be established. A 2-year study on 835 patients with adult periodontitis, recruited from the private offices of both periodontists and general dentists, was carried out (24). All patients were on supportive periodontal therapy (SPT) and had completed definitive periodontal therapy at least one month prior to entry into the study. A CHX chip was placed in pocket sites with PPD ≥ 5 mm. Subsequently the patients continued with routine SPT together with the placement of a CHX chip in pockets with PPD ≥ 5 mm every 3 months. Patients who did not attend the 24-month recall visit, or who failed to attend 2 consecutive time-frame examinations, were excluded from the analyses. The 595 included patients showed a continuous decrease in PPD over the 2 years of 0.95 mm (Fig. 3). After 2 years, 23.2% of patients had at least two pockets showing a reduction in PPD of 2 mm or more and 58.9% of the sites had been reduced to a PPD of <5 mm. Only 2.9% ($n = 57$) of the sites showed an increase in PPD of ≥ 2 mm. Adverse events were mild to moderate in nature and resolved spontaneously without medication. These results indicate that the adjunctive use of the CHX chip is a clinically effective treatment option for dental professionals and their patients for long-term management of chronic periodontitis.

In a randomized, split mouth, single-blind study (25) the effect of the placement of a single PerioChip into residual bleeding pockets with a PPD > 5 mm was examined. The patients were selected from a pool of maintenance patients at least three months after oral hygiene and root debridement therapy. At baseline all the pockets were debrided and PerioChips were placed in the pockets on one side of the mouth while those on the other

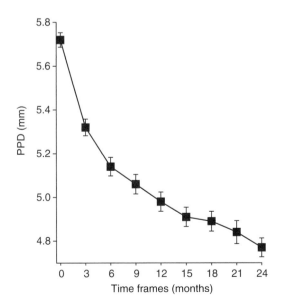

**Figure 3** The mean decrease in probing pocket depths of 595 patients receiving supportive periodontal therapy including PerioChip™ ≥ 5 mm over the 2-year study period. The vertical bars represent the standard deviation from the means.

side received no further treatment. The patients were examined at 1, 3 and 6 months after baseline. The results indicated a significantly greater improvement in PPL, PAL and BOP in the PerioChip treated pockets. This benefit only became apparent at 6 months.

**Adverse events:** Two of the clinical studies report on the adverse events occurring in patients receiving periodontal treatment including the use of the PerioChip (20,24). The adverse events that were treatment related could be included into the categories of toothache or gingival swelling associated with the site of chip placement. Toothache was variously described as dental, gingival, or mouth pain or as being associated with tenderness, aching, throbbing, soreness, discomfort, or sensitivity. These symptoms occurred more frequently with the use of a CHX chip than with a placebo chip. The incidence of treatment-related adverse events is available for the 835 intent-to-treat patients who participated in a 2-year study in which repeated applications of the PerioChip were made at 3-month intervals (24). A total of 300 treatment-related adverse events were reported by 140 of the patients. These 300 events followed a total of 4920 patient visits at which chips were placed, representing an incidence of 6.1%. Bearing in mind that multiple adverse events could be reported by one individual at a single visit, the real incidence would be much lower.

## FUTURE DEVELOPMENTS OF THE TECHNOLOGY

The platform of the PerioChip provides the technology for delivering to the subgingival environment any drug that can be included in the chip formulation. Drugs that can be used for the treatment of periodontal diseases include antibacterial, anti-inflammatory and immunomodulatory agents and drugs that may influence bone resorption. At present we are attempting to develop a chip that can provide the controlled release of nonsteroidal anti-inflammatory drugs to the subgingival environment. Preliminary studies suggest that such a device may have a significant effect on the natural progression of periodontitis. However further studies need to be carried out before any relevant conclusions can be made.

## REFERENCES

1. Flotra L. Different modes of chlorhexidine application and related local side effects. J Periodont Res 1973; 8(Suppl. 12):41–4.
2. Pitcher GR, Newman HN, Strahan JD. Access to subgingival plaque by disclosing agents using mouthrinsing and direct irrigation. J Clin Perio 1980; 7:300–8.
3. Greenstein G. Effects of subgingival irrigation on periodontal status. J Periodont 1987; 58:827–36.

4.  Greenstein G. The role of supra-and subgingival irrigation in the treatment of periodontal diseases. Position paper published by The American Academy of Periodontology. J Periodont 1995; 66:925–32.

5.  Goodson JM, Haffajee A, Socransky SS. Periodontal therapy by local delivery of tetracycline. J Clin Perio 1979; 6:83–92.

6.  Dunn RL, Perkins BH, Goodson JM. Controlled release of tetracycline from biodegradable fibres. J Dent Res 1983; 62:289(abstract).

7.  Goodson JM, Holborow D, Dunn RL, Hogan P, Dunham S. Monolithic tetracycline-containing fibres for controlled delivery to periodontal pockets. J Periodont 1983; 54:575–9.

8.  Addy M, Rawle L, Handley R, Newman HN, Coventry JF. The development and in vitro evaluation of acrylic resin strips and dialysis tubing for local drug delivery. J Periodont 1982; 53:693–9.

9.  Friedman M, Golomb G. New sustained release dosage form of chlorhexidine for dental use. J Periodont Res 1982; 17:323–8.

10. Soskolne A, Golomb G, Friedman M, Sela MN. New sustained release dosage form of chlorhexidine for dental use II. use in periodontal therapy. J Periodont Res 1983; 18:330–6.

11. Donbrow M, Friedman M. Timed release from polymeric films containing drugs and kinetics of drug release. J Pharm Sci 1975; 64:76–80.

12. Stabholz A, Sela MN, Friedman M, Golomb G, Soskolne A. Clinical and microbiological effects of sustained release chlorhexidine in periodontal pockets. J Clin Perio 1986; 13:783–8.

13. Elkayam R, Friedman M, Stabholz A, Soskolne AW, Sela MN, Golub L. Sustained release device containing minocycline for local treatment of periodontal disease. J Control Rel 1988; 7:231–6.

14. Elkayam R, Friedman M, Stabholz A, Soskolne AW, Azoury R. Sustained release device of tetracycline for dental use, structure and kinetics of drug release in vitro and in vivo. Proc Int Conf Pharm Tech 1989; 2:346–54.

15. Stabholz A, Elkayam R, Friedman M, Sela MN, Azoury R, Soskolne AW. Clinical and microbiological evaluation of sustained release device of tetracycline in periodontal pockets. Proc Int Conf Pharm Tech 1989; 2: 336–45.

16. Stabholz A, Soskolne WA, Friedman M, Sela MN. The use of sustained release delivery of chlorhexidine for the maintenance of periodontal pockets: 2-year clinical trial. J Periodont 1991; 62:429–33.

17. Steinberg D, Friedman M, Soskolne A, Sela MN. A new degradable controlled release device for treatment of periodontal disease: In vitro release study. J Periodont 1990; 61:393–8.

18. Soskolne WA, Chajek T, Flashner M, et al. An in vivo study of the chlorhexidine release profile of the PerioChip in the gingival crevicular fluid, plasma and urine. J Clin Perio 1998; 25:1017–21.

19. Soskolne WA, Heasman PA, Stabholz A, et al. Sustained local delivery of chlorhexidine in the treatment of periodontitis: A multi-center study. J Periodont 1997; 68:32–8.

20. Jeffcoat MK, Bray KS, Ciancio SG, et al. Adjunctive use of a subgingival controlled-release chlorhexidine chip reduces probing depth and improves

attachment level compared with scaling and root planing alone. J Periodont 1998; 69:989–97.

21. Jeffcoat MK, Placanis KG, Weatherford TW, Reese M, Geurs NC, Flashner M. Use of a boidegradable chlorhexidine chip in the treatment of adult periodontitis: clinical and radiological findings. J Periodont 2000; 71:256–62.

22. Grisi DC, Salvador SL, Figueiredo LC, Novaes AB Jr, Grisi MFM. Effect of controlled release chlorhexidine chip on clinical and microbiological parameters of periodontal syndrome. J Clin Perio 2002; 29:875–81.

23. Mizrak T, Guncu GN, Caglayan F, Balci TA, Aktar GS, Ipek F. Effect of a controlled-release chlorhexidine chip on clinical and microbiological parameters and prostaglandin E2 levels in gingival crevicular fluid. J Periodont 2006; 77:437–43.

24. Soskolne WA, Proskin HM, Stabholz A. Probing depth changes following 2 years of periodontal maintenance therapy including adjunctive controlled release of chlorhexidine. J Periodont 2003; 74:420–7.

25. Heasman PA, Heasman L, Stacey F, McCraken GI. Local delivery of chlorhexidine gluconate (PerioChip™) in periodontal maintenance patients. J Clin Perio 2001; 28:90–5.

## Part III: Oral Technologies

# 12

# Modified-Release Delivery Systems for Oral Use

R. B. Walker

*Faculty of Pharmacy, Rhodes University, Grahamstown, South Africa*

## INTRODUCTION

The oral route of drug delivery is considered the most convenient and is widely used for drug product development purposes. It has been estimated that approximately 84% of all sales of the top selling commercially available products are delivered via the oral route (1). Therefore it is obvious that drug discovery efforts will necessarily focus on the identification and development of compounds that are readily deliverable via the oral route and will have the most appropriate pharmacokinetic and pharmacodynamic profiles where possible. However the successful development of molecules with these ideal properties is unlikely and many compounds show pharmacokinetic and/or bioavailability deficiencies that may or may not be addressed during lead optimization (2). Consequently there is a need for product life-cycle management of existing molecules in order to maximize returns on the investments made, during the development phases of a drug product. Many of the strategies used by pharmaceutical companies to develop a further market niche for their products include consideration of using different delivery systems and technologies to ensure differentiation including extended, modified, controlled, or rapid release systems among others. The use of molecules with established efficacy will allow reduced development costs thereby providing less expensive therapies for the worldwide market.

Despite the fact that many oral drug delivery systems are available for use there are a number of challenges facing a formulation scientist when considering the oral route as a viable portal for drug delivery when developing a sustained release drug delivery system.

Over and above the physico-chemical properties of the molecule that must be taken into account when developing a drug product there are numerous physiological challenges that must be addressed. The successful development of delivery systems are primarily focused on pH related solubility and stability, gastric emptying rates, sites and rates of absorption, variable gastric transit times, the presence or absence of food, the variable presence of efflux transporters and CYP3A4 along the gastrointestinal tract (GIT), different fluid volumes and compositions that a product may be exposed to following administration. Many of these issues and challenges highlighted above were reported in the first edition of this book (2) and are also addressed in other texts and the literature (3–6) and will not be discussed in any great detail in this chapter other than in specific chapters in this section in which technologies are described that are designed to overcome some of the challenges associated with oral drug delivery or address unmet medical needs.

In the context of this chapter the term "modified release" includes sustained release technologies, gastro-retentive systems, dose-sipping technologies, microparticulate systems and tablets, or capsule systems. In this chapter technologies are discussed that are swallowed for the intention of drug release in the upper regions of the gastro intestinal tract. Technologies that offer the possibility of specifically targeting the colon are described elsewhere in this book (Part IV).

## CURRENT TECHNOLOGIES AND FUTURE DIRECTIONS IN ORAL DRUG DELIVERY

There are many new technologies that have been developed yet their potential for commercialization has yet to be established since there are numerous regulatory hurdles to be overcome. These hurdles include the need for establishing the safety and efficacy of such drug delivery systems. To this end the FDA have established guidelines for the development and evaluation of extended, sustained and modified-release dosage forms (7,8) and the proceedings of an American Association of Pharmaceutical Scientists/Food and Drug Administration (AAPS/FDA) workshop on the scientific foundations for regulating drug product quality (9) provide an excellent overview in this respect including the need for attempting to establish an appropriate in vivo/in vitro correlation.

In general, while there are many new polymers and platform technologies available for use that are continually reported in the literature, a conservative approach to delivery system design prevails and is governed by what are regarded as safe excipients and by what can be manufactured on a large enough scale to be commercially available.

Oral drug absorption can be affected by the dosage form and the manner in which it is presented to the GIT such as, for example, whether the system is a single or multiple unit technology or whether it disintegrates or not (10). Furthermore the type of delivery system can and does impact the mechanism of drug release from such systems, thereby impacting on the in vivo release profile of an active pharmaceutical ingredient and its subsequent absorption (10).

Advancements in manufacturing equipment and technologies, polymer and regulatory sciences have largely driven the recent developments in oral modified-release technologies (2). Despite these advances in technology the approaches to the modification of drug release that are currently used are somewhat similar to those used over the last three decades and delivery systems for sustained or modified release can be broadly classified as membrane, matrix, or hybrid systems (10).

Within each of these categories various opportunities exist for the development of novel and innovative technologies to achieve the desired release characteristics. For example, membrane systems, in general, include a core in which the active pharmaceutical ingredients (API) is located and which is surrounded by a membrane which is usually the rate-controlling element of the technology. Such systems include coated pellets or beads, microcapsules or coated capsules, and tablets and can release drug by mechanisms such as osmotic pumping or solution diffusion. Matrix systems on the other hand are designed by dispersing or dissolving an API in a matrix material that may or may not be soluble or susceptible to erosion. Monolithic matrices are generally simple to manufacture, are still commonly used and release API by a number of different mechanisms including diffusion, dissolution, swelling and/or erosion, and by changes in geometry. Combinations of polymeric materials may also be used to produce matrix technologies. Hybrid technologies include features of both membrane and matrix systems and as such may be technologically challenging to manufacture. However the ideal features of both membrane and matrix systems may be used to produce a dosage form with the desired release characteristics.

Polysaccharide hydrocolloids such as guar gum (11,12) and cellulose-based technologies such as hydroxypropyl cellulose (HPC) (13–15) and hydroxypropyl methylcellulose (16–18), e.g., are extensively investigated for modified-release systems primarily due to their availability and simplicity of use. Two recent additions of cellulosic materials that have been added to the arsenal of the formulator to overcome the potential disadvantage of lack of control or zero-order drug release from monolithic matrix systems include Aqualon® T10 ethyl cellulose and Klucel® and these excipients are described in Chapter 13.

Aqualon T10 ethyl cellulose is a highly compressible and crystalline material that can be used for the control of diffusion in matrices and specifically for devices with complex geometries, thereby permitting accurate and precise control of drug release from such systems. Klucel HPC consists of fine particles of HPC of intermediate weight that allow for precise targeting of erosion rates and/or diffusion versus erosion mechanisms based purely on molecular weight of the polymer independent of the API under investigation. Of further benefit is the fact that these materials are readily available commercially, are generally recognized as safe (GRAS) listed, comply with *U.S. Pharmacopoeia* (USP), *European Pharmacopoeia* (EP), and *Japanese Pharmacopoeia* (JP) standards and are currently under investigation in clinical trials if not already used in commercial products in the United States of America or Europe.

Chitosan derived from chitin is a nontoxic, bioabsorbable polymer that has been investigated for a broad range of drug delivery applications (19) in addition to specific application in sustained or modified-release delivery systems (20,21). Chapter 14 describes a novel application of chitosan in combination with polyethylene glycol (PEG) for the production of SQZgel™ tablets that permit once or twice daily dosing and that are designed to enhance patient compliance, reduce peak to trough blood levels, and eliminate regimens of 4–6 doses daily. SQZgel is a cationic hydrogel that is able to form a stable hydrogel at acidic and neutral pH and that exhibits pH-dependent swelling and shrinking. The technology is a combination of a pH sensitive core comprised of chitosan and PEG in specific proportions and a nonbiodegradable micro-porous coating that can be used to modulate release of API for up to 24 hours on the basis of coating thickness and porosity. Delivery systems, in which SQZgel is used, can be manufactured using conventional manufacturing techniques which make it a potentially useful technology for the production of modified-release oral dosage forms.

A particularly interesting and novel group of excipients that can be used for oral drug delivery are the thiolated polymers and their potential use and application is described in Chapter 15. Thiomers are constructed by the covalent attachment of low molecular mass thiol functional group bearing compounds onto polymeric backbones of well known, established and safe polymers such as chitosan or poly(acrylic acid). The functionality of thiolated polymers is diverse and they have been used to enhance permeation (22) and mucoadhesion (23), facilitate controlled drug release (24), and more recently have been shown to inhibit enzymes and efflux transport mechanisms (25,26). The use of thiomer technology for the delivery of hydrophilic macromolecules and efflux pump substrates is particularly interesting since the thiolated polymer is also able to inhibit such transport mechanism. Advantages of the technology, among which ease of manufacture and low toxicity are extensively summarized in the monograph (see Chapter 15).

One of the major challenges facing drug delivery scientists is the increasing need to develop delivery systems for API with limited or poor aqueous solubility. While the use of salts, complexation, and solubilization are useful up to a point the main aim of any platform should ensure constant drug release in order to facilitate absorption. The use of solid dispersions provides an alternate approach to enhancing bioavailability (27) and the Meltrex® technology described in Chapter 16 is based on this principle. The Meltrex technology has been designed to prepare solid dispersions with defined controlled-release characteristics using a single solvent-free manufacturing process (28). Furthermore the process can used to formulate both amorphous and crystalline API into a solid dispersion regardless of particle size or polymorphic form. The technology uses pharmaceutically acceptable polymers and excipients and products manufactured using the Meltrex process have been approved by European regulatory authorities and by the FDA.

An alternate approach that can be used to overcome solubility-related challenges in the formulation of poorly soluble API is described in Chapter 17 in which the Threeform system is described. The Threeform technology has been previously described (29) and overcomes the challenges associated with formulation of crystalline or polymorphic API as these molecules are transformed into an amorphous form of constant size and that is stabilized by use of a mixture of polymers such as polyvinyl pyrrolidone and cellulose ethers of various viscosities. Drug release is controlled by diffusion and erosion of the matrix, the rate of which is in turn determined by the composition of the mixture of polymers used. In addition a coating material may be applied to the system which can further modify release profiles.

Chapter 25 further addresses the issue of delivery of drugs with poor aqueous solubility by describing the preparation and advantages of solid lipid nanoparticles (SLN), nanostructured lipid carriers (NLC), and lipid drug conjugates (LDC) manufactured using a high pressure homogenization technique (30). The lipid nanoparticle systems SLN, NLC, and LDC are simple carrier technologies that provide new options for oral drug delivery using excipients, surfactants, and stabilizers that have an acceptable regulatory status for oral use. Furthermore the benefits of using lipids for enhancing bioavailability, dissolution rates, and saturation solubilities provide further evidence of the usefulness of such systems for the delivery of vital API. Additional advantages of SLN, NLC, and LDC are that they can be used as carrier technologies to produce tablets and pellets thereby enabling the formulation and oral delivery of drugs that would otherwise be precluded for use due to their poor water solubility.

In addition to low solubility, poorly permeable or BCS Class III drugs (31) pose a significant formulation challenge for achieving effective oral drug delivery. The gastro-intestinal permeation enhancement technology (GIPET™) described in Chapter 21 is a platform technology that addresses this challenge by ensuring the absorption of such poorly permeable drugs across the small intestine in therapeutically relevant concentrations. GIPET is a platform technology designed to enhance the oral bioavailability of a variety of poorly absorbed compounds. The GIPET platform includes two technologies. The first is GIPET I, which uses medium chain fatty acids, salts and derivatives and can be formulated as tablets and the second, GIPET II is a microemulsion-based technology that can be filled into gelatin capsules. All dosage forms are comprised of the enhancer system and the API in an appropriate matrix, which are formulated as physical mixtures thereby retaining the chemical integrity of the API. The subsequent application of an enteric coating protects the API from gastric acidity and permits the release of API at the site of absorption in the small intestine. An added advantage is that technologies based on the GIPET can be readily scaled to commercial production using conventional pharmaceutical manufacturing equipment.

As science and technology has developed more information on the biopharmaceutic processes associated with drug liberation and absorption have become available and the extent of drug absorption from various regions of GIT have been found to be rate and site dependent. Consequently various approaches have been investigated to retain dosage forms in the upper GIT, particularly in the stomach thereby prolonging the period over which a delivery system may release an API above or at the site of absorption (32,33). Mechanisms that have been used include dosage forms that float (34) and that may swell and/or expand (35–37) among others. A new floating capsule system has been shown to be effective in the delivery of amoxicillin alone or in combination with clavulanic acid and is described in Chapter 18. The fairly complex technology relies on the use of a poorly soluble coating that enables the contents of a capsule to float in the stomach and the gastroretentive characteristics of the floating capsule have been shown using gamma scintigraphic studies (Chapter 18). A different approach to gastric retention is described as a gastro-intestinal retention system (GIRES™) and is detailed further in Chapter 22.

The GIRES system operates as both an expandable and floating technology system that enables prolonged and reliable gastro retention. The GIRES system allows for predictable and reliable oral delivery with a system that is small enough to ingest yet is retained in the stomach in the presence or absence of food and in essence is a gas-generating, inflatable, gastroretentive system which is enclosed in a hard gelatin capsule.

Two modified-release drug delivery technologies that address the needs of specific patient populations such as pediatric, geriatric, or patients with condition that preclude them from swallowing or are comatose are described in Chapters 19 and 20. Thin film oral dosage forms are described in Chapter 19 and at least 15 products in which these technologies are used are commercially available for the delivery of API intended for both local and systemic activity. Thin film technologies were originally developed for the confectionary market but as they offer fast and accurate dosing in a safe, efficacious manner that is convenient their use in drug delivery has become more prevalent and they are particularly useful for treating pediatric patients who are unwilling or unable to swallow tablets. The technology described in Chapter 20 overcomes the challenges of delivering large doses to patients by use of a proprietary drinking straw system as opposed to currently used suspension and solution technologies. The SIP® system or dose sipping technology (DST®) is a delivery technology in which granules for suspension are retained in a drinking straw and provide medication via a straw without the need for reconstitution prior to administration. The technology can be handled by most children over the age of two years, with ease. Each individually packaged drinking straw contains a single dose of small, coated granules containing the prescribed amount of API in a suitably taste masked formulation. API delivery from a DST system can be achieved using between 50 and 150 ml of fluid drunk either using the straw or directly from the glass following ingestion of the entire contents of the straw. Clarosip® and Riclasip® are commercially available dose sipping technologies containing clarithromycin and amoxicillin/clavulanic acid, respectively. These two technologies provide an exciting opportunity for improving drug delivery to young patients.

In an effort to overcome the challenges of establishing optimal absorption of a drug following administration of single unit or monolithic sustained drug delivery devices multiparticulate delivery systems have been developed. Multiparticulate technologies are purported to have several advantages including but not limited to the avoidance of dose dumping should a single device fail, predictable gastric emptying (first order) and reduced food effects, uniform distribution of the devices in the GIT, avoidance of high local drug concentrations thereby minimizing GIT irritation, the potential for increased bioavailability due to a large available surface area for dissolution or diffusion, lower inter- and intraindividual variation in bioavailability.

Multiple unit delivery systems are usually comprised of coated and/or layered particles, spheres or pellets, granules, or even crystals. The individual units can be manufactured by granulation, spray coating or layering of nonpareils, or extrusion spheronization (38,39). The particles that are formed may be filled into capsules or compressed into tablets as required. Microparticles and microcapsules may also be manufactured using coacervation, interfacial polymerization, or solvent evaporation techniques.

A novel microparticulate system, Micropump® technology, in which multiple units are used for drug delivery is described in detail Chapter 23. The Micropump technology has been developed for the oral delivery of one or more drug components simultaneously (40) and has been applied to the delivery of a number of drugs including aspirin, acyclovir, metformin, and more recently carvedilol. Each microparticle core contains the API as either crystals, granules, or layered core which is subsequently coated with a material that controls drug release and the resultant units are between 200 and 800 μm in size. The Micropump technology exists as either Micropump I for continuous sustained release of API or Micropump II for delayed release of API at a precise location in the small intestine.

A simple novel modified emulsification/solvent evaporation method for the fabrication of delayed- and extended-release microparticles has been developed and is described in Chapter 24. Conventional manufacturing techniques are used to produce a stable emulsion of the polymer/drug solution in an immiscible liquid paraffin/surfactant phase. Spherical, monodisperse microparticles of <50 μm in diameter are formed following evaporation of solvent at room temperature. Microparticles have been formed from polymer blends including, e.g., acrylic polymers such as Eudragit® L55, L, S, RS, and cellulosic polymers such as cellulose acetate phthalate and ethylcellulose. The application of this technology to the delivery of prednisone is described further in the chapter.

## CONCLUSIONS

Future drug delivery technologies must necessarily take into account the physico-chemical nature of the API to be delivered and must be manufacturable on a large enough scale to be economically viable. The use of lipids, nanostructured materials, amorphous forms of API, and solid dispersions on a micro- or nano-scale may well be the technology of the future. However several aspects of the safety and toxicity of these systems will have to be revisited before they can be exploited commercially. The use of excipients that promote interaction of the modified-release delivery technology with the biosystem such as increased adhesion to membranes or inhibition of efflux transport mechanisms may become a useful and more prevalent strategy to improve bioavailability in the future. Furthermore the current lack of commercially available delivery systems for the oral administration of high molecular weight, soluble but poorly permeable compounds such as proteins and peptides is indicative of the substantial hurdles that must be overcome to deliver these molecules in a safe and effective manner. In order to develop delivery systems for these types of candidates in the future multiparticulate, self-emulsifying, or permeation enhancers may be necessary.

There are increasing regulatory challenges and hurdles that drug developers must overcome in order to bring new chemical entities to market. It may not be surprising therefore to see pharmaceutical manufacturers using modified-release technologies as part of their product lifecycle management strategies in the future. In this way, successful API candidates may be delivered using modified-release technologies that promote higher bioavailability may permit the administration of lower doses with the additional benefits of an improved pharmacological or pharmacodynamic profile with fewer side effects.

## REFERENCES

1. Furness G, Introductory Comment, OnDrugDelivery, Newtimber, United Kingdom, August 2007, 3.
2. Charman SA, Charman WN. Oral modified-release delivery systems in modified release drug delivery technology. In: Rathbone MJ, Hadgraft J, Roberts MS, eds. Drugs and the Pharmaceutical Sciences. New York: Marcel Dekker, 2003: 1–10.
3. Florence AT, Atwood D, eds. Physicochemical Principles of Pharmacy, 4th ed. London, United Kingdom: Pharmaceutical Press, 2006: 329–45.
4. Zhang Y, Benet LZ. The gut as a barrier to drug absorption: combined role of cytochrome P450 3A and P-glycoprotein. Clin Pharmacokin 2001; 40(3): 159–68.
5. Bogman K, Zysset Y, degen L, et al. P-glycoprotein and surfactants: effect on intestinal talinolol absorption. Clin Pharmacol Ther 2005; 77(1):24–32.
6. Dressman JB, Lenneräs H, eds. Oral Drug Absorption: Prediction and Assessment. New York: Marcel Dekker, 2000.
7. Guidance for Industry. Extended Release Oral Dosage Forms: Development, evaluation and Application of In Vitro/In Vivo Correlations. U.S. Department of Health and Human Services, Food and Drug Administration, Center for Drug Evaluation and Research (CDER), September 1997. http://www.fda.gov/cder/guidance/1306fnl.pdf
8. Guidance for Industry. SUPAC-MR: Modified Release Solid Oral Dosage Forms Scale-Up and Postapproval Changes: Chemistry, Manufacturing, and Controls; In Vitro Dissolution Testing and In Vivo Bioequivalence Documentation. U.S. Department of Health and Human Services, Food and Drug Administration, Center for Drug Evaluation and Research (CDER), June 1997. http://www.fda.gov/cder/guidance/1214fnl.pdf
9. Amidon GL, Robinson JR, Williams RL, eds. Scientific Foundations for Regulating Drug Product Quality. Alexandria, VA: AAPS Press, 1997.
10. Lee PI. Oral ER technology: mechanism of release. In: Amidon GL, Robinson JR, Williams RL, eds. Scientific Foundations for Regulating Drug Product Quality. Alexandria, VA: AAPS Press, 1997.
11. McCall TW, Baichwal AR, Staniforth JN. TIMERx oral controlled-release drug delivery system in modified release drug delivery technology. In: Rathbone MJ, Hadgraft J, Roberts MS, eds. Drugs and the Pharmaceutical Sciences. New York: Marcel Dekker, 2003: 11–9.
12. Altaf SA, Friend DR. MASRx and COSRx sustained release technology in modified release drug delivery technology. In: Rathbone MJ, Hadgraft J, Roberts MS, eds. Drugs and the Pharmaceutical Sciences. New York: Marcel Dekker, 2003: 21–33.
13. Johnson JL, Holinej J, Williams MD. Influence of ionic strength on matrix integrity and drug release from hydroxypropyl cellulose compacts. Int J Pharm 1993; 90:151–9.
14. Aldermann DA. Sustained release compositions comprising hydroxypropyl cellulose ethers, US Patent 4,704,285, 1987.
15. Lee DY, Chen C-M. Delayed pulse release hydrogel matrix tablet. US Patent 6,103,263, 2000.

16. Rodriguez CG, Bruneau N, Barra J, Alfonso D, Doelke E. Hydrophilic cellulose derivatives as drug delivery carriers: influence of substitution type on the properties of compressed matrix tablets. In: Wise DL, ed. Handbook of Pharmaceutical Controlled Release Technology. New York: Marcel Dekker Inc., 2000: 1–30.

17. Reynolds TD, Mitchell SA, Balwinski KM. Investigation of the effect of tablet surface area/volume on drug release from HPMC controlled-release matrix tablets. Drug Dev Ind Pharm 2002; 28(4):457–66.

18. Williams RO III, Reynolds TD, Cabelka TD, Sykora MA, Mahaguna V. Investigation of excipient type and level on drug release from controlled release tablets containing HPMC. Pharm Dev Tech 2002; 7(2):181–93.

19. Illum L. Chitosan and its use as a pharmaceutical excipient. Pharm Res 1998; 15:1326–31.

20. Rege PR, Shukla DJ, Block LH. Chitinosans as tableting excipients for modified release delivery systems. Int J Pharm 1999; 181:49–60.

21. Nunthanid J, Laungtana-Anan M, Sriamornsak P, et al. Characterization of chitosan acetate as a binder for sustained release tablets. J Control Release 2004; 99:15–26.

22. Bernkop-Schnürch A, Kast CE, Guggi D. Permeation enhancing polymers in oral delivery of hydrophilic macromolecules: thiomer/GSH systems. J Control Release 2003; 93(2):95–103.

23. Grabovac V, Guggi D, Bernkop-Schnürch A. Comparison of the mucoadhesive properties of various polymers. Adv Drug Deliv Rev 2005; 57(11):1713–23.

24. Bernkop-Schnürch A, Scholler S, Biebel RG. Development of controlled drug release systems based on thiolated polymers. J Control Release 2000; 66:39–48.

25. Bernkop-Schnürch A, Walker G, Zarti H. Thiolation of polycarbophil enhances its inhibition of intestinal brush border membrane bound aminopeptidase N. J Pharm Sci 2001; 90(11):1907–14.

26. Werle M, Hoffer M. Glutathione and thiolated chitosan inhibit multidrug resistance P-glycoprotein activity in excised small intestine. J Control Release 2006; 111(1–2):41–6.

27. Chiou WL, Riegelman S. Pharmaceutical application of solid dispersion systems. J Pharm Sci 1971; 60:1281–302.

28. Breitenbach J. Melt extrusion: from process to drug delivery technology. Eur J Pharm Biopharm 2002; 54:107–17.

29. Kerč J. Three-phase pharmaceutical form-Threeform-with controlled release of amorphous active ingredient for once-daily administration in modified release drug delivery technology. In: Rathbone MJ, Hadgraft J, Roberts MS, eds. Drugs and the Pharmaceutical Sciences. New York: Marcel Dekker, 2003: 115–23.

30. Muller RH, Jacobs C, Kayser O. DissoCubes—a novel formulation for poorly soluble and poorly bioavailable drugs in modified release drug delivery technology. In: Rathbone MJ, Hadgraft J, Roberts MS, eds. Drugs and the Pharmaceutical Sciences. New York: Marcel Dekker, 2003: 135–49.

31. Amidon G, Lennernas H, Shah VP, Crison JR. A theoretical basis for a biopharmaceutic drug classification: the correlation of in vitro drug product dissolution and in vivo bioavailability. Pharm Res 1995; 12(3): 413–20.

32. Streubel A, Siepmann J, Bodmeier H. Drug delivery to the upper small intestine window using gastroretentive technologies. Curr Opin Pharm Sci 2006; 6: 501–8.
33. Singh BN, Kim KH. Floating drug delivery systems: an approach to oral controlled drug delivery via gastric retention. J Control Release 2000; 63: 235–59.
34. Deshpande AA, Shah NH, Rhodes CT, et al. Development of a novel controlled-release system for gastric retention. Pharm Res 1997; 14:815–9.
35. Urquhart J, Theeuwes F. Drug delivery system comprising a reservoir containing a plurality of tiny pills. US Patent 4,434,153, 1984.
36. Mamajek RC, Moyer ES. Drug-dispensing device and method. US Patent 4,207,890, 1980.
37. Klausner EA, Lavy E, Friedman M, Hoffman A. Expandable gastroretentive dosage forms. J Control Release 2003; 90:143–62.
38. Conine JW, Hadley HR. Preparation of small solid pharmaceutical spheres. Drug Cosmet Ind 1970; 106:38–41.
39. Reynolds AD. A new technique for the production of spherical particles. Manuf Chem Aerosol News 1970; 41:40–3.
40. Autant P, Selles J-P, Soula G. FR Patent 2 725 623, 1996.

# 13

# Advances in Cellulose Ether-Based Modified-Release Technologies

Thomas J. Dürig

*Aqualon, a Business Unit of Hercules Incorporated, Hercules Research Center, Wilmington, Delaware, U.S.A.*

## INTRODUCTION AND HISTORY

Cellulose ethers are the most commonly used materials for the design and fabrication of oral modified-release dosage forms. This family of polymers includes hypromellose, hydroxypropyl cellulose, hydroxyethyl cellulose, sodium carboxymethyl cellulose, and ethyl cellulose (EC). The cellulose ethers are widely used primarily due to their long history of safe and effective use in the development and manufacture of modified-release technologies. Indeed, as early as 1968 a detailed account of drug release mechanisms from a hypromellose-based matrix tablet was reported (1). However, despite decades of use in what are now fairly standard applications, such as drug polymer matrix systems, innovations are required to produce highly functional materials and polymer systems to meet the demands for improved performance and reliability of current technologies in addition to developing the next generation of advanced modified-release technologies. In our laboratories we have taken a rational approach to advancing cellulose-based materials and technologies through fundamental structure-function studies. In this monograph we highlight two such examples viz., highly compressible, high crystallinity EC, Aqualon® T10 EC for enhanced matrix diffusion control, especially in compressed devices with complex geometries and modified-release grades of hydroxypropyl cellulose, Klucel® hydroxypropyl cellulose, that permits precise targeting of erosion rates and/or diffusion versus erosion mechanisms based purely on molecular weight.

# HIGH ETHOXYL, LOW VISCOSITY ETHYL CELLULOSE, AQUALON T10 ETHYL CELLULOSE

## Description of the Technology

EC is one of a select few water insoluble polymers that can be used to manufacture compressed controlled-release dosage forms. In the absence of polymer swelling ability, EC compactibility is the key element in such systems, since drug-release kinetics will depend largely on the porosity of the hydrophobic compact. Recently, a new, highly compressible form of EC, Aqualon T10 EC, has been developed. T10 EC derives its compactibility from a unique combination of a high degree of substitution (ethoxyl content 50–51%) and low molecular weight with a resultant solution viscosity of between 8 and 10 cps (2). The increased compactibility of T10 EC results in significant differences in the release profiles of drugs from matrix and compression-coated tablets. Moreover, a distinct advantage was observed for powder handling, flow characteristics, and tablet-weight uniformity when T10 EC–containing dosage forms were compared to those manufactured using micronized EC, another form of EC marketed for direct compression purposes (3,4).

## Research and Development

Results of differential scanning calorimetry (DSC) and polarized X-ray diffraction (PXRD) analysis reveal that EC has both amorphous and crystalline regions. The higher compactibility of T10 EC was associated with a high ethoxyl content; low molecular weight (low viscosity) was correlated with a significantly higher crystallinity and higher melting points, while the amorphous regions had lower glass transition temperatures (Table 1). Compaction simulator studies show that the net effect of this unique solid

**Table 1** Effect of Ethoxyl Content and Viscosity on Selected Solid State Properties of Ethyl Cellulose

| Ethoxyl (%) | Viscosity (cps) | Crystallinity (%) | Melting point (°C) | $T_g$ (°C) | Crushing force (kP)[a] |
|---|---|---|---|---|---|
| 50.4 | 9 | 24.6 | 257.0 | 122.1 | 20.9 |
| 50.8 | 9 | 28.5 | 261.1 | 124.6 | 18.8 |
| 50.0 | 50 | 15.3 | 246.6 | 130.7 | 14.6 |
| 49.6 | 94 | 17.8 | 261.0 | 129.5 | 16.1 |
| 48.0 | 10 | 9.1 | 210.0 | 131.0 | 14.7 |
| 48.5 | 94 | 7.9 | 224.3 | 133.5 | 11.5 |
| 47.5 | 10 | 8.2 | 178.6 | 135.1 | 12.3 |

[a]275 mg pure EC tablets compressed on a Betapress at 25 kN.

state structure is a marked reduction in postcompaction elastic recovery of the polymer (Fig. 1).

Less energy of compaction is therefore lost due to postcompaction axial expansion of T10 EC, resulting in denser compacts with lower porosity. This has a significant effect on drug diffusion from nonswelling, porosity-controlled matrix tablets (Fig. 2). In addition, the reduced visco-elasticity results in lower strain rate sensitivity (10% versus typically 20–25% for other EC types). This makes T10 EC a more robust material that is easily scalable from laboratory scale to large scale, high-speed tablet presses.

While the good powder flow and optimized compaction properties of T10 EC are advantageous for the design of monolithic diffusion matrices, these properties are also crucial for more complex compressed devices such as compression-coated coated tablets and multilayer tablets. Studies on compression-coated tablets designed for pulsatile release (Fig. 3) revealed that the greater compactibility of T10 EC results in an increased resistance to coating failure, and allows greater control of lag times (Fig. 4). For a given model formulation compression-coated with T10 EC the lag time can be systematically varied from 3 to ~16 hours by increasing the coating compression force from 5 to 25 kN and a linear correlation between compression force and lag time was observed ($r^2 = 0.98$). For other grades of EC, lag times varied between 0 and 2 hours over the corresponding pressure range (Table 2).

## Regulatory and Commercial Status

T10 EC has GRAS status and complies with USP, EP, and FCC requirements for EC (5). It is commercially available as a high-performance material for

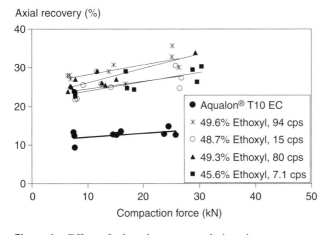

**Figure 1**   Effect of ethoxyl content and viscosity on postcompaction axial recovery. High-ethoxyl, low-viscosity T10EC has lowest axial recovery.

% Drug released

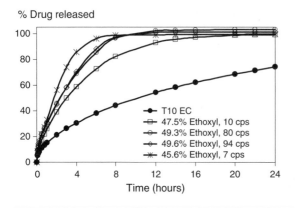

Figure 2 Effect of EC ethoxyl content and viscosity on acetaminophen release from binary drug-EC (1:3) blends. One percent stearic acid was added as lubricant. *Abbreviation*: EC, ethyl cellulose.

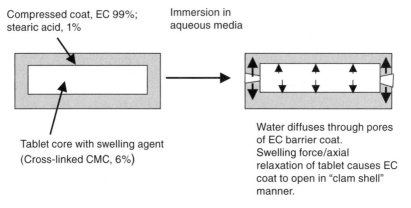

Figure 3    Schematic of compression-coated pulsed-release system.

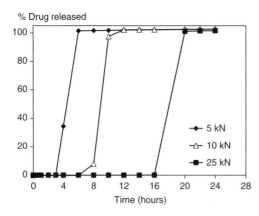

Figure 4    Effect of compression force on pulsed-release lag time; 0.25 inches flat, round 100 mg theophylline cores compression-coated with 200 mg of T10 EC: stearate (99:1) using 0.375 inches flat, round beveled edge tooling formulation. *Abbreviation*: EC, ethyl cellulose.

**Table 2**  Effect of Ethoxyl Percentage of Ethyl Cellulose (EC) and Viscosity on Lag Times from Compression-Coated Pulsatile-Release Systems

| EC type | Coat-compression force (kN) | Lag time (hr) |
|---|---|---|
| T10 EC (51% ethoxyl, 9.2 cps) | 5 | 3.8 |
| T10 EC (51% ethoxyl, 9.2 cps) | 10 | 6.0 |
| T10 EC (51% ethoxyl, 9.2 cps) | 25 | 16.0 |
| 48.0 ethoxyl, 10.0 cps | 25 | 2.0 |
| 49.6 ethoxyl, 94.0 cps | 25 | 0.5 |
| 49.3 ethoxyl, 88.0 cps | 25 | 0.3 |
| 45.6 ethoxyl, 7.1 cps | 25 | 0 |
| 45.7 ethoxyl, 83.0 cps | 25 | 0 |

modified-release applications. A number solid oral dosage forms containing T10 EC as a rate controlling excipient are currently in clinical trials.

## KLUCEL® HYDROXYPROPYL CELLULOSE FOR MOLECULAR WEIGHT–CONTROLLED EROSION AND DIFFUSION SYSTEMS

### Description of Technology

Hydroxypropyl cellulose (HPC) and hypromellose (HPMC) are the most commonly used water-soluble cellulose ethers for oral controlled-release systems. Similar in many respects to HPMC, fine particle, high molecular weight HPC is well known for its efficiency in controlled-release applications (6–8) has outstanding compactibility (9). Fine particle size HPC has traditionally been available as high and low molecular weight (MW) grades designated as Klucel Pharm hydroxypropyl cellulose, grades HXF and EXF, with a typical mean particle size of between 80 and 100 μm. Recently new fine particle grades of Klucel HPC have been developed and that have intermediate MW. These grades have been designated as MXF, GXF, JXF, and LXF. In sharp contrast to HPMC of similar intermediate MW, these HPC grades allow for the precise control of drug release and erosion with rates increasing in an inversely proportional manner to polymer molecular weight. Due to the hydrophobic association of methoxyl functional groups in HPMC polymers, MW-based control of release at similar molecular weights are not possible (4,5). The fine particle size grades of HPC polymer and associated viscosities described in this monograph are summarized in Table 3.

### Research and Development

Studies on three formulations in which drugs of widely differing solubility and dose revealed that varying the MW of fine particle size HPC effectively regulated drug release rates. The formulations used included as model drugs an intermediate dose BCS class II compound (nifedipine), papaverine HCl as a low dose system in which strong pH-dependent solubility is exhibited (high solubility in acidic media, but insoluble in neutral and alkaline conditions) and a high dose BCS class I compound, theophylline. Release rates for all three systems were effectively regulated by varying the MW of the fine particle size HPC. Figures 5 and 6 depict the release profiles of nifedipine and reveal that that after a short lag time the release is linear and closely correlated with the rate of erosion rate of the different formulations.

The rate of erosion of a polymeric system is driven by the rate of disentanglement of polymer chains from a hydrated tablet surface. As the solubility of low MW HPC is higher than that for high MW HPC there will be greater surface erosion from low MW HPC systems. The physical differences attributable to MW are depicted in Figure 7 and show that volume increases (swelling) for the higher MW grades HXF and MXF, whereas the lower MW grades, EXF and JXF, show a volume decrease as a consequence of rapid surface erosion. For the intermediate grade material, GXF (370 kDa) the volume remains relatively constant, indicating that a balance between erosion and swelling events exists.

For an insoluble drug such as nifedipine the rate of drug dissolution from a delivery system is the rate limiting factor in drug absorption. In the low and medium MW grade delivery systems in addition to the limited diffusion of dissolved drug through the tablet matrix, the liberation of undissolved drug particles is promoted by surface erosion. These particles are then able dissolve more rapidly in the bulk fluid of the dissolution test or in the gastrointestinal tract.

The MW-controlled erosion of HPC can also be exploited for drugs, such as papaverine HCl that exhibit pH dependent solubility. Figure 8 shows that regardless of the MW of HPC used in the matrix, drug release is controlled by diffusion and swelling in acidic conditions, which is attributed

**Table 3** Grades of Fine Particle Size HPC Polymer Described in This Chapter

| Klucel® Pharm HPC grade | Nominal molecular weight (kDa) | Apparent viscosity (mPa sec) |
|---|---|---|
| EXF | 80 | 300–600 at 10% |
| LXF (new) | 110 | 75–150 at 5% |
| JXF (new) | 140 | 150–400 at 5% |
| GXF (new) | 370 | 150–400 at 2% |
| MXF (new) | 850 | 4000–6500 at 2% |
| HXF | 1150 | 1500–3000 at 1% |

*Abbreviation*: HPC, hydroxypropyl cellulose.

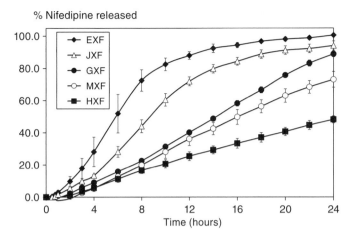

**Figure 5** Effect of fine particle Klucel HPC MW on nifedipine dissolution. Formulation: 20% nifedipine, 30% HPC, 49.5% MCC, and 0.5% magnesium stearate. *Abbreviations*: HPC, hydroxypropyl cellulose; MW, molecular weight.

to the high solubility of papaverine in acid media. When the dissolution medium pH is changed to 6.8 during dissolution testing, the solubility of papaverine decreases resulting in negligible further release of the compound from the high MW, low eroding matrix systems. For the low MW grades JXF and GXF drug release continues due to erosion of the polymer. Following the change of pH to 6.8, the release and erosion profiles from systems

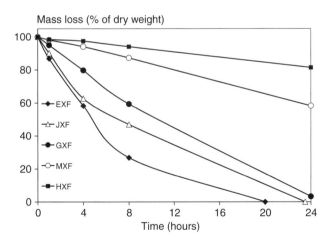

**Figure 6** Effect of fine particle grade Klucel HPC MW on matrix erosion. Formulation: 20% nifedipine, 30% HPC, 49.5% MCC, and 0.5% magnesium stearate. *Abbreviations*: HPC, hydroxypropyl cellulose; MCC, microcrystalline cellulose; MW, molecular weight.

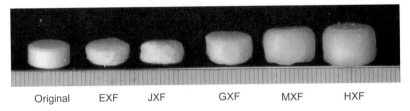

Original    EXF    JXF    GXF    MXF    HXF

**Figure 7** Effect of fine particle grade Klucel HPC on erosion and swelling behavior of nifedipine matrix tablets subjected to dissolution testing for 4 hours. Formulation: 20% nifedipine, 30% HPC, 49.5% MCC, and 0.5% magnesium stearate. *Abbreviations*: HPC, hydroxypropyl cellulose; MCC, microcrystalline cellulose.

manufactured using the GXF and JXF grades are nearly super imposable demonstrating control of erosion and drug release. The use of these grades can reduce the pH dependence of matrix systems containing weak bases without the need for additional buffering agents to be included in the tablet.

Erosion control through the selection of an appropriate MW of HPC is also suitable for systems in which a drug of intermediate solubility and high content is required to be formulated. Figure 9 shows that for 70% w/w theophylline tablets, the erosion and drug release profiles are nearly super imposable for the low and intermediate MW grades (EXF, JXF, and GXF), indicating that erosion is the rate limiting process for drug release from these systems. For the higher MW HPC grades MXF and HXF, the drug release

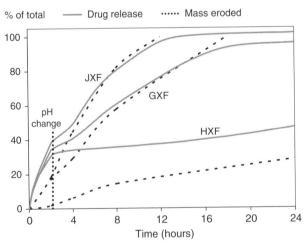

**Figure 8** Effect of MW of HPC on drug release and erosion of low dose papaverine tablets. Formulation: 5% Papaverine HCl, 30% HPC, and 64.5% MCC, were wet granulated before compression. All formulations were lubricated with 0.5% magnesium stearate. *Abbreviations*: HPC, hydroxypropyl cellulose; MW, molecular weight; MCC, microcrystalline cellulose.

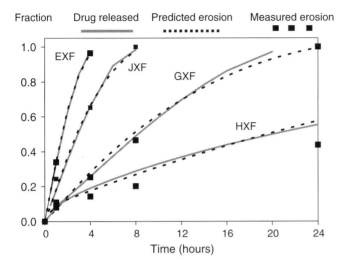

**Figure 9**   Effect of MW of HPC on fractional drug release, predicted erosion and actual erosion of 70% theophylline tablets. *Abbreviations*: HPC, hydroxypropyl cellulose; MW, molecular weight.

profiles and predicted erosion profiles are faster than the actual erosion profiles, suggesting that drug diffusion through the highly swollen gel layers contribute significantly to drug release.

## Regulatory and Commercial Status

Klucel Pharm HPC is USP, EP, and JP compliant and also meets the FCC requirements (10). The different grades of Klucel Pharm HPC are all commercially available and a number of solid oral dosage forms comprising Klucel Pharm HPC are marketed in the USA, Europe, and other countries.

## REFERENCES

1.  Lapidus H, Lordi NG, Drug release from compressed hydrophilic matrices. J Pharm Sci 1968; 57:292–1301.
2.  Dürig T, Hall RH, Salzstein RA, Highly compressible ethyl cellulose for tableting. US patent 6,592,901, 2001.
3.  Skinner GW, Harcum WW, Dürig T. Ethyl cellulose in compression coated tablets: implications for time-controlled pulsed-release dosage forms. AAPS Pharm Sci 2002; 4(4):Abstract T3278.
4.  Skinner GW, Harcum WW, Dürig, T. Ethyl cellulose in direct compression modified release tablets: Impact of polymer structure and formulation variables. AAPS Pharm Sci 2002; 4(4):Abstract T3281.

5. Dahl TC. Ethyl cellulose. In: Kibbe AH. ed. Handbook of Pharmaceutical Excipients, 3rd ed. Washington, DC: Amercican Pharmaceutical Association and Pharmaceutical Press, 2000: 195–200.

6. Johnson JL, Holinej J, Williams MD. Influence of ionic strength on matrix integrity and drug release from hydroxypropyl cellulose compacts. Int J Pharm 1993; 90:151–9.

7. Alderman DA. Sustained release compositions comprising hydroxypropyl cellulose ethers. US Patent 4,704,285, 1987.

8. Lee DY, Chen C-M. Delayed pulse release hydro gel matrix tablet. US Patent 6,103,263, 2000.

9. Joneja, SK, Harcum WW, Skinner GW, Barnum PE, Guo JH. Investigating the fundamental effects of binders on pharmaceutical tablet. Drug Dev Ind Pharm 1999; 25:1129–35.

10. Harwood RJ. Hydroxypropyl cellulose. In: Kibbe AH. ed. Handbook of Pharmaceutical Excipients, 3rd ed. Washington, DC: American Pharmaceutical Association and Pharmaceutical Press, 2000:244–8.

# 14

# SQZgel™

Ramesh C. Rathi, Jong Bark, and Kirk D. Fowers
*Protherics, PLC, Salt Lake City, Utah, U.S.A.*

## INTRODUCTION

Chitosan is a nontoxic and bioabsorbable polymer that has been investigated for a broad range of drug delivery applications (1–4). SQZgel™ are tablets that are a blend of chitosan and polyethylene glycol (PEG) and are used as a controlled-release oral formulation. The technology was developed by MacroMed, Inc. that was recently acquired by Protherics, PLC and is based on a pH sensitive inner core surrounded by a nondegradable microporous coated tablet (5,6). SQZgel tablets permit once or twice daily dosing and are designed to enhance patient compliance, reduce peak to trough blood levels, and eliminate the requirement of 4–6 doses daily.

A variety of drug delivery systems have been developed that exhibit pH-dependent drug release and have been designed to function in a variety of different locations within the body, i.e., periodontal and oral cavities and along the entire gastrointestinal tract (GIT) (7–11). The use of covalently crosslinked pH-sensitive hydrogels that swell under acidic conditions and shrink at neutral pH are well known (12–16). The development of a stable hydrogel that is pH-sensitive and that is not chemically modified or crosslinked to facilitate hydrogel formation is novel and creates a material that is suitable for drug delivery over a wide range of pH (17,18).

SQZgel forms a stable hydrogel at both acidic and neutral pH and exhibits pH-dependent swelling and shrinking. SQZgel is an example of a cationic hydrogel with pH-dependent swelling properties that has been proposed as a candidate for use in developing drug delivery systems. SQZgel is a modified version of the naturally occurring polysaccharide, chitin. The chitin is partially deacetylated under alkaline conditions to produce chitosan. Deacetylation is an essential step in order to produce the desired physical characteristics that allow the formation of a stable hydrogel with the desired viscosity and cationic characteristics that allow the tablet core to swell in an acidic environment (stomach) and to shrink in a neutral environment (small and large intestine) within a specific time frame (Fig. 1) (19).

## Product Concept

The desired functionality of the tablet core that is imparted by the specific blend of chitosan and PEG was developed through the selection of specific chitosan characteristics. In particular the characteristics that impart pH dependent swelling, a specific viscosity and that form a stable hydrogel in an aqueous environment ranging from acidic to neutral pH were considered. Blends of chitosan of different molecular weight, viscosity and degree of deacetylation were evaluated. Each blend tested, exhibited pH dependent swelling of up to 60-times the weight of the starting material, but only select formations exhibited the formation of stable hydrogels with the desired swelling/shrinking characteristics. The chitosan (15 g/L) which met the desired criteria was found to have a MW of approximately 150,000, a degree of deacetylation of between 80–85% and a viscosity of approximately 100 cps in 1% v/v acetic acid. Once an appropriate blend had been developed, a selection of active pharmaceutical ingredients (API) was incorporated into the core of the tablet containing a range of concentrations of the SQZgel blend and the in vitro release characteristics examined. The ultimate selection of an appropriate concentration of SQZgel for a given active compound and formulation was based on the drug loading and the desired release profile characteristics.

## Technology Overview

The SQZgel technology is a combination of a pH-sensitive core and a nonbiodegradable micro-porous coated tablet. The pH-sensitive core

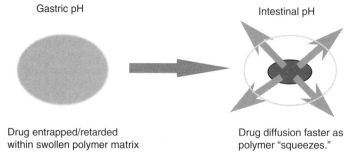

Gastric pH                                    Intestinal pH

Drug entrapped/retarded                    Drug diffusion faster as
within swollen polymer matrix              polymer "squeezes."

**Figure 1**  Schematic representation of the effect of pH on a diltiazem oral dosage form manufactured using SQZgel™.

comprises a blend of chitosan and PEG, which allows controlled release of API, in particular water-soluble APIs for up to 24 hours following administration. The ultimate release profile that is generated is a result of a combination of the composition of the inner SQZgel core and the microporous coating that can be modulated in terms of coating thickness and porosity. Therefore in order to achieve a specific and desire release profile the optimal combination of SQZgel content and membrane permeability must be evaluated and selected.

A select few combinations of chitosan and PEG were shown to for stable hydrogels in both acidic and neutral environments. Outside of these combinations, the hydrogels were unstable or were not formed. The formation of a stable hydrogel is necessary to control the release of the drug as it swells in the acidic environment of the stomach and shrinks at neutral pH encountered in the small intestine. Since SQZgel exhibits swelling up to 60 times its weight in water, nonbiodegradable, rigid tablets were selected to maintain a specific core size during the swelling and shrinking of the SQZgel and to drive the release of drug. The shrinking of the tablet core was shown to occur in a linear fashion in a simulated intestinal environment over the expected period of transit through the GIT. The release properties imparted by the swelling and shrinking of SQZgel maintain a near zero-order release profile for the duration of release of API from these systems. The tablets remain intact and continuous release of API is achieved during transit of the technology through the GIT.

Advantages of the technology include the ability to achieve a high drug loading, the use of standard tablet manufacturing techniques and suitability of the technology for the delivery of highly water soluble drugs. SQZgel tablets can be prepared with drug loading in excess of 90% w/w, which allows for much smaller tablets to be manufactured. Furthermore the formulation and manufacture of dosage forms with low-potency high dosage API that would be difficult as matrix based oral tablets, is facilitated. The core of the tablet is ideally suited for highly water soluble drugs and selection of the appropriate core/coating allows controlled release over the desired time and concentration range. In addition standard tableting approaches reduce the cost and need for development of technology specific equipment for the preparation of SQZgel based tablets.

## Research and Development

Research has been performed on chitosan products in pharmaceutical applications including films for wound dressing (20–22), as mucoadhesives (23–26), for parenteral drug delivery (27–30) and for oral dosage forms (31–33). The goal in the development of SQZgel was to produce a material that would provide controlled oral delivery based on the swelling and shrinking properties of the SQZgel core and the microporous coated tablet.

Initial studies focused on the characterization of chitosan, which is a partially deacetylated form of chitin a major component of the exoskeleton of crustaceans (19). Deacetylation of chitin was conducted at elevated temperatures under alkaline conditions to produce chitosans with a range of chemical and physical properties (34). The degree of deacetylation yields chitosan with varied molecular weights, viscosity and proportions of positively charged functional groups (35). Preliminary studies were conducted to identify the appropriate molecular weight, viscosity, and degree of deacetylation that would allow formation of stable films under acidic and neutral pH conditions (36). The desired properties that were identified as important included an appropriate degree of water absorption, rapid swelling at acidic pH, and a linear decrease in swelling once subjected to neutral pH. Furthermore the formation of a stable hydrogel, i.e., a gel that does not dissolve in an aqueous environment under the conditions expected during dosage form transit through the GIT was a key consideration.

The swelling properties of SQZgel blends manufactures as films was examined under simulated gastric conditions, simulated intestinal conditions in addition to simulated gastric conditions followed by exposure of the films to simulated intestinal pH conditions and the resultant swelling ratios are depicted in Figure 2.

Swelling occurs rapidly at acidic pH, but decreases linearly over approximately and 8-hour period at neutral pH. The linear decrease in the swelling ratio over an 8-hour period was selected as an appropriate profile to allow the controlled release of API during transit of the dosage form through GIT.

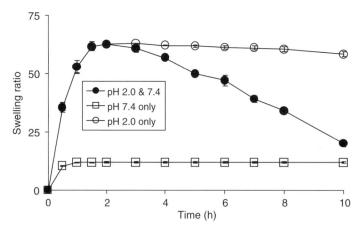

**Figure 2** Swelling ratio of SQZgel™ films following exposure to solutions of pH 2.0, pH 2.0 for 2 hours followed by pH 7.4, and pH 7.4 only ($n = 12$).

Once the optimal SQZgel blend had been determined, proof of concept studies were conducted using a nonporous tablets with 1.3 mm holes drilled into each side of the dosage form. Tablets containing a combination bus-pirone and SQZgel polymer were manufactured and the in vitro release of buspirone investigated under simulated gastric and/or intestinal conditions. The resultant in vitro release profiles are depicted in Figure 3.

At neutral pH approximately 85% of buspirone was released in 2 hours which is due to the low degree of swelling of the SQZgel whereas in a swollen state it takes approximately 24 hours for 85% of the drug to be released from the system. These data demonstrate the potential for retar-dation of drug release when the SQZgel technology exists in a swollen state.

Subsequently SQZgel tablet cores were prepared containing buspirone and were coated with a micro-porous nondegradable coating containing a pore forming agent. The contribution of the SQZgel blend to control of drug release was examined at core tablet concentrations of between 0% and 5% w/w of the SQZgel. An identical micro-porous coating was applied to all cores in all cases. The in vitro release rate profiles were generated by exposing tablets to simulated gastric fluid for 2 hours after which they were transferred to simulated intestinal fluid and monitored for a further 10 hours. The resultant release rate profiles are depicted in Figure 4.

The tablets containing 0%, 1%, 2%, 3%, and 5% SQZgel released 80% of the buspirone in approximately 4, 5.5, 6.5, 7, and 12 hours, respectively. Furthermore additional modulation of drug release can be achieved by altering the composition and characteristics of the microporous coating used to coat the SQZgel/drug tablet core.

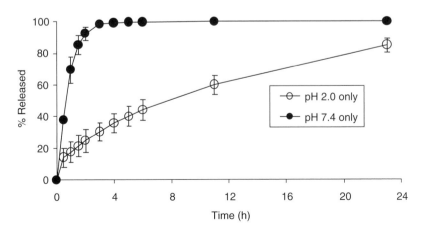

**Figure 3** In vitro release profiles for buspirone from SQZgel^{TM} tablets at gastric pH (2.0) and intestinal pH (7.4) ($n = 3$).

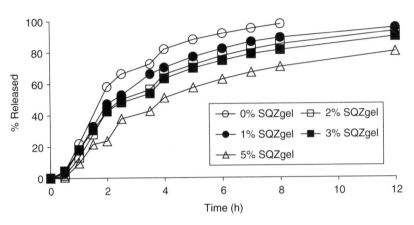

**Figure 4**   In vitro release profiles for buspirone from SQZgel™ tablets of different content at gastric pH (2.0) for 2 hours followed by intestinal pH for 10 hours ($n = 10$).

## Preclinical and Clinical Development of SQZgel

In addition to the evaluation of buspirone, studies have been conducted using diltiazem and tramadol in a canine model and the SQZgel/Tramadol product (Doloryn) was used in a single-dose pharmacokinetic study in humans.[*] Blood levels of diltiazem following administration of a SQZgel/diltiazem tablet revealed that diltiazem serum levels were equivalent when compared to those observed following hourly administration of diltiazem solutions and in which the total dose administered was equivalent (Protherics data on file). SQZgel/diltiazem tablets also exhibited equivalent in vitro release of diltiazem in comparison to commercially available formulations of diltiazem in oral dosage forms manufactured using matrix technologies and in which all tablets contained the same dose. Although the release profiles were equivalent for the four dosage forms tested, the SQZgel tablets were considerably smaller in size. The advantages of smaller tablets include the ease of swallowing and the ability to formulate low potency drugs effectively. The former consideration may be a factor in older patient populations where swallowing is difficult whereas the latter consideration would allow for the manufacture of oral dosage forms where alternative tableting techniques would produce tablets too large to swallow. Furthermore the tablets are prepared using standard tableting equipment and therefore costs of production are not excessive. However oral dosage formulations that use SQZgel technology are proprietary and cannot be disclosed.

The single dose pharmacokinetics of diltiazem in fasted dogs ($n = 5$) following administration of SQZgel/diltiazem tablets and Dilacor-XR were

---

[*] SQZgel™ and Doloryn™ are registered trademarks of Protherics, PLC.

investigated. The diltiazem concentrations were analyzed over a 48-hour period and $C_{max}$ and AUC were calculated for both products and the data are summarized in Table 1. Initial studies included in the development of Doloryn$^{TM}$ included pharmacokinetic modeling following administration in a canine model for fed versus fasted animals, high-fat diet and repeat or multiple dosing studies. Further development of Doloryn included evaluation of multiple dosing of 200 and 400 mg doses, combination tablets containing 150 or 350 mg controlled release and a 50 mg immediate release overcoat and a pharmacokinetic comparison of these technologies to 50 or 100 mg doses of Ultram administered four times a day. $C_{max}$ and steady state levels for the controlled-release formulation were maintained at the target level between the levels measured for the 50 and 100 mg four times a day dosing regimens in the canine model. The canine studies demonstrated plasma levels that are expected to provide the desired analgesia, based on comparison with immediate release formulations of tramadol, while maintaining a near zero-order release profile with a lower $C_{max}$. The sustained release profile and lower $C_{max}$ are common and desirable features of controlled-release formulations. A human pharmacokinetic study of Doloryn was subsequently conducted to determine the pharmacokinetic performance in human subjects and the release profile exhibited near zero-order release of tramadol and appearance of its primary metabolite, which exhibits greater activity than the parent compound. Levels were sustained above the theoretical required analgesic levels over a 24-hour period with a lower $C_{max}$, confirming the results of the canine study.

## Regulatory Strategy

Chitosan is the sole component of the SQZgel technology that has as yet not received regulatory approval. Although chitosan is widely used as a food supplement and questions regarding its safety have been addressed it is still under development and has not as yet been approved for use in pharmaceutical applications (9,23). A number of drug delivery systems using chitosan for parenteral and oral applications are currently at various stages of preclinical and clinical development. An additional factor that may limit regulatory concerns with respect to the use of chitosan is that the SQZgel/drug core is contained in a nonbiodegradable tablet that will pass through the

**Table 1** Pharmacokinetic Comparison of SQZgel$^{TM}$/Diltiazem Versus Dilacor-XR in a Canine Model

| Dosage form | $C_{max}$ (ng/mL) | AUC$_{t=48\,hr}$(hr-ng/mL) |
|---|---|---|
| SQZgel$^{TM}$/diltiazem (240 mg) | 386 ± 160 | 6242 ± 1605 |
| Dilacor-XR (240 mg) | 406 ± 265 | 5949 ± 2894 |

GIT intact. Based on this design, the exposure to the SQZgel blend within the GIT is negligible and the amount of chitosan contained in each tablet is orders of magnitude below the amounts included in food supplements. SQZgel tablets containing new or reformulated active agents should follow standard approval strategies and preclinical GLP safety/toxicity studies.

## Competitive Advantage

The technology has a number of key advantages when compared to other technologies available for oral drug delivery. Drug loading in the core tablet often exceeds 90% w/w in comparison to matrix technologies that are limited to approximately 50% drug loading. Whereas matrix technologies have demonstrated wide spread utility there are numerous examples of active agents that would benefit from administration in smaller tablets, such as acyclovir (1000 mg/day), verapamil (120–480 mg/day), flavoxate (100–800 mg/day), ribavarin (400–800 mg/day) in addition to low potency drugs in development. Patient compliance would improve with smaller, easier to swallow tablets, especially in geriatric and patient populations where swallowing is difficult. Additional advantages include the use of standard tableting techniques for the production of the tablets and the proprietary nature of the technology that would expand the patent protection of formulations created using SQZgel technology.

## Outlook

SQZgel is a widely applicable oral delivery technology that works well for both high potency low drug loading and low potency high drug loading applications. The development of controlled-release formulations will continue to improve patient compliance and the near zero-order release profiles minimizes peak to trough variations in blood levels thereby improving therapeutic responses for patients consequently providing safe and effective therapy. The next steps in developing the technology further include conducting repeat dosing studies of Doloryn to elucidate pharmacokinetic parameters and steady state concentrations for tramadol and the selection of additional API to broaden experience with this unique technology.

## REFERENCES

1. Agnihotri SA, Mallikarjuna NN, and Aminabhavi TM. Recent advances on chitosan-based micro- and nanoparticles in drug delivery. J Control Release 2004; 100:5–28.
2. Illum L. Chitosan and its use as a pharmaceutical excipient. Pharm Res 1998; 15:1326–31.

3.  Muzzarelli R, Baldassarre V, and Conti F, et al. Biological activity of chitosan: ultrastructural study. Biomaterials 1988; 9:247–52.
4.  Ratner BB. Biomedical applications of hydrogels: review and critical appraisal. In: Williams DF, ed., Biocompatibility of Clinical Implant Materials II. Boca Raton, FL: CRC Press, 1981: 146.
5.  Zentner GM, Bark JS, and Liu F. Polymer blends that swell in an acidic environment and deswell in a basic environment. US Patent, 6,537,584, March 25, 2003.
6.  Zentner GM, Bark JS, and Liu F. Polymer blends that swell in an acidic environment and deswell in a basic environment. US Patent, 6,730,327, May 4, 2004.
7.  Deshpande AA, Shah NH, Rhodes CT, and Malick W. Development of a novel controlled-release system for gastric retention. Pharm Res 14:815–9, 1997.
8.  Liu H, Yang XG, and Nie SF, et al. Chitosan-based controlled porosity osmotic pump for colon-specific delivery system: screening of formulation variables and in vitro investigation. Int J Pharm 2006; 332:115–24.
9.  Prabaharan M, and Mano JF. Chitosan-based particles as controlled drug delivery systems. Drug Deliv 2005; 12:41–57.
10.  Kato Y, Onishi H, and Machida Y. Application of chitin and chitosan derivatives in the pharmaceutical field. Curr Pharm Biotechnol 2003; 4:303–9.
11.  Hejazi R, and Amiji M. Chitosan-based gastrointestinal delivery systems. J Control Release 2003; 89:151–65.
12.  Colonna C, Genta I, and Perugini P, et al. 5-Methyl-pyrrolidinone chitosan films as carriers for buccal administration of proteins. AAPS Pharm Sci Tech 2006; 7:70.
13.  Park H, Park K, and Kim D. Preparation and swelling behavior of chitosan-based superporous hydrogels for gastric retention application. J Biomed Mater Res A 2006; 76:144–50.
14.  Kulkarni AR, Hukkeri VI, and Sung HW, et al. A novel method for the synthesis of the PEG-crosslinked chitosan with a pH-independent swelling behavior. Macromol Biosci 2005; 5:925–8.
15.  Chen SC, Wu YC, Mi FL, Lin YH, Yu LC, and Sung HW. A novel pH-sensitive hydrogel composed of N,O-carboxymethyl chitosan and alginate crosslinked by genipin for protein drug delivery. J Control Release 2004; 96:285–300.
16.  Dini E, Alexandridou S, and Kiparissides C. Synthesis and characterization of cross-linked chitosan microspheres for drug delivery applications. J Microencapsul 2003; 20:375–85.
17.  Berger J, Reist M, Mayer JM, Felt O, Peppas NA, and Gurny R. Structure and interactions in covalently and ionically crosslinked chitosan hydrogels for biomedical applications. Eur J Pharm Biopharm 2004; 57:19–34.
18.  Noble L, Gray AI, Sadiq L, and Uchegbu IF. A non-covalently cross-linked chitosan based hydrogel. Int J Pharm 1999; 192:173–82.
19.  Mussarelli R. Chitin in Nature and Technology. New York: Plenum Press, 1986.
20.  Ishihara M, Obara K, and Nakamura S, et al. Chitosan hydrogel as a drug delivery carrier to control angiogenesis. J Artif Organs 2006; 9:8–16.

21. Denkbas EB, Ozturk E, and Ozdemir N, et al. Norfloxacin-loaded chitosan sponges as wound dressing material. J Biomater Appl 2004; 18:291–303.
22. Mi FL, Wu YB, and Shyu SS, et al. Control of wound infections using a bilayer chitosan wound dressing with sustainable antibiotic delivery. J Biomed Mater Res 2002; 59:438–49.
23. Sharma S, Kulkarni J, and Pawar AP. Permeation enhancers in the transmucosal delivery of macromolecules. Pharmazie 2006; 61:495–504.
24. Wittaya-areekul S, Kruenate J, and Prahsarn C. Preparation and in vitro evaluation of mucoadhesive properties of alginate/chitosan microparticles containing prednisolone. Int J Pharm 2006; 312:113–8.
25. Varshosaz J, Sadrai H, and Heidari A. Nasal delivery of insulin using bio-adhesive chitosan gels. Drug Deliv 2006; 13:31–8.
26. Gavini E, Hegge AB, and Rassu G, et al. Nasal administration of carbamazepine using chitosan microspheres: in vitro/in vivo studies. Int J Pharm 2006; 307:9–15.
27. Panchagnula R, Dhanikula RS, and Dhanikula AB. An ex vivo characterization of Paclitaxel loaded chitosan films after implantation in mice. Curr Drug Deliv 2006; 3:287–97.
28. Kim JH, Kim YS, and Kim S, et al. Hydrophobically modified glycol chitosan nanoparticles as carriers for paclitaxel. J Control Release 2006; 111:228–34.
29. Springate CM, Jackson JK, and Gleave ME, et al. Efficacy of an intratumoral controlled release formulation of clusterin antisense oligonucleotide complexed with chitosan containing paclitaxel or docetaxel in prostate cancer xenograft models. Cancer Chemother Pharmacol 2005; 56:239–47.
30. Bhattarai N, Ramay HR, Gunn J, Matsen FA, and Zhang M. PEG-grafted chitosan as an injectable thermosensitive hydrogel for sustained protein release. J Control Release 2005; 103:609–24.
31. Thongborisute J, Takeuchi H, and Yamamoto H, et al. Properties of liposomes coated with hydrophobically modified chitosan in oral liposomal drug delivery. Pharmazie 2006; 61:106–11.
32. Prego C, Torres D, and Alonso MJ. The potential of chitosan for the oral administration of peptides. Expert Opin Drug Deliv 2005; 2:843–54.
33. Nunthanid J, Laungtana-Anan M, and Sriamornsak P, et al. Characterization of chitosan acetate as a binder for sustained release tablets. J Control Release 2004; 99:15–26.
34. Sabnis S, and Block LH. Chitosan as an enabling excipient for drug delivery systems. I. Molecular modifications. Int J Biol Macromol 2000; 27:181–6.
35. Rege PR, Shukla DJ, and Block LH. Chitinosans as tableting excipients for modified release delivery systems. Int J Pharm 1999; 181:49–60.
36. Ren D, Yi H, Wang W, and Maet X. The enzymatic degradation and swelling properties of chitosan matrices with different degrees of N-acetylation. Carbohydr Res 2005; 340:2403–10.

# 15

# Thiolated Polymers for Controlled Release

## M. Werle

*ThioMatrix GmbH, Research Center Innsbruck, Innsbruck, Austria*

## A. Bernkop-Schnürch

*Department of Pharmaceutical Technology, Leopold-Franzens University Innsbruck, Innsbruck, Austria*

## INTRODUCTION

Thiolated polymers or designated thiomers are mucoadhesive polymers, which contain thiol functional groups on side chains. The low molecular mass thiol group compounds are covalently bonded to a polymeric backbone. The polymeric backbone is comprised of well-established and safe polymers such as chitosan or poly(acrylic acid). It has been demonstrated in various studies, that thiomers exhibit mucoadhesive (1), permeation enhancing (2), controlled release (3), as well as enzyme (4) and efflux pump inhibitory properties (5). These features make thiomer technologies potentially useful for noninvasive delivery including the oral, nasal, buccal, and vaginal routes. Thiomers can be directly compressed to into tablets or to produce solutions for administration. Thiomer-based micro- and nanoparticles have been developed, and this monograph describes the technology, its applicability for controlled release and the current research and development and intellectual property status of the technology.

## HISTORICAL DEVELOPMENT

The first thiomers were synthesized in the late 1990s (6) in order to improve the oral bioavailability of hydrophilic macromolecules such as therapeutic peptides and proteins. Initially, the technology was based on a strategy to prolong the residence time of drug delivery systems on mucosal membrane surfaces, which led to improved drug absorption and uptake (7). Further investigations showed that the thiolation of polymers does not only lead to improved mucoadhesiveness, but also to additional improvements for the noninvasive delivery of hydrophilic drugs, such as permeation enhancement. Recently, it has been found that thiomers are capable of inhibiting efflux pumps, which suggests that the technology may be a promising tool for the delivery of efflux pump substrates (5). Nowadays, research groups investigate composite thiomer delivery systems based on thiomeric systems in combination with other novel technologies such as nanotechnology (8,9).

## DESCRIPTION OF THE TECHNOLOGY

Thiomer technology is based on the covalent attachment of low molecular mass thiol functional group bearing compounds on polymeric backbones (Fig. 1). The free thiol groups of the thiomeric system have the potential to form disulfide bonds with cysteine rich subdomains of the mucus which consequently leads to improved mucoadhesion of the polymer (10). Generally there are two mechanisms by which this can occur including thiol/disulfide exchange reactions or simple oxidation of the free thiol groups as shown in Figure 2. In addition, in situ cross linking as depicted in Figure 3 leads to a further improvement of the mucoadhesive properties of these materials. Whereas the mucoadhesive effects of other polymers are generally

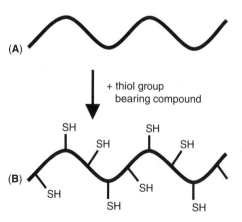

**Figure 1**   Schematic representation of thiomers with low molecular mass thiol group bearing compounds that are covalently bound to a polymer (**A**) to produce a thiomer (**B**).

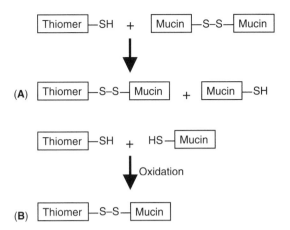

(A)

(B)

**Figure 2** Different mechanisms of disulfide bond formation between thiomers and cysteine-rich subdomains of mucus. (**A**) Thiol/disulfide exchange reaction. (**B**) Oxidation of free thiol groups.

mediated by interpenetration and ionic interactions or the formation of hydrogen bonds of the polymer with the mucus, thiomers form covalent bonds with the mucus. A variety of thiomers has been described and includes anionic polymers such as poly(acrylic acid) derivatives or cationic polymers such as chitosan. Examples of low molecular mass thiol-bearing compounds that have been used for thiomer synthesis are glutathione and cysteine (11,12). By way of example, the chemical structure of the thiomer chitosan-thiobutylamidine (Chito-TBA) is depicted in Figure 4.

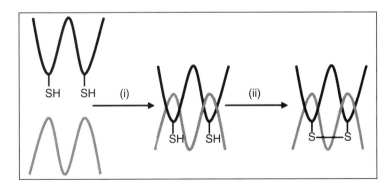

**Figure 3** Schematic representation of improved mucoadhesion mediated by in-situ cross-linking: (i) The thiomer (40) interpenetrates into the mucus gel layer (41); (ii) formation of intra- and intermolecular disulfide bonds between free thiol groups of the thiomers.

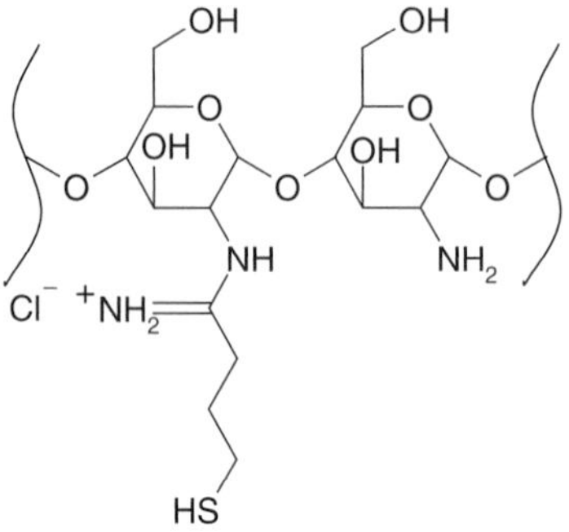

**Figure 4** Schematic representation of the presumed chemical substructure of the thiomer chitosan-TBA (chitosan-4-thiobutylamidine) conjugate.

Thiomers are multifunctional polymers that display additional features, other than their mucoadhesive properties that are important for oral drug delivery. Permeation enhancement is one of these features, and the effect has been demonstrated to be a function of the ability of the thiomeric compounds to open tight junctions between cells of the gastrointestinal mucosa, which is of particular importance for the delivery of hydrophilic molecules that are transported via the paracellular route (13).

A further important feature of thiomer use is based on the cohesive properties of thiomeric materials. The cohesive properties of thiomers allow for the controlled and or sustained release of a drug from a thiomeric polymeric matrix. The cohesive properties of these materials are based on the formation of inter- and intramolecular disulfide bonds, which result in the formation of a tightened three-dimensional polymeric network. Thiomer-based drug delivery systems have been demonstrated to provide an almost zero-order release kinetic for model drugs such as insulin (14). Rapid drug release can also be achieved when using thiomer-based micro- and nanoparticles (15). Mucoadhesive drug delivery systems that are used for mucosal drug delivery should also display cohesive properties as illustrated in Figure 5. Moreover, the combination of a cohesive and mucoadhesive matrix characteristics and the ability of these materials to open tight junctions are important considerations in dosage form design, so as to avoid unintended absorption of potential toxic compounds from the site of mucoadhesion (Fig. 6). The use of mucoadhesive and cohesive polymers results in the opening of tight junctions in restricted areas demarcated by the area of adhesion of the delivery system at the point at which drug release and absorption takes place. The mucoadhesive/cohesiveness of thiomers thereby avoid the unintended absorption of compounds such as low molecular mass auxiliary materials or xenobiotics. Such compounds may be absorbed when using solutions containing excipients or auxiliary agents that improve drug uptake along the entire gastrointestinal tract (Fig. 6).

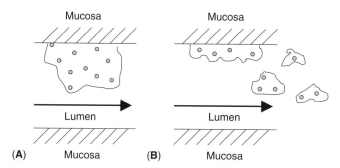

**Figure 5** Importance of cohesiveness in mucoadhesive drug delivery systems. (**A**) Drug delivery system with combined mucoadhesive and cohesive properties and in which the drug (*gray circles*) remain at a specific intestinal site. (**B**) Because of the lack of cohesive properties, the drug does not remain at the specific intestinal site despite the mucoadhesive properties of the delivery system.

Thiomers are capable of inhibiting proteolytic enzymes by mechanisms similar to that exhibited by poly(acrylic acid) derivatives. Enzyme inhibition by these materials is mediated by complexation of cations such as calcium or zinc that are important co-factors of most proteolytic enzymes. It has been demonstrated, that thiolation of poly(acrylic acid) leads to an improvement of zinc binding and inhibition of the abundant membrane bound protease amino peptidase N due to a so called "far-distance" inhibitory effect (4). Furthermore, thiomers can inhibit carboxypeptidase A, B, and chymotrypsin (12).

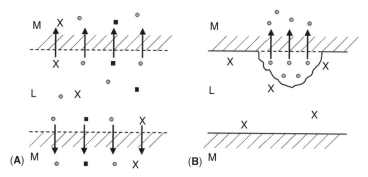

**Figure 6** Protective effect of a mucoadhesive/cohesive polymeric matrix: (**A**) not only the drug (*gray circles*) but also the low molecular mass permeation enhancers (*black squares*) and xenobiotics (X) are transported from the lumen (L) across the mucosa (M). When using mucoadhesive/cohesive polymeric matrices (**B**), permeation enhancement takes place at a restricted area, so that only the drug is transported and the polymeric matrix prevents unintended transport of xenobiotics.

Recently it has been shown that thiomers can also inhibit efflux pumps such as P-glycoprotein or MRP2 (5,16,17), however the mechanism of inhibition is currently not known. Since thiomers do not enter cells, blocking of ATP binding sites can be excluded as a potential cause of the inhibitory effects of these polymers. Efflux pump inhibition may be mediated by altering the integrity of cell membrane lipids and/or interaction of free thiol groups of the thiomers with cysteine residues of the efflux pump channel.

## RESEARCH AND DEVELOPMENT

### Feasibility Studies

Several feasibility studies demonstrating the efficacy of thiomer-based delivery systems have been conducted and thiomer technologies have been shown to improve the bioavailability of drugs following oral (18,19), nasal (20), buccal (21), and vaginal (22) administration. Extensive research focusing on the in vitro investigation of the mucoadhesive, permeation enhancing and protease as well as efflux pump inhibitory properties of thiomers have also been undertaken (2,5,23,24). In addition it has been demonstrated that thiomers can also improve the oral uptake of lipophilic efflux pump substrates such as saquinavir (25). The potential for use of thiomers for ocular drug delivery has been investigated (26) and additional information regarding in vitro and in vivo data obtained following thiomer use is described herein.

### Fabrication of Thiomer Technology

Generally the fabrication of thiomers is performed in aqueous solution and consists of three major steps. Initially a low molecular mass thiol group bearing compound is coupled to a polymeric backbone using a coupling agent such as N-(3-dimethylaminopropyl) N-ethylcarbodiimide hydrochloride. Secondly the thiomer is purified either by dialysis or precipitation to remove excess unbound low molecular mass thiol compound and/or the coupling agent. Finally the polymer is dried, usually via lyophilization. Following fabrication, the resultant thiomers are characterized according to the amount of thiol groups, free unbound thiol groups, and disulfide bonds present.

All educts for synthesis are commercially available and a variety of thiomers have been synthesized and characterized. The synthesis and isolation of thiomers is relatively simple. Factors that are known to influence the synthetic procedure of thiomers are, e.g., pH and concentration ratio of polymer in solution, coupling agent and thiol group bearing compound that are used for the fabrication of these materials.

## Major Obstacles and Solutions

The availability of a broad variety of different thiomers offers an advantage in that suitable delivery systems can be developed and tailored for many drug candidates. The obstacles identified thus far include, e.g., the potential for ionic interactions between the polymer and active pharmaceutical ingredient of choice since in order to control release cationic drugs should be combined with anionic thiomers and vice versa. Another potential difficulty is the potential for interactions between free thiol functional groups of the polymer and disulfide bonds of peptide/protein drugs. These challenges are considered to be primarily of theoretical interest since the successful delivery of several peptides/proteins using thiomers has been accomplished. There are several reports that demonstrate that thiomers exhibit cell toxicity which is in the same range as the toxicity of widely used nontoxic unmodified polymers (27). It is clearly evident that detailed studies will be necessary prior to successful regulatory approval of thiomer delivery systems.

## Scale-Up Challenges and Manufacturing Issues

GMP-material is already available for certain thiomers. One of the aims of the scale-up process is to produce uniform batches of thiomers with a clearly defined number of thiol functional groups and disulfide bounds. The production of stable and uniform thiomer-based nanoparticulate system is more challenging. Stability problems of nanoparticles are generally an important issue and it is believed that such delivery systems will not be launched on the market within the next few years.

## In Vitro Studies

There is plethora of literature (1–5) that describes the predominance of the mucoadhesive, permeation enhancing and protease/efflux pump inhibitory properties of thiomers in comparison to corresponding unmodified polymers in vitro. The mucoadhesive properties of different thiomers are summarized in Table 1. The mucoadhesive studies were performed using the rotating cylinder method and it has been demonstrated, that the mucoadhesive properties were up to 100-fold improved in comparison to the unmodified polymer (28). The in vitro permeation enhancing effect of thiomers is determined either by using freshly excised intestinal tissues of animals such as rats or guinea pigs as depicted in Figure 7, or by use of cell monolayers such as Caco-2 cell lines. The in vitro permeation in presence of certain thiomers can be improved up to about 40-fold, as shown with porcine buccal mucosa for the pituitary adenylate cyclase-activating polypeptide (PACAP) (29). In vitro data describing the synthesis and characterization (11), drug release (3), cohesive properties (30), protease inhibition (4), and efflux pump inhibition (5) of thiomers have been published.

**Table 1**   Comparison of the Mucoadhesive Properties of Various Thiomers Determined Using the Rotating Cylinder Method

| Thiomer | Degree of modification [μmol/g] | Adhesion time [h] | Improvement ratio[a] | Reference |
|---|---|---|---|---|
| Chitosan-TBA | 682 | >160 | >94 | (42) |
| PAA-Cys | 695 | 22 | 13 | (31) |
| PAA-GSH | 354 | 21 | 14 | (43) |
| Chitosan-TEA | 140 | 24 | 8.9 | (44) |
| Chitosan-thioglycolic acid | 27 | 4 | 5 | (45) |
| Polycarbophil-Cys | 12 | >10 | 2.1 | (46) |
| Sodium-carboxy-methylcelluolse-Cys | 22 | 3 | 1.2 | (46) |

[a]Improvement ratio, adhesion time of thiomer/adhesion time of corresponding unmodified polymer. *Abbreviations*: Cys, cysteine; GSH, glutathione; PAA, poly (acrylic acid); TBA, thiobutylamidine; TEA, thioethylamidine.

## In Vivo Studies

In vivo studies demonstrating the potential of thiomers as drug delivery technologies for different model compounds have so far been performed in mice (31), rats (16,32,33), dogs (unpublished), and pigs (21,33). In addition the efficacy of an ocular thiomer delivery system has been evaluated in human volunteers (26). By way of example the effect of thiomers on the plasma concentration time curve of the P-glycoprotein substrate rhodamine 123 following oral administration in rats is depicted in Figure 8 and data demonstrating an increase in low molecular weight heparin plasma levels when administered to rats in thiomer minitablets is depicted in Figure 9. In addition the observed absolute oral bioavailability of heparin from these tablets was 20 ± 9% (19).

## Examples of Drug and Clinical Applications of Thiomer Technology

Generally, there are three classes of compound for which thiomer technology may be used namely, hydrophilic drugs that are transported via the paracellular route and include various class III drugs such as calcitonin (32), insulin (31), cystine-knot micro proteins (34), heparins (19), or human growth hormone (35); efflux pump substrates, the efficacy for which thiomer technology has been demonstrated for model compounds such as rhodamine 123 (16) and sulforhodamine (17) in addition to approved molecules such as saquinavir (25) and paclitaxel (36); therapeutic plasmid DNA or

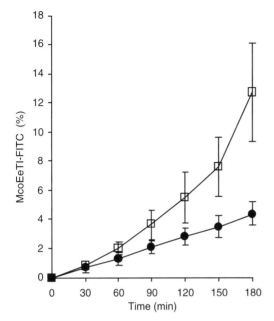

**Figure 7** Permeation of cystine-knot micro protein McoEeTI-FITC through freshly excised rat intestinal tissue in the presence (□) and absence (●) of thiomers ($n = 3$) (mean $\pm$ SD). *Source*: Adapted from Ref. 32.

siRNA. ThioMatrix is focusing on the development of drug delivery systems for calcitonin, human growth hormone, and paclitaxel. Moreover, numerous feasibility studies and co-developments with small, medium, and big pharmaceutical companies focusing on the development of oral, buccal, and vaginal drug delivery systems based on the thiomer technology for a variety of drug candidates are also currently in progress.

## REGULATORY ISSUES

GMP-material of certain thiomers is already available. Thiomer technology is protected worldwide by various patents (37,38). Mucobiomer GMBH (www.mucobiomer.com) holds all patent rights for ocular use and implants and ThioMatrix GMBH (www.thiomatrix.com) holds patent rights for all other applications.

## TECHNOLOGY POSITION AND COMPETITVE ADVANTAGES

Thiomer technology has been found to be "highly promising" by Bromberg (39). Two polymers that are frequently used for oral drug delivery systems are chitosan and poly(acrylic acid) or derivatives thereof. Thiomers based on these polymers offer advantages of improved cohesive properties,

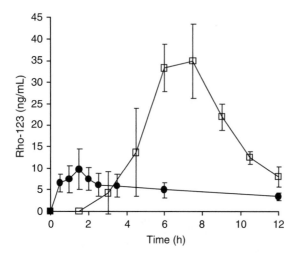

**Figure 8** Plasma concentration–time profiles of rhodamine-123 following oral administration of 1.5 mg as a solution (●) and in chitosan-TBA/GSH tablets (□); ($n$ = 5) (mean ± SD). *Abbreviations*: GSH, glutathione; TBA, thiobutylamidine. *Source*: Adapted from Ref. 13.

mucoadhesive properties, permeation enhancement in addition to more pronounced protease and efflux pump inhibition in comparison to unmodified polymers. Thiomer production is relatively simple and toxicity studies have

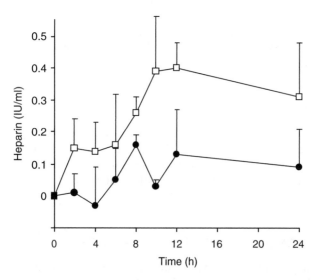

**Figure 9** Plasma concentration profiles of orally administered low molecular weight heparin in poly(acrylic acid)-cysteine minitablets (□) and poly(acrylic acid) minitablets (●) in rats ($n$ = 5) (mean ± SD) *Source*: Adapted from Ref. 16.

**Table 2**  Advantages of Thiomers in Comparison to the Unmodified Parent
Polymer

| Properties | Improvement ratio/comments[a] | References |
|---|---|---|
| Mucoadhesive properties | > 100-fold<br>Due to the formation of disulfide bonds with the mucus, all thiomers display enhanced mucoadhesive properties | 29,42 |
| Permeation enhancement | > 39-fold<br>A 39-fold improvement of the pituitary adenylate cyclase-activating polypeptide (PACAP) through porcine buccal mucosa was achieved with the thiomer chitosan-thiobutylamidine (Chito-TBA). A drug delivery system containing Chito-TBA and GSH improved buccal PACAP permeation even 78-fold in pigs. Improved drug permeation mediated by thiomers has also been observed by using intestinal and nasal tissues as well as monolayers | 30<br>35,47,25 |
| Efflux pump inhibition | Up to 100% inhibition<br>A complete inhibition of efflux pumps mediated by Chito-TBA was achieved in vitro. In vivo studies in rats showed an improved efflux pump substrate uptake after oral administration in presence of thiomer delivery systems | 5<br>16,17,25 |
| Protease inhibition | It has been demonstrated that thiolated polycarbophil is a more potent inhibitor of amino peptidase N than unmodified polycarbophil. Other proteolytic enzymes that can be inhibited by thiomers are carboxypeptidase A and B as well as chymotrypsin. | 4,12,24 |
| Cohesive properties | > 70-fold<br>Due to improved cohesive properties the disintegration time of $PAA_{450}$-Cys tablets could be more than 70-fold prolonged compared to the unmodified polymer | 31 |
| In situ gelling properties | ∞-fold<br>It has been demonstrated for various thiomers that there is a clear correlation between the total amount of polymer-linked thiol groups and the increase in the viscosity of the formed gel. Thiomers that do not disintegrate any more have been developed | 48,49 |

[a]Improvement ratio = values gained with thiomers/values gained with the corresponding unmodified polymers.
*Abbreviations*: Chito-TBA, chitosan-thiobutylamidine; Cys, cysteine; GSH, glutathione; PAA,
poly (acrylic acid); PACAP, pituitary adenylate cyclase-activating polypeptide.

shown that thiomers do not exhibit greater toxicity than the widely used polymers, chitosan and poly(acrylic acid) which are considered safe. Thiomer technology appears to be especially useful for the delivery of hydrophilic macromolecules and efflux pump substrates and the advantages of thiomer technology are summarized in Table 2.

## CONCLUSION AND FUTURE DIRECTIONS

Currently, researchers are focusing on the development of novel thiomers, thiomer-based nanoparticulate delivery systems, thiomer-based gene delivery systems, and on the evaluation of thiomers for the delivery of efflux pump substrates. In particular extensive investigations into the use of thiomers in the emerging field of nanotechnology are underway and there is great potential for use of thiomer technologies in the field of oral efflux pump inhibition. In recent years the potential use of thiomers as delivery vehicles for therapeutic genes has also been evaluated. However the main focus of ongoing research is still the development of delivery systems for hydrophilic macromolecules, such as for example therapeutic peptides and proteins. Therefore research efforts are focusing on the improvement of established thiomers and their evaluation for applicability to delivery of novel drug candidates.

## REFERENCES

1. Grabovac V, Guggi D, Bernkop-Schnürch A. Comparison of the mucoadhesive properties of various polymers. Adv Drug Deliv Rev 2005; 57(11): 1713–23.
2. Bernkop-Schnürch A, Kast CE, Guggi D. Permeation enhancing polymers in oral delivery of hydrophilic macromolecules: thiomer/GSH systems. J Control Release 2003; 93(2):95–103.
3. Bernkop-Schnürch A, Scholler S, Biebel RG. Development of controlled drug release systems based on thiolated polymers. J Control Rel 2000; 66:39–48.
4. Bernkop-Schnürch A, Walker G, Zarti H. Thiolation of polycarbophil enhances its inhibition of intestinal brush border membrane bound aminopeptidase N. J Pharm Sci 2001; 90(11):1907–14.
5. Werle M, Hoffer M. Glutathione and thiolated chitosan inhibit multidrug resistance P-glycoprotein activity in excised small intestine. J Control Rel 2006; 111(1–2):41–6.
6. Bernkop-Schnürch A, Schwarz V, Steininger S. Polymers with thiol groups: a new generation of mucoadhesive polymers? Pharm Res 1999; 16:876–81.
7. Longer MA, Ch'ng HS, Robinson JR. Bioadhesive polymers as platforms for oral controled drug delivery. III: Oral delivery of chlorothiazide using a bioadhesive polymer. J Pharm Sci 1985; 74:406–11.

8. Schmitz T, Bravo-Osuna I, Vauthier C, Ponchel G, Loretz B, Bernkop-Schnürch A. Development and in vitro evaluation of a thiomer-based nanoparticulate gene delivery system. Biomaterials 2007; 28(3):534–1.

9. Bernkop-Schnürch A, Weithaler A., Albrecht K, Greimel A. Thiomers: preparation and in vitro evaluation of a mucoadhesive nanoparticulate drug delivery system. Int J Pharm 2006; 317(1).

10. Leitner VM, Walker GF, Bernkop-Schnürch A. Thiolated polymers: evidence for the formation of disulphide bonds with mucus glycoproteins. Eur J Pharm Biopharm 2003; 56(2):207–14.

11. Kafedjiiski K, Föger F, Werle M, Bernkop-Schnürch A. Synthesis and in vitro evaluation of a novel chitosan-glutathione conjugate. Pharm Res 2005; 22(9): 1480–8.

12. Bernkop-Schnürch A, Thaler S. Polycarbophil-cysteine conjugates as platforms for oral (poly)peptide delivery systems. J Pharm Sci 2000; 89:901–9.

13. Clausen AE, Kast CE, Bernkop-Schnürch A. The role of glutathione in the permeation enhancing effect of thiolated polymers. Pharm Res 2002; 19:602–8.

14. Clausen AE, Bernkop-Schnürch A. In vitro evaluation of matrix tablets based on thiolated polycarbophil. Pharm Ind 2001; 63:312–7.

15. krauland AH, Bernkop-Schnürch A. Thiomers: development and in vitro evaluation of a peroral microparticulate peptide delivery system. Eur J Pharm Biopharm 2004; 57:181–7.

16. Föger F, Schmitz T, Bernkop-Schnürch A. In vivo evaluation of an oral delivery system for P-gp substrates based on thiolated chitosan. Biomaterials 2006; 27(23):4250–5.

17. Grabovac V, Bernkop-Schnürch A. Thiolated polymers as effective inhibitors of intestinal MRP2 efflux pump transporters. Sci Pharm 2006; 74(2).

18. Guggi D, Krauland AH, Bernkop-Schnürch A. Systemic peptide delivery via the stomach: in vivo evaluation of an oral dosage form for salmon calcitonin. J Control Rel 2003; 92:125–35.

19. Kast CE, Guggi D, Langoth N, Bernkop-Schnürch A. Development and in vivo evaluation of an oral delivery system for low molecular weight heparin based on thiolated polycarbophil. Pharm Res 2003; 20(6):931–6.

20. Krauland AH, Guggi D, Bernkop-Schnurch A. Thiolated chitosan microparticles: a vehicle for nasal peptide drug delivery. Int J Pharm 2006; 307(2):270–7.

21. Langoth N, Kahlbacher H, Schoffmann G, et al. Thiolated chitosans: design and in vivo evaluation of a mucoadhesive buccal Peptide drug delivery system. Pharm Res 2006; 23(3):573–9.

22. Valenta C, Kast CE, Harich I, Bernkop-Schnürch A. Development and in vitro evaluation of a mucoadhesive vaginal delivery system for progesterone. J Control Rel 2001; 77:323–32.

23. Bernkop-Schnürch A. Thiomers: a new generation of mucoadhesive polymers. Adv Drug Deliv Rev 2004; 57(11):1569–82.

24. Valenta C, Marschutz M, Egyed C, Bernkop-Schnürch A. Evaluation of the inhibition effect of thiolated poly(acrylates) on vaginal membrane bound aminopeptidase N and release of the model drug LH-RH. J Pharm Pharmacol 2002; 54(5):603–10.

25. Föger F, Kafedjiiski K, Hoyer H, Loretz B, Bernkop-Schnürch A. Enhanced transport of P-glycoprotein substrate saquinavir in presence of thiolated chitosan. J Drug Targ 2006; 15(2):132–9.
26. Hornof MD, Weyenberg W, Ludwig A, Bernkop-Schnürch A. A mucoadhesive ocular insert: development and in vivo evaluation in humans. J Control Release 2003; 89:419–28.
27. Guggi D, Langoth N, Hoffer MH, Wirth M, Bernkop-Schnürch A. Comparative evaluation of cytotoxicity of a glucosamine-TBA conjugate and chitosan-TBA conjugates. Int J Pharm 2003; 278(2):353–60.
28. Roldo M, Hornof M, Caliceti P, Bernkop-Schnürch A. Mucoadhesive thiolated chitosans as platforms for oral controlled drug delivery: synthesis and in vitro evaluation. Eur J Pharm Biopharm 2004; 57(1):115–21.
29. Langoth N, Bernkop-Schnürch A, Kurka P. In vitro evaluation of various buccal permeation enhancing systems for PACAP (pituitary adenylate cyclase-activating polypeptide). Pharm Res 2005; 22(12):2045–50.
30. Leitner VM, Marschütz MK, Bernkop-Schnürch A. Mucoadhesive and cohesive properties of poly(acrylic acid)-cysteine conjugates with regard to their molecular mass. Eur J Pharm Sci 2003; 18(1):89–96.
31. Caliceti P, Salmaso S, Walker G, Bernkop-Schnürch A. Development and in vivo evaluation of an oral insulin-PEG delivery system. Eur J Pharm Sci 2004; 22:315–23.
32. Guggi D, Kast CE, Bernkop-Schnürch A. In vivo evaluation of an oral salmon calcitonin-delivery system based on a thiolated chitosan carrier matrix. Pharm Res 2003; 20(12):1989–94.
33. Bernkop-Schnürch A, Pinter Y, Guggi D, et al. The use of thiolated polymers as carrier matrix in oral peptide delivery—proof of concept. J Control Release 2005; 106(1–2):26–33.
34. Werle M, Kafedjiiski K, Kolmar H, Bernkop-Schnürch A. Evaluation and improvement of the properties of the novel cystine-knot microprotein McoEeTI for oral administration. Int J Pharm 2007; 332(1–2):72–9.
35. Leitner VM, Guggi D, Bernkop-Schnürch A. Thiomers in noninvasive polypeptide delivery: in vitro and in vivo characterization of a polycarbophil-cysteine/glutathione gel formulation for human growth hormone. J Pharm Sci 2004; 93(7):1682–91.
36. Föger F, Malaivijtnond S, Thanakul W, Huck C, Bernkop-Schnürch A, Werle M. Effect of a thiolated polymer on oral paclitaxel absorption and tumor growth in rats. J Drug Targ (in press) 2008.
37. Mucobiomer GmbH, ThioMatrix GmbH, Austria, WO03020771. 2003.
38. Bernkop-Schnürch A. ThioMatrix GmbH, Austria, EP1126881, AU760929, CA2348842, CN1325312T.
39. Bromberg LE. Intelligent polyelectrolytes and gels in oral drug delivery. Current Pharm Biotechnol 2003; 4:339–49.
40. Reddy P, Slack JL, Davis R, et al. Functional analysis of the domain structure of tumor necrosis factor-alpha converting enzyme. J Biol Chem 2000; 275:14608–14.
41. Powell MF, Grey H, Gaeta F, Sette A, Colon S. Peptide stability in drug development: a comparison of peptide reactivity in different biological media. J Pharm Sci 1992; 81(8):731–5.

42.  Bernkop-Schnürch A, Guggi D, Pinter Y. Thiolated chitosans: development and in vitro evaluation of a mucoadhesive, permeation enhancing oral drug delivery system. J Control Release 2004; 94(1):177–86.

43.  Kafedjiiski K, Werle M, Föger F, Bernkop-Schnürch A. Synthesis and in vitro characterisation of a novel poly(acrylic acid)-glutathione conjugate. Drug Del Sci Techn 2005; 15(6):411–7.

44.  Kafedjiiski K, Krauland AH, Hoffer MH, Bernkop-Schnürch A. Synthesis and in vitro evaluation of a novel thiolated chitosan. Biomaterials 2005; 26: 819–26.

45.  Kast CE, Bernkop-Schnürch A. Thiolated polymers—thiomers: development and in vitro evaluation of chitosan-thioglycolic acid conjugates. Biomaterials 2001; 22:2345–52.

46.  Bernkop-Schnürch A, Steininger S. Synthesis and characterisation of mucoadhesive thiolated polymers. Int J Pharm 2000; 194(2):239–47.

47.  Bernkop-Schnürch A, Obermair K, Greimel A, Palmberger TF. In vitro evaluation of the potential of thiomers for the nasal administration of Leu-enkephalin. 2006; 30(4):417–23.

48.  Greindl M, Föger F, Bernkop-Schnürch A. In vivo evaluation of thiolated poly (acrylic acid) as a new drug absorption modulator for MRP2 efflux pump substrates. Pharm Res 2006; (under review).

49.  Bernkop-Schnürch A, Hornof M, Zoidl T. Thiolated polymers—thiomers: synthesis and in vitro evaluation of chitosan-2-iminothiolane conjugates. Int J Pharm 2003; 260(2):229–37.

50.  Hornof MD, Kast CE, Bernkop-Schnürch A. In vitro evaluation of the viscoelastic behavior of chitosan—thioglycolic acid conjugates. Eur J Pharm Biopharm 2003; 55(2):185–90.

# 16

# Two Concepts, One Technology: Controlled-Release Solid Dispersions Using Melt Extrusion (Meltrex®)

Jörg Breitenbach and Jon Lewis

*SOLIQS Drug Delivery Unit, Abbott GmbH & Co. KG, Ludwigshafen, Germany*

## INTRODUCTION

Improvements in the solubility, dissolution rate and absorption properties of active pharmaceutical ingredients (API) remain challenging aspects in the development of pharmaceutical products. New drug delivery technology development therefore focuses on enhancing the bioavailability of the API, overcoming solubility barriers throughout the body and on the provision of an optimum release profile for the API so as to control the duration of action in the body and to reduce side effects. These considerations are important for the development of formulations for new chemical entities and in improving the formulations of established products for the purposes of product life-cycle management.

Melt extrusion has proved to be an ingeniously simple way of combining the embedding of amorphous drug substance with a defined release profile and can modify profile kinetics from extended release to zero-order. Abbott has used melt extrusion to produce the Meltrex® technology for the purposes of producing controlled-release dispersions. Drugs with poor solubility have been shown to have higher bioavailability when formulated as solid dispersions (1). The mechanism of dissolution of molten matrices is highly dependent on the choice and combination of polymeric excipients used to produce the matrix and the effects of molecular weight of polymers on dissolution profiles has been described with respect to solid dispersions

(2,3). A further factor that can affect the release rate of an API from drug delivery technologies is the form of the API in the technology and which can be either a crystalline or amorphous form in which particles are suspended in the polymer matrix or perhaps even dissolved. In the latter case the API is an intrinsic part of the matrix thus influencing its wettability and ultimate release characteristics. The release characteristics may range from being predominantly diffusion- to erosion controlled.

## HISTORICAL DEVELOPMENT

Whereas extrusion of wet masses is a standard technology in the field of pharmaceutical production (4), melt extrusion has been mainly used in the polymer engineering sphere of practice. Melt extrusion for the manufacture of pellets (5,6) and other pioneering work (7) have revealed limitations of melt extrusion and its application to the controlled-release of polymer-embedded drugs. Meltrex represents significant progress in developing the use of melt extrusion processes for application to drug delivery technology development.

The use of solid dispersions to control release rates (8) can be of particular value when poor absorption from the lower gastrointestinal tract is a function of the poor water solubility of an API. In addition, solid dispersions can also offer benefits such as reducing gastric irritation (9) or by circumventing issues of polymorphism and differing solubilities due to the use of crystalline API, by dissolving the API in the polymer matrix. Processing advantages include the possibility of direct shaping of the dosage form without dust formation and cross contamination in addition to the possibility of the production of smaller tablets.

Solid dispersion systems for drugs have been discussed extensively with particular respect to their methods of preparation, the need to optimize the drug/carrier loads and the need to maximize dissolution and absorption rates. Examples can be found in the following cases: Suitable polymers that have been used to prepare solid dispersions include polyvinylpyrrolidone (10) or its copolymers (11), poly(ethylene-covinylacetate) (5), poly(ethylene-oxide), cellulose-ethers (12), and acrylate (13). The basic prerequisite for the use of any polymer in the Meltrex process is its thermoplasticity which may, however, be influenced by the use of plastizers and the API itself may fulfil this role. There are many possible permutations and combinations of excipients that can be used in the polymer matrix and therefore defined controlled-release profiles can be tailor-made to suit specific applications for specific APIs.

## DESCRIPTION OF MELTREX TECHNOLOGY

Meltrex technology has been developed over a number of years with the intention of combining the preparation of solid dispersions with defined controlled-release characteristics into a single solvent-free manufacturing process (14,15) which can be used to produce product with API in either an amorphous or crystalline form. The Meltrex process can be used to formulate crystalline drug substances into solid dispersions regardless of their particle size or polymorphic form.

Figure 1 depicts a schematic diagram of an extruder that is the core element of the Meltrex manufacturing process. This equipment consists of a hopper, barrels, screws, kneaders, dies, and a kneading device. Feed screws and a kneading paddle are incorporated into the two con-rotating screws in such a way that their type and arrangement can be changed according to particular requirements, e.g., the viscosity of the plastified mass or the sensitivity towards oxidation or hydrolysis of the API. The temperatures of all barrel blocks are independently controlled and can range from 30°C up to 250°C, depending on the choice of polymer matrix, the thermal stability and other physicochemical properties of the API and the desired pharmacokinetic and in vivo performance of the final product. The molten polymeric matrix acts as the solvent for the API and no additional solvents are used. Furthermore oxygen and moisture can be completely excluded from the process thereby allowing for the processing of unstable API.

The residence time of the material being manufactured in the extruder is short and is typically about 2 minutes. The extrusion process moves the molten mass continuously through the extrusion channel, thereby avoiding heat stress on both the API and the polymeric matrix.

Another core element of the Meltrex process is the ability to shape, online, the molten strand that is expelled from the extruder. The mass is forced through two calender rollers, which can then produce tablets of various shapes and sizes or as a thin film (Xellex®). Granules can also be

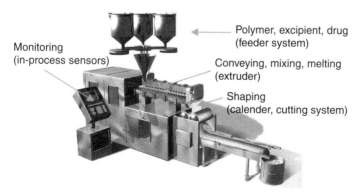

Product can be either tablet, granulate, pellet, film, or sheet

**Figure 1**  Schematic of a typical pharmaceutical extruder.

produced for subsequent milling and compressing into conventional tablets. The ultimate release profile for the API is an intrinsic property of the extrudate and this profile is retained during milling and compression should granules be required for the manufacture of a specific delivery system.

The final core element of the Meltrex process lies in the selection of an appropriate polymer and excipients to provide solid dispersions that will result in the desired release profiles in vivo. A laboratory screening system, SoliScreen®, has been developed and which can predict, with a high level of confidence, the probability of being able to produce a stable solid dispersion of an API in a particular polymer matrix. In addition the system is able to predict the likely drug load which may be achieved using the Meltrex process.

## RESEARCH AND DEVELOPMENT

A number of solid dispersion formulations have been developed and manufactured using the Meltrex process (16–19) with drug loads ranging from 30% up to 60% w/w.

Two recent developments illustrate the capability of the Meltrex process to produce solid dispersions with defined release rates for ibuprofen (19) or a combination of lopinavir and ritonavir (20,21). Abbott Laboratories reformulated their leading HIV protease-inhibitor combination product, Kaletra using the Meltrex process as part of the life-cycle management of the product. The active ingredients, lopinavir and ritonavir, in this fixed dose combination product are poorly water soluble and have poor bioavailability when administered as pure API. The original Kaletra product was manufactured as a soft-gel capsule formulation with each capsule containing 133 mg lopinavir/33 mg ritonavir and an inconvenient dosing regimen for adults of six capsules per day.

The Meltrex combination formulations were designed to match the in vitro release profiles for both API's in an attempt to ensure that bioequivalence between the tablets and capsule was possible (Fig. 2) (20,21). The Kaletra tablets, made using Meltrex technology are manufactured to a label claim of 200 mg lopinavir/50 mg ritonavir per tablet in a solid dispersion. The advantage of the higher drug load is an adult dosing regimen of only four tablets per day. Additional benefits for patients that may lead to enhanced compliance when using the new formulation include reduced food effects and that there is no need for refrigeration of the product prior to or after dispensing. Furthermore lower inter-patient variation and reduced gastrointestinal side-effects have also been reported in Phase I studies in healthy volunteers (21). The FDA granted fast-track approval of Kaletra tablets in the United States in October 2005.

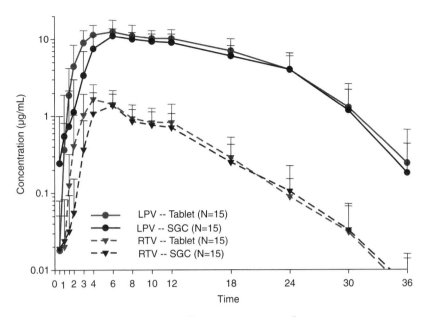

**Figure 2**   Comparison of Kaletra® tablets vs. Kaletra® soft gel capsules following single dose administration of 800 mg lopinavir/200 mg ritonavir.

Ibuprofen was formulated as a solid dispersion tablet to produce a fast onset of action (19). This was readily achieved, despite the relatively low melting point of ibuprofen and the resultant bioavailability curves are depicted in Figure 3. This product has now been approved in most of the EU countries.

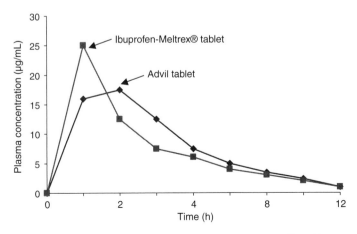

**Figure 3**   Comparison of 200 mg ibuprofen-Meltrex® tablets vs. 200 mg Advil tablets following a single oral dose ($n = 24$).

## REGULATORY ISSUES

Products manufactured using the Meltrex process have been approved by European regulatory authorities and by the U.S. FDA. The process is a mature engineering technology which lends itself to comprehensive documentation, thus satisfying the requirements of regulatory authorities. The polymers and excipients used are all pharmaceutically-acceptable materials permitting ease of use and ready modification of existing formulation to allow for more efficient dosage forms to be approved.

## REFERENCES

1. Chiou WL, Riegelman S. Pharmaceutical application of solid dispersion systems. J Pharm Sci 1971; 60:1281–302.
2. Ford J. The current status of solid dispersions. Pharma Acta Helv 1986; 61: 69–88.
3. Nogami H, Nagai T, Kondo A. Dissolution kinetics of polyvinylpyrrolidone. Chem Pharm Bull 1970; 18:1185–7.
4. Vervaet C, Baert L, Remon JP. Extrusion-spheronisation—a literature review. Int J Pharm 1995; 116:131–46.
5. Follonier N, Doelker E, Cole ET. Various ways of modulating the release of diltiazem hydrochloride from hot-melt extruded sustained release pellets prepared using polymeric materials. J Control Rel 1995; 36:243–50.
6. Follonier N, Doelker E, Cole ET. Evaluation of Hot-Melt-Extrusion as new technique for the production of polymer based pellets for sustained release capsules containing high loadings of freely soluble drugs. Drug Dev Ind Pharm 1994; 20:1323–39.
7. Adel El-Egakey M, Soliva M, Speiser P. Hot extruded dosage forms. Pharma Acta Helv 1971; 46:31–52.
8. Ozeki T, Yuasa H, kanaya Y. Application of the solid dispersion method to the controlled release medicine. IX. Difference in the release of flurbiprofen from solid dispersions with poly(ethylene oxide) and hydroxypropylcellulose and the interaction between medicine and polymers. Int J Pharm 1997; 155: 209–17.
9. Khan MA, Shojaei AH, Karnachi AA, Reddy IK. Comparative evaluation of controlled-release solid oral dosage forms prepared with solid dispersions and coprecipitates. Pharm Technol 1999; 5:58–72.
10. Tantishaiyakul V, Kaewnopparat N, Ingkatawornwong S. Properties of solid dispersions of piroxicam in polyvinylpyrrolidone. Int J Pharm 1999; 181: 143–51.
11. Zingone G, Moneghini M, Rupena P, Vojnovic D. Characterization and dissolution study of solid dispersions of theophylline and indomethacin with PVP/ VA copolymers. STP Pharma Sci 1992; 2:186–92.
12. Yano K, Kajiyama A, Hamada M, Yamamoto K. Constitution of colloidal particles formed from a solid dispersion system. Chem Pharm Bull 1997; 45: 1339–44.

13. Abd A, El-Bary A, Geneidi AS, Amin SY, El-Ainan AA. Preparation and pharmacokinetic evaluation of carbamazepine controlled release solid dispersion granules. J Drug Res Egypt 1998; 22:15–31.

14. Breitenbach J. Melt extrusion: from process to drug delivery technology. Eur J Pharm Biopharm 2002; 54:107–17.

15. Nakamichi K, Yasura H, Fukui H, et al. A process for the manufacture of nifedipine hydroxypropyl-methyl cellulose phthalate solid dispersions by means of a twin screw extruder and appraisal thereof. Yakuzaigaku 1996; 56:15–22.

16. Breitenbach J, Liepold B, Mägerlein M, et al. Modified release metoprolol tablets by melt extrusion and on-line calendering. Proc Int Symp Control Rel Bioact Mater 1999; 26:941–2.

17. Breitenbach J, Schrof W, Neumann J. Confocal Raman spectroscopy: analytical approach to solid dispersions and mapping of drugs. Pharm Res 1999; 16:1109–13.

18. Breitenbach J, Mägerlein M. Melt-extruded molecular dispersions. Pharm Extrusion Tech 2003; 133:245–60.

19. Klueglich M, Ring A, Scheuerer S, et al. Ibuprofen extrudate, a novel, rapidly dissolving ibuprofen formulation: relative bioavailability compared to ibuprofen lysinate and regular ibuprofen, and food effect on all formulations. J Clin Pharmacol 2005; 45:1055–61.

20. J. Breitenbach. Melt extrusion can bring new benefits to HIV therapy the example of Kaletra® tablets. Am J Drug Del 2006; 4(2):61–4.

21. Klein CE, Chiu YL, Awni W, et al. The tablet formulation of lopinavir/ritonavir provides similar bioavailability to the soft gelatin capsule formulation with less pharmacokinetic variability and diminished food effect. J Acquir Immune Defic Syndr 2007; 44(4):407–10.

# 17

# Threeform—Technology for Controlled Release of Amorphous Active Ingredient for Once-Daily Administration

Janez Kerč

*Lek Pharmaceuticals d.d., Sandoz Development Center Slovenia, Ljubljana, Slovenia*

## INTRODUCTION

Pharmaceutical forms containing a crystalline active ingredient have the essential disadvantage that, due to the possible presence of the crystalline active ingredient in several polymorphous modifications, the release rate of the active ingredient depends on the polymorphous modification and the crystal size, and thus on the specific surface area of the active ingredient. The dissolution rate of a crystalline substance is not constant, and it changes depending on various shapes and size distribution of the crystals of the active ingredient.

A novel three-phase pharmaceutical dosage form, Threeform—oral delivery system has been developed to provide for the controlled release of amorphous active pharmaceutical ingredients (API) and to facilitate once-daily dosing. It has been used primarily to develop once-daily dosing systems for low soluble compounds such as nifedipine. At least three polymorphic forms of nifedipine are known (1) whose solubilities are dependent to their particle size and specific surface area. In Threeform technology crystalline nifedipine is transformed into amorphous nifedipine which is released from Threeform with a constant and controlled rate of zero order and wherein the solubility and dissolution rate of the active ingredient are independent on its starting polymorphic form and crystallinity.

In addition, the new technology was applied to other API's such as venlafaxine for which controlled-release delivery is necessary over a prolonged period of time. In contrast to nifedipine, venlafaxine (in the form of hydrochloride salt) is a highly soluble drug and the challenge was to sustain the release of a high-dose drug over a prolonged time as close to first-order release as possible. Patent Number US 6,042,847 and EP 0 827 397 B1 were granted for the technology and formulation on March 28, 2000 and September 5, 2001, respectively (2).

## HISTORICAL DEVELOPMENT

The advantages of controlled-release products are well known (3) in the pharmaceutical field and include the ability to maintain a desired blood level of an API over an extended period of time. The rationale for controlled-release systems is to increase patient compliance by reducing the number of doses needed to achieve the same clinical results as multiple administrations of an immediate-release formulation of the same drug. The minimization of dosing may be achieved through a variety of methods, such as oral controlled-release formulations, transdermal formulations, and inhalation formulations. However, oral controlled-release formulations are probably the most effective and convenient administration route for a wide range of active drug substances.

A disadvantage of the currently available oral extended-release dosage forms is that the API is usually incorporated in its crystalline form, which leads to the possibility that a crystalline API can occur in several polymorphic forms. Since the release rate of an API depends on polymorphism and crystal size, the specific surface area of the API and its corresponding dissolution rate is not constant and may change depending on the shape and size distribution of the API crystals.

## DESCRIPTION OF THE TECHNOLOGY

In the Threeform oral drug delivery system the API, even if it is crystalline, is transformed into an amorphous form that is stabilized by use of a mixture of polymers that is comprised of the water-soluble polymer, polyvinyl pyrrolidone, and cellulose ethers of various viscosities. The release of the amorphous API from this three-phase pharmaceutical dosage form is controlled by diffusion through a gel layer and erosion of the matrix. The extent of diffusion and/or erosion is determined by the composition of the mixture of polyvinyl pyrrolidone, surfactant, cellulose ethers, and mono-, di-, and triglycerides used. In addition the release may be modified by use of a film coating consisting of an ester of hydroxypropyl methylcellulose with phthalic anhydride or of a copolymerizate based on methacrylic acid and ethyl acrylate, if appropriate.

The amorphous API is stabilized and dispersed in a mixture of polymers at a molecular level and therefore always has the same particle size and specific surface area resulting in a constant release rate, which is dependent only on the formulation composition that is tailored to control the release rate of amorphous API.

A schematic representation of Threeform oral delivery system is shown in Figure 1. The first phase of the three-phase pharmaceutical dosage form comprises an amorphous active ingredient (0), a surfactant (1), polyvinyl pyrrolidone (2), and a cellulose ether (3). The second phase of the system is comprised of cellulose ether (4) and/or a mixture of mono-, di-, and triglycerides (5) and other excipients common to solid dosage forms. The third phase is comprised of a single or double film coating layer. The first film coating consists of an ester of hydroxypropyl methylcellulose with phthalic anhydride or a copolymerizate based on methacrylic acid and ethyl acrylate. The second coating is a nonfunctional coating or a finish coat which may contain a dye and that is used to protect the core from light and usually consists of cellulose ethers as film formers and other additives such as plastisizers, pigments, lakes, talc among others.

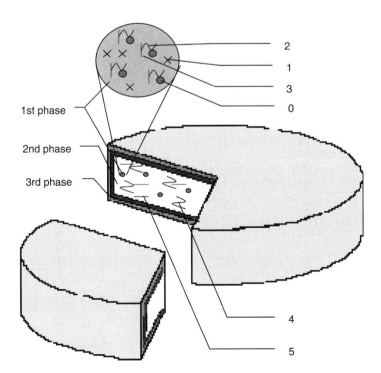

**Figure 1**   Schematic representation of the Threeform technology.

## RESEARCH AND DEVELOPMENT

The Threeform oral delivery system is especially suitable for API that occurs in an amorphous form or in one or more polymorphic forms and that exhibit poor solubility in crystal form. The active ingredient is converted into an amorphous form during the manufacturing process of the three-phase pharmaceutical dosage form. The presence of the amorphous form of the API is confirmed by use of differential scanning calorimetry (DSC) and X-ray diffraction.

In order to show the versatility of the Threeform technology two APIs of vastly different solubility, nifedipine and venlafaxine hydrochloride were used as model compounds. Nifedipine is a vasodilatory calcium antagonist that was used as a low solubility model drug. In addition, nifedipine exists in at least three polymorphic forms (1) each of which exhibit particle size and specific surface area dependent solubility. Venlafaxine hydrochloride, a potent antidepressant drug was used as a high solubility model drug.

### Manufacturing Process

The process used for the manufacture of the Threeform technology is depicted in Figure 2. Initially the first step in the preparation of the Threeform oral delivery system involves dissolving the API, a surfactant (in the case of a low solubility drug) and polyvinyl pyrrolidone in an organic solvent. The resultant solution is then sprayed onto a specific grade of cellulose ether in the fluidized bed drier. As previously mentioned,

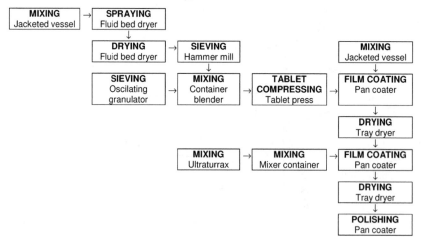

**Figure 2**   Summary of the manufacturing process of the Threeform technology.

the API can be incorporated in any form whether amorphous, crystalline, or polymorphic. During the drying process co-precipitation of the API and polyvinyl pyrrolidone occurs and the API is converted into an amorphous form that is stabilized by polyvinyl pyrrolidone and the cellulose ether.

The second step in the production process is conducted in such a manner that the granulate obtained in the first step is homogeneously mixed with a specific but different grade of cellulose ether and any other adjuvants that are commonly used in the preparation of solid pharmaceutical forms and the blends are then compressed into tablets.

The third and final step of the manufacturing process involves the preparation of the film coating solution by dissolving the polymers in an organic solvent, mixtures of organic solvents, or in mixtures with water. The polymer solution may contain plasticizers such as polyethylene glycol of various molecular weights, triacetine, triethyl citrate, dibutyl sebacate, or other appropriate material. The coating solution is sprayed onto the cores in a coating pan and if necessary a color coating may be applied to protect the tablets from light.

## In Vitro Studies

### Nifedipine

In vitro dissolution testing was conducted using USP Apparatus 2 (4) with a receptor medium of 1000 mL of 0.1 N HCl with 1% w/v sodium lauryl sulfate (0–2 hr) and/or 1000 mL phosphate buffer pH 6.8 with 1% w/v sodium lauryl sulfate (2–24 hr). The paddles were rotated at 75 rpm and the temperature was maintained at 37°C for the duration of the study. Samples were analyzed using UV spectrophotometry at 340 nm (in-house method). The release of nifedipine from the Threeform technology prepared according to the method described above yielded constant and controlled in vitro release profiles (Fig. 3) and appeared to be independent of the amount of API incorporated in the tablets (5,6).

The viscosity, degree and type of substitution of the hydroxypropyl methylcellulose (HPMC) used in the formulation had an effect on the rate and extent of nifedipine release dissolution profile (Fig. 4). Furthermore the combination of HPMC with a viscosity of 4000 cP and fillers such as Ludipress® or Emcompress® resulted in faster dissolution rates for nifedipine after 12 hours of dissolution as the HPMC matrix disintegrated (Fig. 4) (5). Consequently a much larger proportion of HPMC was necessary to form a strong hydrogel matrix with slow erosion rates in order to produce a constant release rate over the 24-hour dissolution test (Fig. 5) (5).

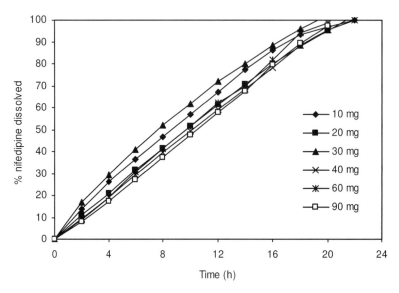

**Figure 3**  Dissolution profiles for nifedipine from tablet cores ($n=6$) representing the first and the second phase of Threeform technology manufactured using different amounts of nifedipine. (SD = 1.8–4.9 for all samples and time points).

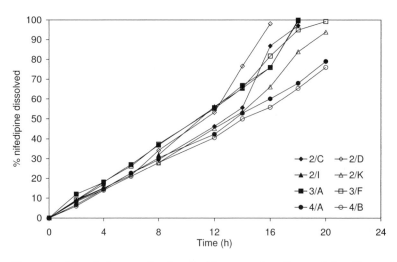

**Figure 4**  Dissolution profiles from tablet cores ($n=4$) containing 60 mg of nifedipine. 2/C: 20% HPMC E4M, 8% Ludipress®; 2/D: 20% HPMC E4M, 8% Emcompress®; 2/I: 20% HPMC K4M, 8% Ludipress®; 2/K: 24% HPMC E4M, 8% Ludipress®; 3/A: 24% HPMC K4M, 8% Ludipress®; 3/F: 20% HPMC K15M, 8% Ludipress®; 4/A:17% HPMC K100M, 8% Ludipress®; 4/B: 17% HPMC K100M, 8% Emcompress®. (SD = 1.9–4.2 for all samples up to 12 hours). *Abbreviation*: HPMC, hydroxypropyl methylcellulose.

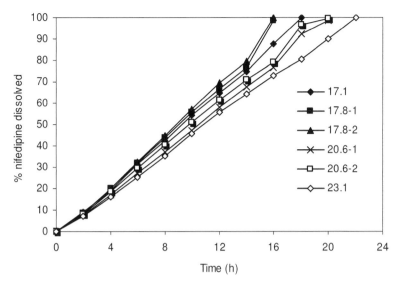

**Figure 5** Dissolution profiles from tablet cores (*n* = 4) containing 60 mg nifedipine and different amounts (% w/w) HPMC K100M (tablet hardness: 1. 7–10kP; 2. 11–13 kP). (SD = 1.5–4.6 for all samples up to 14 hours). *Abbreviation*: HPMC, hydroxypropyl methylcellulose.

Venlafaxine

In vitro dissolution testing was conducted using USP Apparatus 2 (4) with a receptor medium of 900 mL of 0.1N HCl (0–2 hr) and in 900 mL phosphate buffer pH 6.8 (2–24 hr). The paddles were rotated at 75 rpm and the temperature was maintained at 37°C for the duration of the study. Samples were analyzed using UV spectrophotometry at 273 nm (in-house method). The release of the amorphous API from the tablet core is primarily determined by the strength of the high viscosity HPMC hydrogel formed after dropping the tablet into the aqueous dissolution medium. Tablets were prepared with different proportions of Methocel® K100M and increasing the amount of this polymer in the second phase of the tablet core resulted in a decreased dissolution rate (Fig. 6) (7). Drug release from the Threeform technology was found to be reproducible and four batches of the same formula prepared either on a laboratory scale (5C, 6B, 7A) or production scale (11C) were found to produce identical dissolution profiles (Fig. 7) (5).

## In Vivo Studies (Nifedipine)

GMP batches were produced and used for in vivo studies. Fasted, fed and multiple dose (once daily dosing for 6 days) studies were performed in vivo

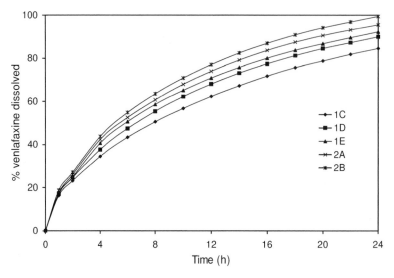

**Figure 6**   Dissolution profiles of venlafaxine hydrochloride from tablet cores ($n = 3$) containing varying amounts of HPMC K100M. 1C:150 mg; 1D: 140 mg; 1E: 130 mg; 2A: 90 mg; 2B: 70 mg. (SD = 0.4–1.2 for all samples and time points). *Abbreviation*: HPMC, hydroxypropyl methylcellulose.

using 40 (90 and 60 mg dose) and 12 (30 mg dose) healthy male volunteers. All volunteers gave informed consent to participation and the study protocol was approved by the Ethics Committee and the Committee for clinical trials at the Ministry of Health. Blood samples were withdrawn at

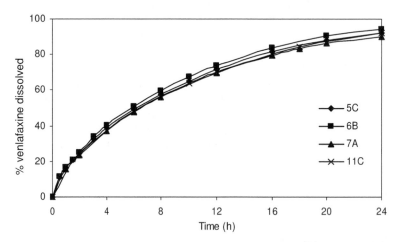

**Figure 7**   Dissolution profiles of venlafaxine hydrochloride from tablet cores ($n = 3$) with the same formula manufactured on a laboratory scale (5C, 6B, 7A) or production scale (11C). (SD = 0.2–1.3 for all samples and timepoints).

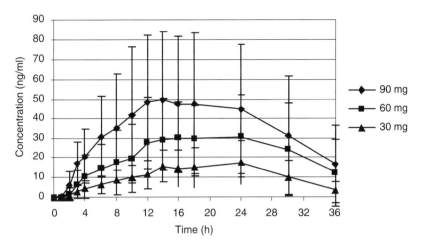

**Figure 8** Mean plasma concentrations for nifedipine following administration of 30 mg, 60 mg, and 90 mg Threeform to healthy volunteers in a fasted study.

predetermined times for up to 60 hours after administration of the nifedipine containing Threeform oral delivery system. Plasma samples were assayed using a gas chromatographic method with an electron capture detector (in-house method).

Following single dose administration of the Threeform nifedipine oral delivery system, plasma concentrations were found to be fairly constant over a 24-hour period in fasted patients and dose linearity was apparent (Fig. 8). Furthermore no peaks that are typically observed when an immediate-release nifedipine dosage form is administered are observed. In addition since nifedipine is used in chronic therapy of arterial hypertension, it is essential that therapeutic concentrations are achieved during multiple dosing and it is evident that steady-state levels are obtained (8).

## CONCLUSION

The ability to deliver a difficult-to-formulate API such as the poorly soluble compound, nifedipine with a unique delivery profile, demonstrates the extensive capability of Threeform oral delivery system. Furthermore, the Threeform oral delivery system can be applied to many other active drug substances that exist in amorphous or different polymorphic forms. In particular, the technology is applicable to compounds intended for chronic therapy because the Threeform oral delivery system is administered once daily and is capable of providing therapeutic concentrations of API over 24 hours, therefore promoting improved patient compliance.

# REFERENCES

1. Eckert T, Müller J. Über polymorphe Modifikationen des Nifedipine aus unterkühlten Schmelzen. Arch Pharm (Weinheim) 1977; 310:116–8.
2. Kerč J, Rebič LB, Kofler B. Three-phase pharmaceutical form with constant and controlled release of amorphous active ingredient for single daily application. US 6,042,847, 2000 and EP 0 827 397 B1, 2001.
3. Charman SA, Charman WN. Oral modified-release delivery systems. In: Rathbone MJ, Hadgraft J, Roberts MS, eds. Modified-Release Drug Delivery Systems. New York, Basel: Marcel Dekker, Inc. 2003: 1–10.
4. USP 30-NF 25, online edition, 2007 The United States Pharmacopeial Convention http://www.uspnf.com/uspnf/display?cmd = jsp&page = chooser
5. Kerč J, Mohar M, Kofler B. Three-phase pharmaceutical form (Threeform) for nifedipine zero order release. Proceedings of 25th International Symposium on Controlled Release of Bioactive Materials, Las Vegas, NE, June 21–26, 1998. Controlled Release Society, 1996; 912–3.
6. Kerč J, Rebič B, Kofler B, Mohar M, Urbančič J. Preparation and evaluation of three-phase pharmaceutical form (Threeform) for nifedipine once daily application. Farm Vestn 1999; 50:273–4.
7. Kerč J, Mohar M. Controlled release solid dosage form utilizing threeform technology. Transactions 31st Annual Meeting and Exposition of the Controlled Release Society, Honolulu, HI, June 12–16, 2004, Controlled Release Society, 2004; 393.
8. Kerč J, Urbančič J. Three-phase pharmaceutical form (Threeform) for nifedipine once daily administration: in vivo studies. Proceedings of 26th International Symposium on Controlled Release of Bioactive Materials, Boston, MA, June 20–25, 1999, Controlled Release Society, 1999; 879–80.

# 18

# Floating Gastroretentive Capsule for Controlled Drug Delivery

Janez Kerč and Jerneja Opara

*Lek Pharmaceuticals d.d., Sandoz Development Center Slovenia, Ljubljana, Slovenia*

## INTRODUCTION

A floating gastroretentive capsule as one component of a new therapeutic system for the peroral delivery of drugs with specific absorption sites in the upper gastrointestinal tract (GIT) has been developed. The technology has been used to produce a formulation containing the antibacterial drug, amoxicillin. However, the new technology can also be adapted for use with various active pharmaceutical ingredients (API) that require extended and controlled delivery over a period of time. Therefore a new peroral amoxicillin/clavulanaic acid therapeutic system that is composed of an immediate release tablet representing an initial dose of both APIs and a controlled release floating capsule containing additional amoxicillin was evaluated using an in vivo bioavailability study. Several pharmacokinetic (PK) parameters for amoxicillin and clavulanic acid were calculated from the plasma levels. The pharmacokinetic parameters investigated included $AUC_{0-t}$, $AUC_{0-\infty}$, $AUC_{0-t}/AUC_{0-\infty}$, $C_{max}$, $T_{max}$, $k_{el}$ and $T_{1/2}$. In addition the time over which ($T_4$ and $T_2$) the plasma concentration of amoxicillin was above the minimum inhibitory concentration (MIC) was calculated from the resultant plasma levels. Enhanced pharmacokinetic parameters of the newly developed therapeutic system containing 1500 mg of amoxicillin and 125 mg of clavulanic acid were confirmed. A prolonged time over MIC ($T_4$ and $T_2$) of amoxicillin in relation to a regular immediate release amoxicillin/clavulanate formulation was also confirmed. The floating gastroretentive capsule and the new therapeutic system are claimed in patent applications WO 2004/058230 and WO 2004/073695 (1,2).

## HISTORICAL DEVELOPMENT

Differences in the extent of drug absorption from various regions of GIT have been extensively studied and absorption was found to be rate and site dependent. A drug with a so-called absorption window in upper GIT is well absorbed in duodenum and jejunum, but absorption decreases and is rate dependent in the ileum. Furthermore a drug may show a limited or no absorption in all colonic regions (3).

Over the last three decades, various approaches have been pursued to increase the retention of peroral dosage forms in the upper GIT, particularly in the stomach (4). Such approaches have included the use of high-density (5–7), floating (8), bioadhesive (9–13), swelling and expanding (14,15), or modified-shape (16–21) systems. In addition, other strategies to delay gastric emptying have attempted to use fatty acid salts (22,23) or sham feeding of indigestible polymers (24–26) that change the motility pattern of the stomach from a fasted to a fed state, thereby decreasing the gastric emptying rates and permitting considerable prolongation of drug release in the stomach.

## DESCRIPTION OF THE TECHNOLOGY

A schematic representation of the coated capsule system that has been developed is shown in Figure 1.

A poorly soluble coating is used to enable floating of the contents of the capsule. The contents of the capsule start to hydrate and swell after the uncoated capsule cap is dissolved and water penetrates into the

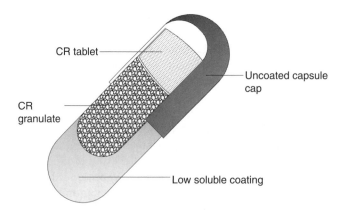

**Figure 1**   Schematic representation of the coated floating capsule technology.

controlled-release tablet and granulate in the capsule body. The function of the tablet is to fix the controlled-release granulate in the capsule body in order to retain the structure of the controlled-release granulate during production, transport, and administration. As water penetrates into the capsule, the sustained release polymer in the tablet and granulate starts to swell and a hydrogel from which the API is released by diffusion forms. The gastroretentive characteristics of the floating capsule have been shown using gamma scintigraphic studies (Lek, unpublished data).

## RESEARCH AND DEVELOPMENT

Amoxicillin is primarily absorbed from the upper small intestine and therefore it is difficult to improve the bioavailability of amoxicillin using conventional sustained release formulations such as, e.g., polymer matrices (Lek, unpublished data). Therefore innovative approaches must be considered to retain the dosage form at or above the absorption site in order to ensure optimal bioavailability is possible.

Consequently the development of a perorally administered therapeutic system that is comprised of an initial dose in immediate release (IR) form of amoxicillin/clavulanic acid and floating controlled release (CR) amoxicillin dosage form that would extend the time over MIC of amoxicillin in vivo was considered a feasible option. Such a system would provide therapeutic advantages of zero-order delivery without the limitations of administration of parenteral infusions.

The new peroral therapeutic system was developed to provide more effective therapy against organisms showing an increasing resistance to amoxicillin, specifically *Streptococcus pneumoniae*. The development of the therapeutic system took into account the characteristic GIT absorption properties of amoxicillin in which the majority of absorption takes place in the upper small intestine and with poor colonic absorption (3). Furthermore amoxicillin exhibits nonlinear absorption kinetics (27).

### Manufacturing Process

#### Amoxicillin Floating Capsule

Empty hydroxypropyl methylcellulose (HPMC) capsule bodies (Vcaps size #00) were film coated with a coating suspension that was comprised of Surelease®:Methocel® E6 in ratios of 60:40 (Sample A) or 70:30 (Sample B) in an O'Hara Labcoat 1 perforated coating pan to a dry amount of 6.5 mg/cm². A mixture of amoxicillin trihydrate, Methocel K100LV, Avicel® PH102 and magnesium stearate was blended (Mixture M) and 180 mg tablets 7.4 mm in diameter were compressed (Tablet T). Furthermore 560 mg of Mixture M was filled into each coated capsule body and Tablet T was placed on top of the mixture and the capsule was closed using an uncoated HPMC cap. Each capsule (A or B) therefore contained 603 mg amoxicillin trihydrate (equivalent to 500 mg amoxicillin). A detailed description of the manufacturing process has been previously described (1,2,28).

### Amoxicillin/Clavulanate IR Tablet

Conventional amoxicillin/clavulanic acid (Amoksiklav®625 mg) including 500 mg of amoxicillin in the form of amoxicillin trihydrate and 125 mg of clavulanic acid in the form of potassium clavulanate were taken from a regular production batch that had been produced and released for sale.

### Therapeutic Systems A and B

Two therapeutic systems, i.e., therapeutic systems A and B were developed and their bioavailability tested in vivo.

Therapeutic system A (1500 mg of amoxicillin and 125 mg of clavulanic acid) included one IR Amoksiklav 625 mg tablet and two floating capsules (Sample A) whereas therapeutic system B (1500 mg of amoxicillin and 125 mg of clavulanic acid) included one IR Amoksiklav 625 mg tablet and two floating capsules (Sample B).

## In Vitro Studies

In vitro floating tests were performed in media comprised of 0.001M HCl and phosphate buffer pH 4.5 at 37°C. The medium (400 mL) was placed into a vessel, heated and mixed (50rpm) on a 10 station magnetic stirrer to 37°C. A single floating capsule was placed on the surface of the medium whilst stirring was maintained at 50 rpm. Capsules were monitored every 0.5 hour for 5 hours for changes in formulation and/or floating characteristics of the dosage form and significant changes were recorded when observed. As expected the composition of the coating materials used to coat the capsule bodies affected the performance of each system and floating capsules coated with Sample A started to break, swell and hydrate faster that those systems manufactured as floating capsules using Sample B.

In 0.001M HCl Sample A started to hydrate within 1 hour and floated until 4 hours when the matrix sank to the bottom of the test vessel. After 5 hours the entire matrix is hydrated and is completely covered. In contrast capsules coated using Sample B hydrate after 2 hours and remained afloat for the entire 5-hour period under investigation.

The processes of floating, hydration, and erosion observed using phosphate buffer pH 4.5 are similar to that observed in 0.001M HCl but occur approximately 2 hours earlier due to better solubility of the coating material in the phosphate buffer. For example Sample A is completely covered in 3.5 hours and Sample B is partially afloat in the middle of the vessel after 5 hours, but shows significant erosion of the matrix.

The dissolution rates of amoxicillin from the floating capsule dosage form were monitored using USP Apparatus II as the dissolution test apparatus with a rotation speed of 75 rpm in 900 mL phosphate buffer pH 4.5 maintained at 37°C. Amoxicillin release during dissolution testing was monitored using ultraviolet (UV) spectrophotometry at a wavelength of 272 nm.

As expected the different composition of the capsule coating suspensions had an influence on the dissolution rate of amoxicillin from the coated capsules. Capsules from Sample A revealed a faster dissolution rate for amoxicillin than coated capsules from Sample B and the dissolution profiles are shown in Figure 2.

The results correlate favorably to the composition of the coating materials used to coat the capsules in which the higher ratio of insoluble ethyl cellulose in Sample B (ratio 70/30) than in Sample A (ratio 60/40) produces a slower release rate of amoxicillin.

The dissolution of amoxicillin and clavulanic acid from a therapeutic system [one IR Amoksiklav 625 mg tablet and two floating capsules (Samples A and B)] were monitored using USP Apparatus II at a rotation speed of 75 rpm in 900 mL phosphate buffer pH 4.5 and a temperature of 37°C. Amoxicillin and clavulanic acid levels in dissolution media were monitored by HPLC with UV detection at 272 nm.

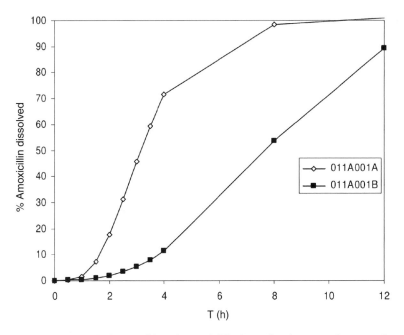

**Figure 2** Dissolution profiles of amoxicillin from floating capsules manufactured as samples A and B in phosphate buffer pH 4.5. *Source*: From Ref. 28.

As was expected, a biphasic dissolution profile was generated for amoxicillin release from either therapeutic system A or B as the amoxicillin was released immediately from the IR tablet and in a sustained manner from the floating capsule. However, a different dissolution profile for system A and B were observed as depicted in Figure 3 in which amoxicillin dissolution from therapeutic system B is slower due to lower solubility of the capsule coating due to a higher ethyl cellulose ratio in the coating suspension than for system A.

### In Vivo Studies

Twelve healthy male volunteers, aged between 18 and 45 participated in the in vivo evaluation of the therapeutic systems. All volunteers gave informed consent to participation and the study protocol was approved by the Ethics Committee and the Committee for clinical trials at the Ministry of Health. The study was conducted in a randomized, single dose, three period, three formulation, and six sequence cross-over design under fed conditions. The wash out period was one week. At the scheduled dosing times, each volunteer was given a peroral dose of an assigned formulation, with 240 mL of water,

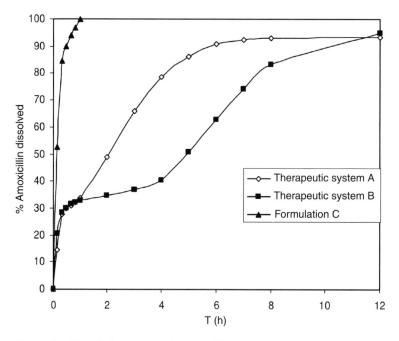

**Figure 3**  Dissolution rates of amoxicillin from therapeutic system A (1500 mg), therapeutic system B (1500 mg), and Formulation C (500 mg) in phosphate buffer pH 4.5. *Source*: From Ref. 28.

according to the randomization list. Blood samples were withdrawn at predetermined intervals up to 24 hours after drug administration (22 samples per
subject per period). Amoxicillin and clavulanic acid in plasma were analyzed
by HPLC and the resultant blood levels were used to calculate $AUC_{0-t}$,
$AUC_{0-\infty}$, $AUC_{0-t}/AUC_{0-\infty}$, $C_{max}$, $T_{max}$, $k_{el}$ and $T_{1/2}$ in addition to $T_4$ and $T_2$.

Both therapeutic systems A and B revealed prolonged absorption times
in comparison to that observed following administration with a standard
Amoksiklav 625 mg tablet (Formulation C) as shown in Figure 4A.

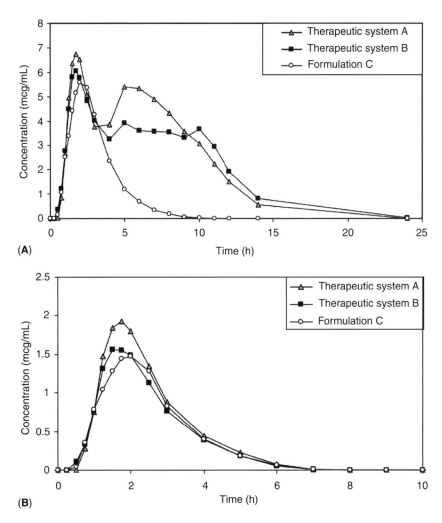

**Figure 4**   Mean plasma concentrations for amoxicillin (**A**) and clavulanic acid (**B**)
for therapeutic systems A, B, and formulation C. *Source*: From Ref. 28.

Since the dose of amoxicillin in therapeutic systems A and B is 1500 mg as compared to 500 mg in formulation C, it was expected that $AUC_{0-t}$ for amoxicillin from the test systems would be equivalent to three times the $AUC_{0-t}$ for a standard Amoksiklav tablet. The resultant ratio for therapeutic system A is 2.9 (A/C) and is 2.7 (B/C) for therapeutic system B as more amoxicillin is unabsorbed. A summary of the pharmacokinetic parameters is listed in Table 1.

The $C_{max}$ ratio and $T_{max}$ for amoxicillin, calculated for floating capsules in the therapeutic systems A and B are 0.88, 6.61 hours and 0.73, 6.52 hours, respectively. These results prove that delayed, sustained and substantial amoxicillin absorption was achieved by use of floating capsules in the systems under investigation.

Clavulanic acid was incorporated in the immediate release component of therapeutic systems A and B and also in formulation C and the resultant pharmacokinetic parameters generated following analysis of plasma samples are similar for all three formulations tested. The plasma concentration versus time curves for all three systems are depicted in Figure 4B.

The ratios of pharmacokinetic parameters for therapeutic system A and B compared to formulation C are summarized in Table 1. The results show that for therapeutic system A, the time above MIC 4 is long enough to provide a high degree of bactericidal efficacy, even with twice daily dosing. Therapeutic system A achieved higher plasma concentrations in comparison with therapeutic system B in addition to a longer time above MIC 4. The impact of the use of floating capsules in both therapeutic systems A and B is significant and the contribution of the IR component of the formulation in both therapeutic systems to the time that plasma levels remain above the MIC is 1.74 hours for MIC 4 and 3.04 hours for MIC 2. Consequently the contribution of the two floating capsules of therapeutic system A to the time that plasma levels remain above the MIC is about 4 hours for MIC 4 and about 6 hours for MIC 2. These data are summarized in Table 2.

This is more than can be expected for a 1000 mg IR dose administered as two immediate release 500 mg tablets of amoxicillin. Furthermore the bioavailability of amoxicillin is dose dependent (29) and significant non-linearity of absorption occurs above doses of 776 mg doses (30). In addition an absorption window exists in the upper small intestine for amoxicillin. The drug is well absorbed in the duodenum and jejunum, but absorption is decreased and rate dependent in the ileum. For drugs that exhibit an absorption window and have a saturable absorption mechanism, the increase in dose has a limited effect on plasma concentrations if the drug is not retained in the GIT at a site above the absorption window. The new therapeutic systems are designed in a way to increase the bioavailability of amoxicillin from delivery systems and formulations with doses in excess of 776 mg.

**Table 1** Mean Values and Ratios of Geometric Means (Arithmetic Means for $T_{max}$) of Amoxicillin and Clavulanic Acid Pharmacokinetic Parameters for Therapeutic Systems A and B and Formulation C

|  | $C_{max}$ (µg/mL) | $T_{max}$ (hr) | $AUC_{0-t}$ (µg/ mL*hr) | $AUC_{0-\infty}$ (µg/ mL*hr) |
|---|---|---|---|---|
| Amoxicillin |  |  |  |  |
| Mean A | 8.27 | 4.25 | 48.16 | 49.75 |
| Mean B | 7.08 | 2.52 | 44.52 | 46.81 |
| Mean C | 7.17 | 1.89 | 16.75 | 17.23 |
| Ratio A/B | 1.17 | 1.59 | 1.08 | 1.06 |
| Ratio A/C | 1.15 | 1.97 | 2.88 | 2.89 |
| Ratio B/C | 0.99 | 1.24 | 2.66 | 2.72 |
| Clavulanic acid |  |  |  |  |
| Mean A | 2.10 | 1.67 | 4.07 | 4.29 |
| Mean B | 1.61 | 1.85 | 3.29 | 3.53 |
| Mean C | 1.78 | 1.82 | 3.27 | 3.51 |
| Ratio A/B | 1.30 | 0.90 | 1.24 | 1.22 |
| Ratio A/C | 1.18 | 0.94 | 1.25 | 1.22 |
| Ratio B/C | 0.91 | 1.04 | 1.01 | 1.01 |

*Source*: From Ref. 28.

## CONCLUSION AND COMPETITIVE ADVANTAGE

The potential of a newly developed gastroretentive floating capsule to deliver drugs with absorption window in upper GIT has been proven. Based on the time that plasma levels remain above the MIC in a bioavailability study in humans has confirmed the enhanced efficacy of an amoxicillin/clavulanic acid therapeutic system containing 1500 mg of amoxicillin and 125 mg of clavulanic acid. Irrespective of the higher dose of amoxicillin and known nonlinear absorption kinetics above doses of 776 mg of amoxicillin, no significant loss of amoxicillin was confirmed for the new therapeutic system where the controlled release of amoxicillin is provided by use of a gastroretentive floating capsule. Furthermore the gastroretentive floating

**Table 2** Mean Time of Amoxicillin Plasma Concentrations above MIC 2 and 4 for Therapeutic Systems A and B and Formulation C

|  | A | B | C |
|---|---|---|---|
| $T_2$ (hr) (% of 12-hr dosing interval) | 9.28 (77%) | 10.64 (89%) | 3.04 (25%) |
| $T_4$ (hr) (% of 12-hr dosing interval) | 6.05 (50%) | 3.81 (32%) | 1.74 (15%) |

*Abbreviation*: MIC, minimum inhibitory concentration.
*Source*: From Ref. 28.

capsule can be adapted to deliver high or low dose APIs with an absorption window in upper GIT or that exhibit nonlinear absorption kinetics.

## REFERENCES

1. Kerč J. Modified release pharmaceutical composition. WO 2004/058230.
2. Kerč J, Opara J, Jenko Osel M. Therapeutic system comprising amoxicillin and clavulanic acid. WO 2004/073695.
3. Barr WH, Zola EM, Candler EL, et al. Differential absorption of amoxicillin from the human small and large intestine. Clinical Pharmacol Ther 1994; 56: 279–85.
4. Singh BN, Kim KH. Floating drug delivery systems: an approach to oral controlled drug delivery via gastric retention. J Control Release 2000; 63: 235–59.
5. Rednick AB, Tucker SJ. Sustained release bolus for animal husbandry. 1970, US 3,507,952.
6. Bechgaard H, Ladefoged K. Distribution of pellets in the gastrointestinal tract. The influence on transit time exerted by the density or diameter of pellets. J Pharm Pharmacol 1978; 30:690–2.
7. Davis SS, Stockwell AF, Taylor MJ, et al. The effect of density on the gastric emptying of single- and multiple-unit dosage forms. Pharm Res 1986; 3:208–13.
8. Deshpande AA, Shah NH, Rhodes CT, et al. Development of a novel controlled-release system for gastric retention. Pharm Res 1997; 14:815–9.
9. Alvisi V, Gasparetto A, Dentale A, et al. Bioavailability of a controlled release formulation of ursodeoxycholic acid in man. Drugs Exp Clin Res 1996; 22: 29–33.
10. Lenaerts VM, Gurny R. Bioadhesive Drug Delivery Systems. Boca Raton, FL: CRC Press, 1990.
11. Lehr CM, Bioadhesion technologies for the delivery of peptide and protein drugs to the gastrointestinal tract. Crit Rev Ther Drug Carrier Syst 1994; 11: 119–60.
12. Ponchel G, Irache JM. Specific and non-specific bioadhesive particulate systems for oral delivery to the gastrointestinal tract. Adv Drug Del Rev 1998; 34: 191–219.
13. Wilson CG, Washington N. The stomach: its role in oral drug delivery. In: Rubinstein MH, ed. Physiological Pharmaceutics: Biological Barriers to Drug Absorption. Chichester: Ellis Horwood, 1989: 47–70.
14. Urquhart J, Theeuwes F, Drug delivery system comprising a reservoir containing a plurality of tiny pills. 1984, US 4,434,153.
15. Mamajek RC, Moyer ES. Drug-dispensing device and method. 1980, US 4,207,890.
16. Cargill R, Caldwell LJ, Engle K, et al. Controlled gastric emptying. I. Effects of physical properties on gastric residence times of nondisintegrating geometric shapes in beagle dogs. Pharm Res 1988; 5:533–6.
17. Caldwell LJ, Gardner CR, Cargill RC. Drug delivery device which can be retained in the stomach for a controlled period of time. 1988, US 4,735,804.

18. Caldwell LJ, Gardner CR, Cargill RC, et al. Drug delivery device which can be retained in the stomach for a controlled period of time. 1988, US 4,758,436.

19. Caldwell LJ, Gardner CR, Cargill RC. Drug delivery device which can be retained in the stomach for a controlled period of time. 1988, US 4,767,627.

20. Fix JA, Cargill R, Engle K. Controlled gastric emptying. III. Gastric residence time of a nondisintegrating geometric shape in human volunteers. Pharm Res 1993; 10:1087–9.

21. Kedzierewicz F, Thouvenot P, Lemut J, et al. Evaluation of peroral silicone dosage forms in humans by gamma-scintigraphy. J Control Release 1999; 58: 195–205.

22. Gröning R, Heun G. Oral dosage forms with controlled gastrointestinal transit. Drug Dev Ind Pharm 1984; 10:527–39.

23. Gröning R, Heun G, Dosage forms with controlled gastrointestinal passage-studies on the absorption of nitrofurantoin. Int J Pharm 1989; 56:111–6.

24. Russell J, Bass P. Canine gastric emptying of polycarbophil: an indigestible, particulate substance. Gastroenterology 1985; 89:307–12.

25. Russell J, Bass P. Canine gastric emptying of fiber meals: influence of meal viscosity and antroduodenal motility. Am J Physiol 1985; 249:G662–7.

26. Leung SH, Irons BK, Robinson JR. Polyanionic hydrogel as a gastric retention system. J Biomater Sci Polym Ed 1993; 4:483–92.

27. Torres-Molina F, Peris-Ribera JE, Garcia-Carboneli MC, et al. Nonlinearities in amoxicillin pharmacokinetics. II Absorption studies in the rat. Biopharm Drug Dispos 1992; 13:39–53.

28. Kerč J, Opara J. A new amoxicillin/clavulanate therapeutic system: preparation, in vitro and pharmacokinetic evaluation. Int J Pharm 2007; 335:106–13.

29. Westphal J.F, Deslandes A, Brogard, JM, et al. Reappraisal of amoxicillin absorption kinetics. J Antimicrob Chemother 1991; 27:647–54.

30. Chulavatnatol S, Charles BG. Determination of dose-dependent absorption of amoxycillin from urinary excretion data in healthy subjects. Br J Clin Pharmacol 1994; 38:274–7.

# 19

# Thin Film Oral Dosage Forms

Scott D. Barnhart

*ARx, LLC, a Subsidiary of Adhesives Research, Inc.,
Glen Rock, Pennsylvania, U.S.A.*

## INTRODUCTION

This chapter describes a thin film oral dosage form, of which a systemically active form has been in commercial production since 2004. The primary advantage of the thin film oral dosage form is that it does not require any liquids or dose measuring device to deliver and ingest an exact dose of an active pharmaceutical ingredient (API). Thin film oral dosage forms disintegrate instantly upon contact with saliva in the oral cavity and the strength of the drug product is pre-defined by the concentration of API in the delivery system and the mass of each unit dose film. Therefore they offer a better opportunity for patient compliance for those individuals who have difficulty or even an aversion to swallowing a traditional tablet or capsule dosage form. Representative groups falling into this category are pediatric and geriatric patient populations. This chapter will discuss the virtues and advantages that make thin films the most portable and convenient oral dosage form of any available today.

## HISTORY

The thin film oral dosage forms have evolved from a need in the marketplace for a fast-dissolving delivery system that would help specific patient populations, such as the geriatric and pediatric groups, who have difficulty in swallowing large solid oral dosage forms such as tablets and/or capsules (1). Fast-dissolving solid tablets were first developed in the late 1970s (2) and have evolved into oral thin film products that were first available as breath strips in the confectionary market in 2001.

In recent years, oral thin films have expanded into the personal care, food, and drug delivery markets. Pharmaceutical companies and consumers have embraced the thin film oral dosage format as a practical option to traditional over-the-counter (OTC) medicines in liquid, tablet, and capsule formats because of the various benefits of using such films. The thin film oral dosage form offers fast, accurate dosing in a safe, efficacious format that is convenient and portable, without requiring the use of water or a spoon. The ease of use and potential for targeted delivery when using thin films also increases the potential for patient compliance specifically in the aforementioned patient population groups.

## FORMULATION

Since the primary use of all thin film oral dosage forms relies on their disintegration in the saliva of the oral cavity, the final film that is used must necessarily be water soluble. In order to prepare a thin film formulation that is water soluble, any of a number of water-soluble excipients or ingredients may be used of which at least one must be a polymer with excellent film-forming properties. It is impractical to take a traditional tablet composition, dissolve the ingredients in a suitable solvent, and cast the resultant liquid into a thin film. The resultant dried layer of such a composition would be a fragile, brittle crystalline solid that would fracture readily into a powder on handling. Representative water-soluble polymers that may be used include the natural gums such as those derived from guar, xanthan, acacia, arabic or tragacanth, polyethylene oxide, derivatives of cellulose, polyvinyl pyrrolidone, polyvinyl alcohol, and acrylic-based polymers. The physicochemical characteristics of the polymer or polymers selected for film formation play a vital role in determining the resultant disintegration time of the cast thin film oral dosage form. A list of examples of how polymer selection and blends thereof can impact disintegration times of resultant thin films is shown in Table 1.

The selection of different film-forming polymers permits the selective production of a thin film oral dosage form that may disintegrate very rapidly for immediate release applications, or that may disintegrate slowly for controlled-release applications. In addition excipients such as flavors and texture enhancers may be included to improve the aesthetic appeal of the formulation.

The use of taste-masking excipients is an important consideration for thin film oral dosage forms. Traditional methods of taste-masking that are applied to other oral dosage forms such as in syrups and soft-chew dosage forms are also appropriate for thin film oral dosage forms. Taste-masking methods that have been successfully used include traditional flavor and

**Table 1**  Effect of Polymer Selection on Disintegration Time

| Formula | Film composition | | | | Disintegration time (sec) $(n = 4)$ |
| | Low MW cellulose | Low MW water-soluble polymer | High MW cellulose A | High MW cellulose B | |
| --- | --- | --- | --- | --- | --- |
| Example A | 1 | — | — | — | 18 |
| Example B | 1 | 0.9 | — | — | 8 |
| Example C | 1 | 1 | — | — | 5 |
| Example D | — | — | 1 | 1 | 24 |

*Abbreviation*: MW, molecular weight.

sweetener combinations, encapsulation or particle coating or complexation with ion exchange resins (3). In the case of taste-masking techniques that result in discrete particles, particle size is a critical parameter for the manufacturing process and is dependent upon the coating method selected. Generally, particles larger than 250 μm may present problems for many coating techniques as they can accumulate in the fluid flow path and this may cause scratches on the surface of thin coating layers.

   Liquid formulations prepared for thin film casting can be in the form of solutions, emulsions, dispersions or suspensions. Dispersions or emulsions for casting may be prepared as oil-in-water phases and emulsions are typically used for the manufacture of aqueous formulations to which an oil-soluble ingredient, such as a flavor may be added. Thin film oral dosage form solutions for casting will require the use of ICH Class 3 solvents in order to benefit from an acceptable industry safety profile. The drying process is a critical operation and the drying process must assure that the Class 3 solvent is removed to acceptable levels provided for by the draft guideline (4).

## MANUFACTURING PROCESS

### Preparation of Liquid Formulation

As previously discussed, liquid formulations prepared for thin film casting can be in the form of solutions, emulsions, dispersions or suspensions and there are well established and standard mixing techniques that are used in the industry for the preparation of these pharmaceutical liquids. However, it is important to note that higher viscosities will be encountered when working with water-soluble film-forming polymers in a formulation.

Consequently, mixing processes must be designed to handle fluid rheologies in the range of 1,000–50,000 cps.

## Preparation of Cast Thin Film

Thin film oral dosage forms may be produced by liquid casting or completely by solid extrusion. The film is produced as a wide web form and wound upon itself to yield what is commonly referred to in the industry as rollstock. The thin film that is cast is relatively wide (30–120 cm) and rolled upon itself for storage prior to subsequent processing. Some manufacturers claim to use a single belt to support the film during manufacture, while other manufacturers rely upon an in-process aid such as a release-coated substrate that may be easily removed from the film. The release-coated substrate is typically disposed of following removal of the thin film prior to unit-dose packaging.

The 100% solids extrusion manufacturing process offers advantages in terms of throughput efficiency and decreased operating cost as compared to liquid cast film lines. A typical medium-sized extrusion process can produce between 550 and 700 kg of film per hour depending upon the diameter of the extrusion screw and barrel length. Extruders may also operate with a much smaller footprint than cast film lines of equal width. Extruders do not use the large-sized dryers that are required to remove the solvents or in-process vehicle that are required when preparing liquid cast films. Extruders also consume less energy than equivalent width liquid cast film lines simply because there is no drying process for 100% solid formulations for extrusion and therefore, no heated ovens are required to maintain the elevated temperatures necessary for removal of solvents that are used in the liquid film casting process. However, the extrusion process may result in exposure of the API to localized, short-term elevated temperatures during which time the drug may degrade. For this reason, most, if not all, processing of commercial thin film oral dosage forms are produced by liquid casting techniques.

Liquid casting techniques for pharmaceutical coatings such as transdermal matrices are well established. The selection of a specific liquid casting technique is based on fluid rheology, the desired mass to be applied, and the required dose uniformity. The various techniques offered by coating equipment suppliers may prove suitable for liquid casting manufacture of thin film oral dosage forms. These techniques include knife-over-roll, reverse roll, slot-die, gravure cylinder, and meyer rod coating. Typical medium-sized liquid casting processes can produce about 15 kg of film per hour depending on the coating width and casting line speed used.

An advantage of liquid casting techniques appears to be the low variability exhibited throughout a manufacturing campaign. A typical relative standard deviation following content uniformity testing of a single thin film lot is in the order of 1–2%. Therefore, the liquid casting technique lends itself to the manufacture of this type of oral dosage form in particular for highly potent compounds and APIs with a narrow therapeutic index.

Synthroid, a compound that is potent and has a narrow therapeutic range, requires the experimental titration of each patient in order to determine the correct strength for chronic ongoing drug therapy. Synthroid is a good example of how low manufacturing process variability would be of benefit when producing a range of strengths, particularly since marketed strengths of synthroid (e.g., 75,88,100,112 µg) may have allowable overlap for the potency specification range.

## Unit Dose Packaging

The final manufacturing process for producing thin film oral dosage forms is unitizing and primary packaging for each dose. The bulk film rollstock is die-cut to the desired size and shape. The flexibility of this manufacturing technique allows for multiple strengths of a given bulk film formulation to be manufactured, simply by changing the area of the die that is used to cut the rollstock. In-process aids such as a release-coated substrate if used during film manufacture are removed prior to packaging.

Unit dose packaging of thin film oral dosage forms is preferred over multi-dose packaging techniques that are used for thin film confectionary products and breath strips. The use of unit dose packaging is one of risk minimization so as to avoid the potential of more than one thin film sticking to another that may result in accidental overdosing. Many manufacturers are able to supply flexible packaging materials suitable for providing a primary package for these delivery systems. It is critical to use packaging films that provide a moisture barrier to avoid the ingress of residual moisture into the packaged thin film oral dosage form, while maintaining the stability of the drug product to its expiration date. Typical flexible film constructions include the use of aluminum foil or Aclar® film as an important component of the complete laminate.

## TESTING

Standard HPLC testing for potency and content uniformity apply to thin film oral dosage forms. Analytical methods are similar to those used for other solid oral dosage forms, taking into account the potential interference of the film-forming polymers during methods development. Additional tests that may be selected to characterize thin film oral dosage forms are film strength, disintegration, and dissolution.

Film strength may be performed using an Instron in extension mode or by use of a texture analyzer in compression mode. Film strength is effectively a tensile test to failure, which is a measurement of the force required to cause the film to break (5–7).

Disintegration and dissolution are required USP tests (8) using the USP disintegration apparatus (9) and USP dissolution apparatus (10), respectively. Disintegration times will vary depending on the formulation (Table 1), but typical disintegration times will range from about 5 to 30 seconds. The conduction of a USP dissolution test can be difficult due to the tendency of thin film oral dosage forms to float in the dissolution media when tested using USP Apparatus 2. Instantly disintegrating, immediate release thin film oral dosage forms tend to dissolve immediately and diffuse through the mesh of the basket of USP Apparatus 1, releasing the formulation components into the dissolution media (10). At this stage in the testing, complete dissolution of the API is controlled by the solubility in the dissolution media and by the amount of time until complete API dissolution.

Sensory analysis to determine the success of masking a bitter API or off notes of a formulation have been conducted through qualified human panels or more recently through in vitro testing using electronic techniques (11–13).

## CLINICAL STUDIES

Local oral mucosal irritation studies may be performed in animals and humans, particularly if novel excipients are used to produce thin film oral dosage forms. The hamster cheek pouch model has proven to be a reasonably useful method of predicting safety in animals prior to human oral mucosal irritation studies.

Bioavailability studies for an erectile dysfunction medication have found that thin film oral dosage forms have superior bioavailability when compared to conventional oral tablet dosage forms. Clinical endpoints also determined the bioavailability of an anti-ulcer oral thin film to be equivalent to that of commercially marketed lyophilized orally disintegrating tablets (ODT) and patient compliance was found to be improved for the thin film oral dosage form compared to the ODT (14).

Table 2 summarizes the commercially available thin film oral dosage forms marketed by the end of 2007. The majority of the products listed in Table 2 are systemically active; however, a few products, such as Chloraseptic™, Orajel®, and Suppress®, are topical analgesics or demulcents that do not produce systemic drug blood levels. Additionally, the polydimethylsiloxane (simethicone) API listed for the Gas-X® product is not systemically absorbed.

## CONCLUSIONS

The drug content as a proportion of the total weight of the formulation, surface area, and thickness determine the strength of the thin film oral

**Table 2** Commercial Thin Film Oral Dosage Form Products at the End of 2007

| Product | Distributor | API | Strength (mg) |
|---------|-------------|-----|---------------|
| Triaminic® | Novartis | Dextromethorphan HBr | 7.5 |
| Triaminic | Novartis | Diphenhydramine HCl | 12.5 |
| Theraflu® | Novartis | Dextromethorphan HBr | 15 |
| Theraflu | Novartis | Diphenhydramine HCl | 25 |
| Triaminic | Novartis | Phenylephrine HCl | 2.5 |
| Triaminic | Novartis | Phenylephrine HCl/ Diphenhydramine HCl | 5/12.5 |
| Triaminic | Novartis | Phenylephrine HCl/ Dextromethorphan HBr | 2.5/5 |
| Gas-X | Novartis | Simethicone | 62.5 |
| Sudafed® | Pfizer | Phenylephrine HCl | 10 |
| Benadryl® | Pfizer | Diphenhydramine HCl | 12.5 |
| Benadryl | Pfizer | Diphenhydramine HCl | 25 |
| Chloraseptic® | Prestige | Benzocaine/Menthol | 3/3 |
| Chloraseptic | Prestige | Vitamin C/Zinc citrate | N/A |
| Suppress® | InnoZen | Menthol | 2.5 |
| Orajel® | Del | Menthol/Pectin | 2/30 |
| Theraflu | Novartis | Phenylephrine HCl/ Diphenhydramine HCl | 10/25 |
| Theraflu | Novartis | Phenylephrine HCl/ Dextromethorphan HBr | 10/20 |

*Abbreviation*: API, active pharmaceutical ingredient.

dosage form. Limitations on surface area are determined by the maximum area that will conveniently fit into the oral cavity. There are compromises that must be made between film thickness and disintegration rates as these properties are indirectly proportional to each other and if the thickness of a thin film oral dosage form is increased the time for complete disintegration of the dosage form will be increased proportionally.

The mass of immediate-release thin film oral dosage forms is in the range of 50–200 mg whereas the mass of a conventional tablet that has been formulated to be rapidly disintegrating will typically be in the region of 200–750 mg. In addition conventional tablet dosage forms are also friable and lyophilized orally disintegrating tablets are very easily fractured. Consequently care must be taken when transporting, dispensing, and handling these dosage forms. An advantage of thin film oral dosage forms is that they are flexible and are nonfriable and handling these dosage forms is similar to carrying a small piece of paper or plastic film. A patient may carry the packaged thin film unit dose in a flexible pouch, inside their pocket, wallet, or purse without damaging the integrity of the dosage form by crushing it.

Clearly the flexible packaging format, in combination with oral thin film unit doses, is appropriate for discreet transport and dispensing of these systems.

Thin film unit dose systems are particularly useful for improving patient compliance in situations such as when treating prisoners, mentally ill individuals, children, or even in veterinary applications.

Therapeutic areas that would benefit from the convenience, portability, and discreetness of thin film oral dosage forms include the treatment of analgesia (e.g., migraine), emesis (e.g., travel), sexual dysfunction, CNS disorders (e.g., anxiety-related disorders), and smoking cessation. Some of these therapeutic categories are currently being treated with orally disintegrating tablets; however, this fact should not preclude other companies from entering a certain therapeutic area using thin film oral dosage form technology. Thin film oral dosage forms provide a platform for extending patent protection of a branded API. Furthermore, patients will continue to look towards more convenient delivery systems for medication in the future and the thin film oral dosage form is a viable alternative to other oral dosage forms intended for human use.

## REFERENCES

1.  Doheny K. You really expect me to swallow these horse pills? Amer Drug 1993; 208:34–5.
2.  Virley P, Yarwood R. Zydis. A novel, fast-dissolving dosage form. Manuf Chemist 1990; 61:36–7.
3.  Ettner N, Grave A. Taste masking: reducing the bitterness of drugs. Pharm Formulation Qual 2006; 8(5):24–7.
4.  Federal Register 1997; 62(85):24301–9.
5.  ASTM D882–83 Standard Test Method for Tensile Properties of Thin Plastic Sheeting, 1983: 454–65.
6.  ASTM D638–84 Standard Test Method for Tensile Properties of Plastics, 1984: 210–24.
7.  ASTM D774/774M-97 Standard Test Method for Bursting Strength of Paper, 1997.
8.  USP 29/NF 24, General Chapter < 1088> In Vitro and In Vivo Evaluation of Dosage Forms, 2006.
9.  USP 29/NF 24, General Chapter <701> Disintegration, 2006.
10. USP 29/NF 24, General Chapter <711> Dissolution, 2006.
11. Takagi S, Toko K, Wada K, et al. Detection of suppression of bitterness by sweet substance using multichannel taste sensor. J Pharm Sci 1998; 87:552–5.
12. Miyanaga Y, Tanigake A, Nakamura T, et al. Prediction of the bitterness of single, binary- and multiple component amino acid solutions using a taste sensor. Int J Pharm 2002; 248:207–18.
13. Keast R, Breslin P. Modifying the bitterness of selected oral pharmaceuticals with cation and anion series of salts. Pharm Res 2002; 19:1019–26.
14. Borsadia S, O'Halloran D, Osborne J. Quick-dissolving films—a novel approach to drug delivery. Drug Deliv Technol 2003; 3(3):46–9.

# 20

# Dose Sipping Technology—A Novel Dosage Form for the Administration of Drugs

Iris M. Ziegler

*Pharmaceutical Development, New Therapeutic Entities, Grünenthal GmbH, Aachen, Germany*

## INTRODUCTION: THE UNMET MEDICAL NEED IN PEDIATRIC THERAPY

Despite the fact that novel delivery systems, such as transdermal therapeutic patches, or formulations for inhalation have been developed that provide specific advantages for patient therapy, the oral route of administration is still the most preffered route of treatment by patients.

However, in cases where large amounts of active pharmaceutical ingredient (API) need to be administered the resultant tablets or capsules tend to become rather bulky dosage forms, which are difficult to swallow for many patients. Antibiotics and analgesics are examples of therapeutic classes of drugs that are frequently administered in high doses of up to several hundred of milligrams of API per dose. In particular small children and elderly people have difficulty in swallowing big dose units, thereby necessitating the use of alternate dosage forms to ensure safe, effective, and compliant administration of the API to such patients.

Antibiotic therapy for pediatric patients usually takes the form of powders or granules for reconstitution and use as either solutions or suspensions. In addition other drugs in multiple dose containers are also presented in this way. There are a few antibiotics that are also available as single dose units in the form of dispersible tablets or sachets containing either powder or granules for oral suspension. The aforementioned dosage forms need to be redispersed in water or other suitable solvent prior to administration, but allow for the ingestion of the medication as an easy to swallow solution or suspension. Dosing from multiple dose containers requires the use of measuring spoons, cups and/or syringes to administer the prescribed amount of a flavored syrup or liquid per dose. The contents of sachets are usually redispersed in a glass of water, sprinkled on food or viscous liquids, and in some cases ingested directly from the sachet without redispersion. The powders or granules available for oral suspension, whether presented as a multiple dose container (bottle), a single dose sachet, or tablets for oral suspension pose several problems that may potentially impact on the safe and effective use of the API in addition to inconveniencing the patient with the possible result of noncompliance. Specifically the aforementioned issues relate to poor dosing accuracy for suspensions from multiple dose containers (1), the bitter taste of most antibiotics and different taste perception of children (2), the need for preservatives for most aqueous suspensions in multiple dose containers (3), and/ or poor in-use stability of some API's in aqueous media requiring overages to ensure a suitable shelf life can be assigned to the product (4).

## THE OPPORTUNITY: GRANULES FOR SUSPENSION IN A DRINKING STRAW

A proprietary drinking straw system (5) presents an alternative to currently existing dosage forms. The SIP® system or dose sipping technology (DST®) is a delivery technology that presents a novel approach for the administration of well-known dosage forms to patients, such as granules for suspension.

Granules for suspension retained in a drinking straw are an easy to administer system, as it allows for the administration of medication through a straw and the technology can be handled without any difficulties by most children over the age of two years. In addition this technology can be effectively used by elderly patients. Each drinking straw contains a single dose of small, coated granules containing the prescribed amount of API in a suitably taste masked formulation. Each drinking straw system is individually packaged and only removed for use prior to administration. On administration the coated granules form a suspension for oral administration in situ, while the patient drinks a beverage using the SIP® system as they would an everyday drinking straw. In this way, there is no need to redisperse the powder or granules prior to administration.

The taste masking of granules ensures that the aesthetic appeal of the medication is determined solely by the beverage selected as the carrier vehicle as no additional sugar, flavors, sweeteners, or other excipients are added to modify the taste. Beverages that are considered suitable are clear liquids served at room temperature, e.g., mineral water, apple juice, Coca-Cola®, lemonades, tea, or homogenized milk. Flavored, carbonated beverages, or fruit juices are preferred due to their favorable palatability and acceptability to children. The acidic pH values (between pH 3 and 5.5) of these beverages further assists taste masking particularly when using enteric polymers that are insoluble at lower pH-values and dissolve at higher pH values. Viscous liquids, beverages containing solids or hot beverages ($>40°C$) are not recommended for use with this delivery system.

Granules of approximately 500 μm in diameter are preferred for use in DST so as to reduce the sensation of grittiness associated with the use of bigger diameter particles. Furthermore, the chances of biting into or onto these tiny granules are reduced assisting the concept of taste masking on ingestion. Due to the small size of the spherical or close to spherical pellets dispersion in the liquid of choice occurs readily on sipping, thereby facilitating the movement of the particles towards the upper end of the straw. Most of the dose will thus be swallowed together with the liquid on the first sip with few or no pellets remaining in the mouth. The few granules, which may remain in the mouth over the course of sipping, will not affect the dose administered or reduce the compliance when using the system, since continued ingestion of the beverage of choice will ensure that the complete dose will ultimately be administered. The standard recommendation for the correct use of the DST system suggests that an adequate amount of liquid (e.g., 50–150 mL) is drunk either using the straw or directly from the glass following ingestion of the entire contents of the straw.

The drinking straw system can be prefilled with various small solid oral dosage forms such as crystals, granules, pellets or micro-tablets thereby revealing the flexibility of the technology. In order to ensure the correct functionality of the system and easy dispersion of the granules the total amount of granules per straw should not significantly exceed 1 g.

The rate of dissolution of the API is independent of the DST system and is determined solely by the characteristics of the multi-particulate dosage forms that are placed into the drinking straw system. The resultant dissolution profiles are also, in part, dependent on API characteristics such as solubility, wetting behavior, stability and may be designed to be rapid and immediate release or delayed and all types of prolonged release or even suitable to produce colon targeted systems. Complex and specific dissolution profiles can be easily generated by filling different types of granules into the DST technology. Furthermore, different APIs in different particulate technologies can be combined in the SIP system for co-administration in a single delivery technology.

## THE IMPROVEMENT: CLAROSIP® AND RICLASIP®

ClaroSip or Neo-ClaroSip®granules for oral suspension contain 125, 187.5, or 250 mg of clarithromycin as completely taste masked micro pellets that are filled into the SIP® system such that a single dose can be administered.

The available dose strengths provide correct dosing for children in the 2–4 year/12–19 kg (125 mg twice daily), the 4–8 year/20–29 kg (187.5 mg twice daily) and the 8–2 year/30–40 kg (250 mg twice daily) age and body weight ranges respectively.

RiclaSip is available as a combination of 7:1 amoxicillin/clavulanic acid enabling the delivery of doses of 200/28.5 mg, 300/42.75 mg and 400/57 mg for treatment of children in the 2–4 year/12–16 kg (200/28.5 mg twice daily), the 4–7 years/17–24 kg (300/42.75 mg twice daily), the 7–10 years/25–32 kg (400/57 mg twice daily) and of 10–12 year/33–37 kg (2 straws of 300/42.75 mg twice daily) age and body weight ranges respectively. Higher per kg amoxicillin doses for patients requiring doses of 43–67 mg/kg as required for acute otitis media require the use of 2 straws of RiclaSip.

Whereas ClaroSip/Neo-ClaroSip contain only one type of granule the RiclaSip is manufactured by filling two types of granule, viz., taste masked amoxicillin and clavulanic acid granules. Due to the small dose and rather indifferent taste of clavulanic acid, no additional taste masking beyond the formation of granules is required for this API. Both types of granule can be combined in different ratios (e.g., 4:1, 7:1, 8:1) and are filled at different dose strengths for each ratio, by adjusting the fill weights of each, separately. Therefore as both API are subjected to separate filling correct dosing of each can be assured despite the substantial difference in dose of API and corresponding pellet weights. Separate filling is necessary since attempts to blend both sizes of granule would result in segregation and subsequent issues in dose uniformity in each straw.

The correct use of the SIP system is depicted by means of a pictogram on the aluminium sachet in which the straw is packaged (Fig. 1). Furthermore the correct use of the technology is described in the product information leaflet (SPC) as described below:

- Open the sachet holding it in an upright position, so that the instructions of the pictogram can be followed.
- Remove the drinking straw system from the sachet in an upright position.
- Remove the cap and hold the straw upright to prevent the contents from falling out.
- Place the drinking straw with its lower end into the preferred beverage, which should be a nonviscous, clear beverage at room temperature, not containing solid particles.
- The total contents of the straw should be sipped at the same time. Biting on granules should be avoided, as this might reduce their taste masking properties. Sipping the dose in several sips may be easier for smaller children, yet most children manage intake of the complete dose in one sip without problems. When pausing, the straw should not be taken out of the beverage.

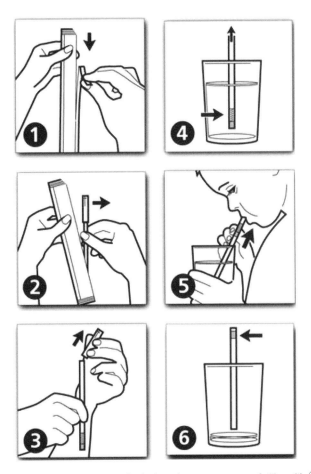

**Figure 1**  Pictogram depicting the correct use of ClaroSip®.

- The completion of the intake of the dose is visualized by the controller, which has moved up together with the granules to the top end. The child should carry on drinking the remaining contents of the glass either using the straw or directly from the glass.
- Thereafter, the empty system should be discarded safely out of the reach of children.

## Dissolution and Bioequivalence

ClaroSip

Clarithormycin delivered using the ClaroSip technology has a similar, pH-dependent in vitro dissolution profile as the innovator granules for oral suspension (Fig. 2). Consequently there is a high possibility that the two products would have similar in vivo behavior during GI-transit in which drug dissolution occurs mainly in the upper part of the small intestine.

The comparative bioavailability or bioequivalence of ClaroSip 250 mg granules for oral suspension in a drinking straw was compared to that of Klacid® 125 mg/5 mL Suspensie (Abbott, Netherlands) in a single centre study with a single-dose, two-treatment, two-period cross over design in 36 healthy male subjects aged between 18 and 45 years, with a 6-day wash-out period between doses. The resultant data are summarized in Table 1. Bioequivalence was demonstrated according to the defined criteria in the CPMP Note for Guidance (6) and as demonstrated in Table 2.

RiclaSip

The innovator amoxicillin/clavulanic acid powder for oral suspension ensures rapid dissolution of the water soluble potassium clavulanate while only some of the poorly soluble amoxicillin trihydrate will have dissolved at the time of administration of the suspension. Due to the rapid dissolution requirements of both actives the taste masked amoxicillin granules and clavulanic acid granules should also demonstrate almost equally rapid dissolution profiles in vitro which as can be seen in Figure 3 is the case. Both types of pellets in the RiclaSip technology fulfil the requirements for rapidly

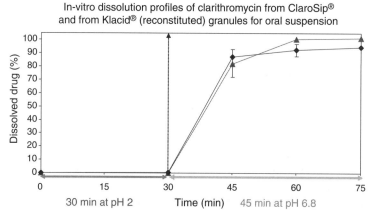

**Figure 2**   Dissolution of clarithromycin from ClaroSip® 250 mg granules for oral suspension in a drinking straw and 10 mL of reconstituted Klacid® 25 mg/ml granules for oral suspension in a biphasic dissolution test using USP Apparatus II with 300 mL of simulated gastric fluid, pH 2 and 1000 ml of simulated intestinal fluid, pH 6.8 at 37°C ($n = 6$).

**Table 1** Pharmacokinetic Parameters Clarithromycin after a Single Oral Dose of 250 mg

| Formulation | Arithmetic mean $C_{max}$ ($\mu$g/L) | Arithmetic mean $AUC_{0-\infty}$ ($\mu$g$\cdot$hr/L) | Median $T_{max}$ (hr) |
|---|---|---|---|
| ClaroSip® 250 mg Granules for oral suspension in a drinking straw | 783.26 | 5574.71 | 3.0 |
| Klacid® 25 mg/ml suspension Granules for oral suspension (10 mL suspension) | 837.94 | 5198.35 | 3.0 |

dissolving products with more than 85% of each API being released within 30 minutes as outlined in the biopharmaceutical classification guidance (7).

The bioequivalence of RiclaSip 400/57 mg granules for oral suspension in a drinking straw (2 × 400/57 mg) was compared to Augmentin® Duo 400/57 (Glaxo SmithKline, U.K.) powder for oral suspension (10 mL containing 800/114 mg) in a single centre study in an open, single-dose, two-treatment, two-period, two sequences cross over design in 48 healthy male subjects aged between 18 and 45 years, with a 7-day wash-out period between doses. The resultant data are summarized in Table 3. RiclaSip 400/57 mg granules for oral suspension in a drinking straw was shown to be bioequivalent for the pharmacokinetic parameters $AUC_{0-\infty}$ and $AUC_{0-t}$ for amoxicillin and for clavulanic acid according to the criteria defined in the current CPMP Note for Guidance (6).

Bioequivalence criteria for $C_{max}$ were fully met for amoxicillin but were at the lower limit for the 90% confidence interval for clavulanic acid (Table 4). The reference product Augmentin powder for oral suspension contains an overage of up to 15% of clavulanic acid (4) to ensure sufficient potency of clavulanic acid at the end of its in-use period, while RiclaSip 400/57 mg granules for oral suspension in a drinking straw contains no such overage.

**Table 2** Ratios and 90% CI of ClaroSip® 250 Granules for Oral Suspension/Klacid® 25 mg/ml Suspension Granules for Oral Suspension (10 mL Suspension) for Selected Pharmacokinetic Parameters of Clarithromycin[a]

| Clarithromycin | Point estimate $T/R$ ratio | 90% CI |
|---|---|---|
| $C_{max}$ (mg/L) | 0.92 | 0.87–0.99 |
| AUC (mg$\cdot$hr/L) | 1.08 | 1.01–1.15 |

[a]Clarithromycin in a crossover study.
*Abbreviation*: CI, confidence interval.

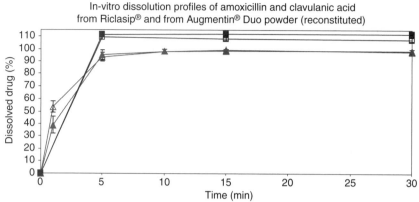

**Figure 3** Dissolution of amoxicillin and clavulanic acid from RiclaSip® 400/57 mg granules for oral suspension in a drinking straw and from 5 mL of reconstituted Augmentin Duo 400/57 mg powder for oral suspension using USP Apparatus II in 900 ml of simulated intestinal fluid pH 6.8 agitated at 75 rpm and maintained at 37°C ($n = 6$).

**Table 3** Pharmacokinetic Parameters of Amoxicillin/Clavulanic Acid 7:1 Granules for Oral Suspension after Oral Dose of 800 mg Amoxicillin and 114 mg Clavulanic Acid

| Formulation | Geometric mean $C_{max}$ (µg/L) | Geometric mean $AUC_{0-\infty}$ (µg·hr/L) | Median $T_{max}$ (hr) |
|---|---|---|---|
| Amoxicillin | 13.04 | 33.83 | 1.25 |
| 2 × RiclaSip® 400/57 mg granules for oral suspension in a drinking straw | | | |
| 10 mL of Augmentin® Duo 400/ 57 mg powder for oral suspension | 13.59 | 34.86 | 1.00 |
| Clavulanic acid | 2.32 | 5.11 | 1.00 |
| 2 × RiclaSip® 400/57 mg granules for oral suspension in a drinking straw | | | |
| 10 mL of Augmentin® Duo 400/ 57 mg powder for oral suspension | 2.73 | 5.83 | 0.75 |

**Table 4**  Ratios and 90% CI (Parametric Approach) of 800/114 mg ($2 \times 400/57$ mg) RiclaSip® Granules for Oral Suspension/Augmentin® Duo 400/57 mg Powder for Oral Suspension for Selected Pharmacokinetic Parameters of Amoxicillin and Clavulanic Acid

|  | Point estimate *T/R* ratio | 90% CI |
|---|---|---|
| Parametric approach | | |
| *Amoxicillin*: | | |
| $C_{max}$ (mg/L) | 0.96 | 0.92–1.00 |
| $AUC_{0-\infty}$ (mg·hr/L) | 0.97 | 0.95–0.99 |
| Nonparametric approach | | |
| *Clavulanic acid*: | | |
| $C_{max}$ (mg/L) | 0.86 | 0.80–0.93 |
| $AUC_{0-\infty}$ (mg·h/L) | 0.89 | 0.84–0.95 |

*Note*: Due to significant deviation from normal distribution of the clavulanic acid data, the non-parametric approach was used for assessment of bioequivalence for this analyte. The reason for this deviation was outlying low concentrations of clavulanic acid following RiclaSip® administration in Subject No. 019.
*Abbreviation*: CI, confidence interval.

## Handling and Correct Use of DST by Healthy and Sick Children

In a handling study the acceptance and handling capability of the technology were tested in different countries with children between 2 and 12 years of age participating in the study. The results of these studies demonstrated the practicality and wide acceptance of DST in children and parents alike. DST is suitable for patients above the age of two years, who are able to use an ordinary drinking straw.

In a clinical study (10) the treatment adherence ("compliance") and treatment satisfaction were investigated in 266 children suffering from upper respiratory tract infections. In these studies clarithromycin was administered using either ClaroSip granules for oral suspension in a drinking straw (175 children) or using an established treatment regimen using a reconstituted oral suspension, Klacid® Forte (87 children) with administration made possible using a dosing syringe. Explorative statistical analyzes demonstrated that sick children can use the system without problems and revealed significant advantages for ClaroSip in all parameters tested, e.g., the treatment adherence (compliance), the willingness of intake, and the ease of handling of ClaroSip from a parents' perspective.

## DESCRIPTION OF THE SYSTEM AND ITS MANUFACTURING PROCESS

A schematic drawing of a filled SIP system and blow ups of the essential components are depicted in Figure 4.

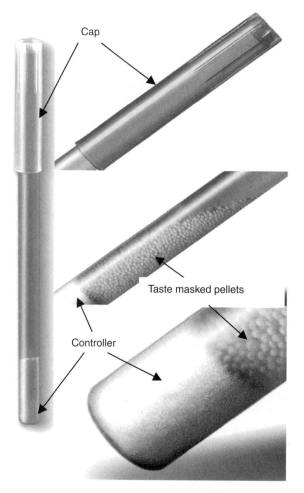

**Figure 4**  Schematic drawing of the SIP® system in which granules for oral suspension are filled into a drinking straw for single dose administration.

Besides the drinking straw itself, which is rounded at both ends and contains the correct amount of taste masked granules for all dose strengths, the cap and the controller are further, essential components for the appropriate functionality of the SIP system.

## The Cap and the Controller

The cap is used to close the system to prevent granules from falling out of the straw during transport and it must be removed prior to use of the system. The controller prevents loss of granules through the bottom end of the drinking straw. When a patient sips liquid into the straw the controller allows liquid to enter the straw to facilitate dispersion of the granules. In contrast to conventional oral suspensions the taste masking coating is protected from contact with the liquid prior to the actual administration of the dose. The contact time of any liquid with the granules is therefore the same time as it takes to swallow the beverage and is much shorter than with other solid oral dosage forms and suspensions. Nevertheless all of these systems are generally recommended to be taken with a suitable amount of liquid to assist dissolution and absorption of the API in and from the gastrointestinal tract.

On sipping the medication the controller will move upwards together with the suspended granules until it reaches the top end of the straw, thereby indicating to the parent or caretaker, that all granules have been administered. Even though it may drop down again when sipping stops, the temporary top position clearly indicates completion of the administration of the complete does. The controller cannot be removed from the system due to the rounded ends of the drinking straw system thereby making it impossible for it to leave the straw as long as the system has not been tampered with. Therefore, parents should not let children play with the system, chew or bite on it prior to, during or after administration of the medication.

## Manufacturing of the Dose Sipping System

The manufacture of ClaroSip granules for oral suspension in a drinking straw is basically comprised of two phases. Initially taste-masked granules for oral suspension are manufactured using standard pharmaceutical technologies, which are commonly used for the manufacture of pharmaceutical dosage forms and includes neither unusual or critical steps, nor novel excipients. In the final phase of the process the granules are filled into the online assembled drinking straw system at the correct weight per dose, using a special assembly machine. The edge of the bottom end of the straw is crimped by means of short thermal treatment. The softened polyolefin is than mechanically shaped to form a smooth, rounded end, which prevents the controller from leaving the straw when pushed down. The controller can be inserted into each straw prior to or after shaping of the lower end, but is only pushed down after crimping of the bottom end of the straw. A second thermal treatment and mechanical shaping is carried out to form the upper end of the straw. Filling of the granules into the drinking straw is performed using the same principles as those used for filling of granules or pellets into hard gelatine capsules. Fill weight variations are comparable to those of hard gelatine capsules and are always well below 10% for fill weights of less than 300 mg and 7.5% for fill weights exceeding 300 mg. The filled drinking straws are then closed with plastic caps.

The manufacturing of RiclaSip granules for oral suspension in a drinking straw is almost identical to that described for ClaroSip except that a separate fill step is added to the process to allow for the addition of the different types of granules. Furthermore, due to the moisture sensitivity of clavulanic acid these pellets need to be manufactured and handled under conditions of low relative humidity and temperature. ClaroSip or RiclaSip granules for oral suspension are individually packed into aluminium sachets immediately after assembly and filling of the drinking straw systems. Appropriate in-process-controls are in place to assure the correct assembly of each drinking straw, the correct filling of granules into the system and that the subsequent packaging steps have been appropriately conducted.

## Materials Used for the SIP System

The drinking straw system used with ClaroSip or RiclaSip is not ingested itself, but is solely a delivery technology that assists in the correct administration of a premeasured dose of granules for oral suspension. The individual components are therefore regarded as primary packaging materials, being in direct contact with the dosage form and the patient during administration of the finished product. All materials used for the system are summarized in Table 5 and fulfil the requirements of the commission directives for materials intended to come into contact with foodstuffs (8,9).

## CONCLUSION

The use of DST and the SIP systems is highly beneficial since the technology is able to ensure accurate dosing and improved compliance in pediatric patients. These advantages are also regarded by health and regulatory

**Table 5** Components, Description, Materials and Dimensions of the Drinking Straw System

| Each SIP® system consists of | Material description | |
|---|---|---|
| | ClaroSip® | RiclaSip® |
| *Straw*: approx. $152 \times 8\,mm^2$ | Polyolefin, translucent white | Polyolefin, translucent blue |
| *Cap*: approx. $51 \times 10\,mm^2$ | Polyolefin, white translucent | Polyolefin, white opaque |
| *Controller*: approx. $9 \times 8\,mm^2$ | Cylindrical, white opaque plug of porous structure formed out of polyolefin | |

authorities to be of substantial importance for the improved administration of antibiotics to children.

## REFERENCES

1. Deicke A, Süverkrüp R. Dose uniformity and redispersibility of pharmaceutical suspensions I. Eur J Pharm Biopharm 1999; 48(3):25–32.
2. Reflection Paper: Formulations of Choice for the Paediatric Population; EMEA/CHMP/PEG/194810/2005; London, 28 July 2006.
3. Note for Guidance on Excipients, Antioxidants and Antimicrobial Preservatives in the Dossier for Application for Marketing Authorisation of a Medicinal Product; CPMP/QWP/419/03; http://www.emea.eu.int/pdfs/human/qwp/041903en.pdf
4. Grießmann K, Breitkreutz J, Schoettler P, et al. Amoxicillintrockensäfte: Dosierungsgenauigkeit und sichere Handhabung. Monatsschrift Kinderheilkunde 2005; 153:735–40.
5. WO 97/03634 Oral Delivery of Discrete Units; Wong et al.; 06 February 1997; US 5,780,058 Oral Delivery of Discrete Units; Wong et al.; 14 July 1998; US 5,989,590 Oral Delivery of Discrete Units; Wong et al.; 23 November 1999; US 6,106,845 Oral Delivery of Discrete Units; Wong et al.; 22 August 2000; US 6,210,713 Oral Delivery of Discrete Units; Wong et al.; 03 April 2001.
6. Note for Guidance on the Investigation of Bioavailability and Bioequivalence; 2001; CPMP/EWP/QWP/1401/98; http://www.emea.eu.int/pdfs/human/ewp/140198en.pdf
7. Guidance for Industry: Waiver of In Vivo Bioavailability and Bioequivalence Studies for Immediate-Release Solid Oral Dosage Forms Based on a Biopharmaceutics Classification System; FDA CDER, Rockville, MD; 2000; http://www.fda.gov/cder/guidance/3618fnl.htm
8. Commission Directive 2002/72/EC relating to plastic materials and articles intended to come into contact with foodstuffs; Official Journal of the European Communities; L 220, 08/2002 pp. 18–58.
9. Commission Directive 97/48/EC amending for the second time Council Directive 82/711/EEC laying down the basic rules necessary for testing migration of the constituents of plastic materials and articles intended to come into contact with foodstuffs; Annex; Official Journal L 222, 12/08/1997 pp. 0010–5.
10. D. Adam; Compliance with a new taste masked oral clarithromycin preparation and efficiency in the treatment of respiratory tract infection in children; G-871, ICCAC, San Francisco 2006.

# 21

# Enhanced Gastroretentive Dosage Form with Minimal Food Effects: GIRES™

**David C. Coughlan and Edel O'Toole**

*Merrion Pharmaceuticals PLC, Trinity College Dublin, Dublin, Ireland*

**Thomas W. Leonard**

*Merrion Pharmaceuticals LLC, Willmington, North Carolina, U.S.A.*

## INTRODUCTION

Numerous classes of drugs could benefit by improved delivery using a gastro-retentive delivery system, including drugs with a short half-life, a selective absorption window, those for local delivery to the gastromtestinal tract, and formulations for which improved pharmacokinetic control are required (1–5). An ideal gastroretentive drug delivery system should be small enough to swallow, to not swell or expand in the esophagus and/or intestines, display controlled-release properties, be sufficiently rigid to remain intact in the stomach, decrease in size or degrade after it has performed its function, while at the same time showing minimal food effects following administration (3). Gastrointestinal retention system (GIRES™, Merrion Pharmaceuticals, PLC, Dublin, Ireland) is a platform technology that addresses these challenges. This chapter briefly describes some in vitro and in vivo human studies that demonstrate the safety and effectiveness of GIRES™.

## HISTORICAL DEVELOPMENT

The factors that affect gastric emptying of an oral dosage form include the density, size, and shape of the dosage form, the concomitant ingestion of food (including its nature, caloric content and frequency of intake), and to biological factors such as gender, age, and disease state (1). Numerous types of gastroretentive delivery systems are in development (2) including floating

(4) and expandable systems (5). Floating systems have a lower bulk density than the gastric contents and remain buoyant in the stomach for a prolonged period of time. A disadvantage of many floating gastroretentive systems is their substantive reliance on the presence of food to retard gastric emptying (4,6) resulting in unreliability and irreproducibility in the observed residence time in the stomach following oral administration (4). In contrast, expandable retentive systems withstand gastric transit by increasing their physical size to greater than that of the pyloric sphincter, which in humans, has an approximate diameter of $12 \pm 7\,mm^2$ (7,8). Expandable systems are the most promising approach to achieving gastroretention following oral administration (3). It is estimated that large objects (>20 mm) are retained in the fasted or fed stomach, while objects less than 10 mm in size are emptied from the stomach (3). Expandable systems must exceed these dimensions in order to prevent premature emptying through the pylorus. In addition, expandable systems must decrease in size or degrade to enable clearance from the stomach after a specified period of time. A significant advantage of using an expandable gastroretentive dosage form is that once they are in an expanded state above the size of the pyloric sphincter, they do not empty from the stomach, irrespective of whether it is in the fed or fasted state (1). Possible drawbacks of gastroretentive systems include the potential for permanent retention in the stomach, or premature clearance of the dosage form from the stomach and inflation directly in the small intestine. In addition, the swelling/expanding and, therefore, retention time of many of these proposed products is often relatively short (2,9,10), while other expandable systems may be difficult to commercialize and may not be cost-effective (2).

GIRES can be classified as both an expandable and a floating delivery system, thereby using the advantages of each type to produce prolonged and reliable gastro retention. GIRES is also able to overcome several of the major limitations of the gastroretentive systems described above. The development of GIRES stemmed from the need for a predictable and reliable oral delivery system that is small enough to ingest orally, yet is retained in the stomach without adverse effects in the presence or absence of food.

## DESCRIPTION OF THE TECHNOLOGY

GIRES is a gas-generating, inflatable, gastroretentive system which is enclosed in a hard gelatin capsule. On contact with gastric fluids the capsule dissolves to release a pouch, which contains an active pharmaceutical ingredient (API) that is formulated with effervescent- and rate-controlling excipients. When gastric fluid penetrates the pouch, gas is generated through effervescence resulting in the inflation of the pouch. The inflation of the pouch results in retention of the system in the stomach, and its geometry prevents it from passing through the pyloric valve. In addition, the system also floats on the stomach contents. Controlled release of the drug from the pouch into the stomach is maintained by the permeation rate of the drug across the film, and the release rate of the drug from the matrix. The pouch is designed to maintain inflation for at least 16 hours, thereby providing an extended gastric retention time. Once the gas-generating excipients are depleted, the pouch deflates and becomes flexible. This deflation allows the pouch to pass through the pyloric sphincter into the proximal part of the small intestine. The pouch does not disintegrate in the gastrointestinal tract (GIT), therefore, it is possible to track the passage of the system through the GIT until elimination occurs. GIRES™ is designed to improve therapy for several classes of compounds, including those that have a short half-life, exhibit a narrow absorption window, require pharmacokinetic control due to narrow therapeutic indices and/or require extended local delivery to the GIT. Furthermore GIRES has the potential to provide controlled delivery of two or more drugs with different pharmacokinetic properties, such as combination antiretroviral therapy.

## RESEARCH AND DEVELOPMENT

### In Vitro Studies

Numerous in vitro studies have been undertaken to evaluate the performance of the components of GIRES. In addition, the feasibility of formulating and including a particular API into GIRES can also be established using these in vitro methods.

The diffusion profiles of several drugs through a GIRES film alone have been evaluated in vitro, using a custom dual chamber permeability apparatus, with the GIRES film clamped in place between the two chambers. During evaluation, the film acted as a barrier to diffusion of the drug across an aqueous drug concentration gradient. The influence of the physicochemical properties of the drug, concentration gradient, and gas generation on diffusion rates of the drug, has been investigated and each of these parameters has been shown to influence the rate of diffusion of drug across the GIRES film (data not shown).

In vitro studies evaluating the release of drug from a GIRES tablet and pouch, as well as the swelling rate of the pouch, have also been undertaken. The release rate of drug from the GIRES tablet, in addition to the rate of gas generation, can be controlled by modification of the gas-generating agent/excipient/drug ratio or the type of excipients used. Control of these factors impact swelling of the GIRES pouch and the drug release rate from the pouch. The inflation of a typical GIRES pouch over the first two hours following administration is depicted in Figure 1.

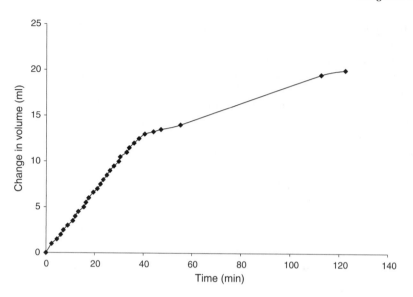

**Figure 1**   Volume of inflation of a typical GIRES pouch following administration.

## In Vivo Biostudies

A pharmacoscintigraphic study of the GIRES system containing a placebo formulation was carried out in healthy human volunteers. The study objectives were to investigate the effect of pouch size or simultaneous administration of two placebo gastroretentive formulations on gastric retention time in the fed state. Gelatine capsules were pre-packed with one GIRES pouch. Several pouches with various internal diameters (i.d.), $20 \times 20 \, mm^2$, $22 \times 25 \, mm^2$, $20 \times 25 \, mm^2$, or $25 \times 25 \, mm^2$ were evaluated. The study was a randomized four-way crossover oral study in healthy volunteers ($n = 8$). There was a washout period of at least four (4) days between study periods. The four treatments were one GIRES capsule with a pouch formulation of i.d. $20 \times 20 \, mm^2$, one GIRES capsule with a pouch formulation of i.d. $22 \times 25 \, mm^2$, one GIRES capsule with a pouch formulation of i.d. $20 \times 25 \, mm^2$, and two GIRES capsules with pouch formulations of i.d. $25 \times 25 \, mm^2$. The formulations were all administered following a standard FDA high fat breakfast. The formulation within the GIRES pouch included a gamma-emitting radionucleotide (Samarium-153) to enable photoscintigraphic analysis. Anterior scintigraphic images were recorded at approximately 10-minute intervals for 12 hours, and then every 20 minutes for a further 4 hours, with a final image being taken at 24 hours following administration.

Typical scintigraphic images obtained are depicted in Figure 2. Gastric emptying and retrieval times of the GIRES pouches are summarized in Table 1. The data from the pharmacoscintigraphic study reveal that under

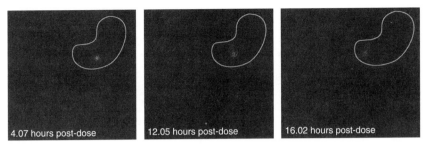

4.07 hours post-dose   12.05 hours post-dose   16.02 hours post-dose

**Figure 2** Typical scintigraphic images obtained in a human volunteer following administration of a GIRES delivery system containing Samarium-153.

fed conditions, the gastric retention time of all GIRES prototypes investigated was longer than 16 hours, and that reducing the pouch size from $25 \times 25\,mm^2$ to $20 \times 20\,mm^2$ i.d. had no impact on gastric retention. Simultaneous administration of two GIRES prototypes showed similar gastric retention characteristics to that observed following administration of a single GIRES prototype. Therefore, it is possible to administer multiple units of the GIRES system to deliver high doses of an API or to administer multiple APIs. All treatments were well-tolerated, with no evidence of intestinal "hold-up" in any case. Intestinal transit times were found to similar for all administration regimens tested.

In vivo studies have also been performed in both the fed and fasted state using GIRES containing an API. These studies compared gastrointestinal transit of the GIRES systems and the extent of drug absorption to an immediate release (IR) reference formulation. The plasma profiles revealed a reduced $C_{max}$ and increased $T_{max}$ (~8 hr) for both the fed and fasted states, compared to the IR reference product. A typical GIRES pharmacokinetic study profile in humans is shown in Figure 3. This study compared the plasma profile of an IR drug formulation with that of two GIRES formulations of the same drug (formulation 1 or 2), administered in both the fasted and fed states. The IR reference was dosed in the fasted state

**Table 1** Human Scintigraphy Study: Gastric Emptying and Retrieval Times of GIRES™ Containing Samarium-153

| Treatment ($n = 8$) | Gastric emptying time (hr) | Pouch retrieval time (hr) |
|---|---|---|
| 1 Pouch ($20 \times 20\,mm^2$) fed state | 16–24 | $43.8 \pm 9.5$ |
| 1 Pouch ($22 \times 25\,mm^2$) fed state | 16–24 | $38.3 \pm 9.9$ |
| 1 Pouch ($20 \times 25\,mm^2$) fed state | 16–24 | $45.2 \pm 16.9$ |
| 2 Pouches ($25 \times 25\,mm^2$) fed state | 16–24 | $41.6 \pm 7.4$ |

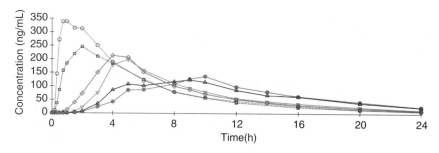

**Figure 3** Typical pharmacokinetic profiles obtained following administration of IR and GIRES™ dosage forms in the fed and fasted states to human volunteers (20 mg drug X, $n$ = 12–14 subjects). ⊖ (dashed)—reference IR fasted (PO); ⊟ (dashed)—reference IR fed high fat (PO); ◇—GIRES formulation 1 fasted (PO); △—GIRES formulation 1 fed high fat (PO); ▽—GIRES formulation 1 fed low fat (PO); ●—GIRES formulation 2 fed high fat (PO).

or following a standard FDA high fat meal. GIRES formulation 1 was dosed either in the fasted state, following a standard FDA high fat meal, or following a low fat meal. GIRES formulation 2 was dosed following a standard FDA high fat meal. All GIRES formulations in this study reduced the $C_{max}$ of the drug while significantly increasing the $T_{max}$ compared to the IR reference. A significant extension of the $T_{max}$ was, therefore, apparent in both the fasted state and the fed state when the drug was formulated as a GIRES dosage form (Fig. 3).

## SAFETY SUMMARY

No system-related adverse events have been observed to date following 182 administrations of GIRES dosage forms to 60 individuals (1 or 2 pouches).

## TECHNOLOGY POSITION/COMPETITIVE ADVANTAGE

GIRES has the potential to offer key competitive advantages as a marketable, cost- and therapeutically effective gastroretentive dosage form. The finished dosage form is provided as a conventional orally administered hard gelatine capsule, thereby improving patient acceptability and potentially, patient compliance. The payload of API and the pouch size used will influence the size of the final product. Furthermore, GIRES as both an expandable and floating gastroretentive dosage form, utilizes key advantages of each of these systems to ensure effective gastric retention. In the fasted stomach, which contains little fluid and where floating will be transient (3), GIRES is still sufficiently activated to ensure swelling is adequate and to prevent the passage of the system through the pyloric sphincter. The timely inflation of GIRES in acid conditions, along with its floatability, ensures consistent, reproducible and significant gastric retention, whilst the effects of food on gastric retention are minimized. In our opinion, GIRES has the longest gastric retention time of any system under development, and is the most inert to the effects of food, thereby offering a competitive advantage over other gastroretentive dosage forms (1,3,10).

## REFERENCES

1.  Streubel A, Siepmann J, Bodmeier. Drug delivery to the upper small intestine window using gastroretentive technologies. Curr Opin Pharm 2006; 6:501–8.
2.  Bardonnet PL, Faivre V, Pugh WJ, Piffaretti JC and Falson F. Gastroretentive dosage forms: Overview and special case of Helicobacter pylori. J Control Release 2006; 111:1–18.
3.  Davis SS. Formulation strategies for absorption windows. Drug Discovery Today 2005; 4:249–57.
4.  Singh BN, Kim KH. Floating drug delivery systems: an approach to oral controlled drug delivery via gastric retention. J Control Release 2000; 63: 235–59.
5.  Klausner EA, Lavy E, Friedman M, Hoffman A. Expandable gastroretentive dosage forms. J Control Release 2003; 90:143–62.
6.  Mazer N, Abisch E, Gfeller JC, et al. Intragastric behavior and absorption kinetics of a normal and "floating" modified-release capsule of isradipine under fasted and fed conditions. J Pharm Sci 1988; 77(8):647–57.
7.  Salessiotis N. Measurement of the diameter of the pylorus in man I. Experimental project for clinical application. Am J Surg 1972; 124:331–3.
8.  Timmermans J, Moes AJ. The cutoff size for gastric emptying of dosage forms. J Pharm Sci 1993; 82(8):854.
9.  Klausner EA, Lavy E, Barta M, Cserpes E, Friedman M, Hoffman A. Novel gastroretentive dosage forms: evaluation of gastroretentivity and its effect on levodopa absorption in humans. Pharm Res 2003; 20(9): 1466–73.
10. Kagan L, Lapidot N, Afargan M, et al. Gastroretentive Accordion Pill: Enhancement of riboflavin bioavailability in humans. J Control Release 2006; 113:208–15.

# 22

# Advancing Gastrointestinal Permeation Enhancement Formulations into the Clinic: GIPET™

## David C. Coughlan and Edel O'Toole
*Merrion Pharmaceuticals PLC, Trinity College Dublin, Dublin, Ireland*

## Thomas W. Leonard
*Merrion Pharmaceuticals LLC, Willmington, North Carolina, U.S.A.*

## INTRODUCTION

Poorly permeable drugs remain a significant formulation challenge for achieving therapeutically-effective oral drug delivery. Gastrointestinal Permeation Enhancement Technology (GIPET™, Merrion Pharmaceuticals PLC) is a platform technology that addresses this challenge by safely delivering drugs across the small intestine in therapeutically-relevant concentrations. This monograph provides an evaluation of GIPET, with particular emphasis on the use of a simple, inexpensive, preclinical feasibility model to advance formulations into clinical testing.

## HISTORICAL DEVELOPMENT

The absorption of poorly permeable Class III drugs (1), which include most peptides, can potentially be improved by use of approaches that enhance the ability of the compound to cross the gut/epithelial membranes. By the mid-1990s it was well known that millimolar concentrations of medium chain fatty acids and related compounds could boost the flux of hydrophilic agents across membranes in in vitro experiments (2,3). However, enhanced permeation using isolated tissue mucosae or perfused rodent intestinal segments using solutions of active and excipients has no direct relationship to a marketable formulation for human patients. Attempts to promote oral absorption of poorly absorbed drugs over the past 15 years have not, for the most part, been commercially successful. The reasons for such failure include the inability to deliver consistent therapeutic levels of drug, safety issues associated with new chemical compounds used as enhancers, and the high cost of goods due to the poor efficacy of the enhancer system, which results in the need for incorporation of large amounts of active pharmaceutical ingredient (API) in the dosage form. The lack of reliable and predictive in vivo animal models and the inability to convert technology into practical, solid oral dosage forms have also been impediments to commercial success. The development of GIPET was driven by the need for solid dosage form presentations with oral enhancement techniques.

## DESCRIPTION OF THE TECHNOLOGY

GIPET is a platform technology designed to enhance the oral bioavailability of a variety of poorly absorbed compounds. The GIPET platform includes GIPET I, which uses medium chain fatty acids, salts and derivatives, formulated as tablets, and GIPET II, a microemulsion-based system in a hard or soft gelatine capsule. Importantly, the GIPET excipients are food additives that are generally regarded as safe (GRAS) in the European Union and the United States, and they appear on the GRAS list in the Code of Federal Regulations, 21 CFR 170.3. GIPET dosage forms are enteric-coated tablets or capsules that are comprised of the enhancer system and the API in an appropriate matrix. GIPET systems are formulated as physical mixtures and the chemical composition of the API does not change in any way. The enteric coating protects the API from gastric acidity and permits the release of the dosage form contents in the small intestine. This maximizes the relative concentrations of API and enhancer at the site of absorption. The targeted co-release of API and enhancer is inherent in GIPET formulations and provides optimum conditions for therapeutically effective oral drug delivery.

## RESEARCH AND DEVELOPMENT

Human intestinal monolayers have limited value in predicting the in vivo application of absorption promotors (4). An animal model is needed that approximates the performance of the GIT and associated systems in humans in order to advance a preclinical concept to a dosage form suitable for human use.

### GIPET Feasibility Dog Model

An in vivo model has been developed in beagle dogs that is able to predict performance of a particular drug/GIPET combination in humans. Dogs are surgically implanted with vascular access ports (VAP) and each VAP is connected to a cannula which is inserted into the duodenum. Drug/ GIPET™ (GIPET I or GIPET II) combinations are instilled into the cannulated dog. Plasma drug levels are subsequently measured and bioavailability is determined relative to a control that is either a parenteral or a simple solution administered to the same dog colony. The feasibility model has been shown to be an inexpensive, rapid, minimally invasive technique for advancing the oral formulation of poorly absorbed drugs with GIPET into the clinic.

There are several additional advantages to using the GIPET feasibility model. In the first instance there is minimal drug substance requirement for initial feasibility studies, which is particularly important in the case of a new chemical entity or a high value therapeutic compound. Second, the inherent variability introduced by the model itself is minimized by use of the same dogs for each phase of any crossover studies. Finally, the feasibility model mimics the enteric coated co-release of API/GIPET in the duodenum, an important factor in enabling the model to be reflective of results in later stage development. The model, therefore, enables the selection of a lead API/GIPET system for formulation development and for advancing the drug into the clinical phases of drug development. Some API/GIPET case studies are described and comparisons of human clinical data with preclinical dog data are made.

## Alendronate/GIPET Feasibility and Clinical Studies

Alendronate sodium (Fosamax®, Merck & Co., Whitehouse Station, NJ) is approved as both once-daily and -weekly tablets for the treatment and prevention of post-menopausal osteoporosis in women and in men requiring an increase in bone mineral density. Approximately 0.65% of an oral dose of alendronate is absorbed and approximately half of that is excreted in the urine (5). Bisphos-phonates are normally not administered as enteric-coated products as the use of enteric systems further reduces the oral bioavailability. Fosamax tablets must be taken in the morning with a full glass of water on an empty stomach to ensure that some drug is absorbed, and patients are required to remain upright for 30 minutes to an hour following administration to minimize esophageal erosion due to gastric irritation caused by unabsorbed drug. The complex dosing regime severely decreases compliance (6). In addition, to achieve high doses, bisphosphonates are administered parenterally [pamidronate, (Aredia®, Novartis) and zoledronic acid, (Zometa®, Novartis)] when used in the treatment of metastatic bone cancer (7).

The resultant pharmacokinetic parameters obtained from an alendronate preclinical feasibility dog study, a human intubation study and a human oral study are summarized in Table 1. The urinary excretion results obtained in the dog study are indicative of the trends shown in the

**Table 1** Dog and Human Bioavailability Data: Alendronate-GIPET I

**Feasibility model dog study 7mg/kg**

| | Alendronate (unenhanced) (oral, n=8) | Alendronate (unenhanced) (ID, n=8) | High GIPET I (oral, n=8) | High GIPET I (ID, n=8) | Low GIPET I (ID, n=8) |
|---|---|---|---|---|---|
| % Excreted | 1.27 ± 0.79 | 1.30 ± 0.75 | 3.31 ± 3.01 | 4.52 ± 3.28 | 3.48 ± 2.61 |
| CV % | 61.8 | 57.7 | 90.8 | 72.6 | 74.8 |
| Cum amt (mg) | 0.84 ± 0.53 | 0.92 ± 0.52 | 2.27 ± 2.07 | 3.21 ± 2.23 | 2.76 ± 2.09 |
| CV% | 62.5 | 56.7 | 91.0 | 69.5 | 75.7 |
| Absolute F (%) | 2.66 ± 1.67 | 3.00 ± 2.36 | 6.18 ± 6.13 | 9.97 ± 6.89 | 8.49 ± 7.23 |
| CV% | 62.9 | 78.7% | 99.2 | 69.2 | 85.1 |

**Human intubation study**

| | 10 mg Fosamax® (oral, n=12) | Low GIPET I (IJ, n=12) | Medium GIPET I (IJ, n=12) | High GIPET I (IJ, n=12) | Low GIPET II (IJ, n=6) | High GIPET II (IJ, n=6) |
|---|---|---|---|---|---|---|
| % Excreted | 0.61 ± 1.11 | 3.77 ± 3.16 | 6.64 ± 4.97 | 7.66 ± 3.72 | 2.61 ± 2.50 | 8.38 ± 5.49 |
| CV % | 181.3 | 83.9 | 74.9 | 48.6 | 96.0 | 65.6 |
| Cum Amt (mg) | 0.06 ± 0.11 | 0.38 ± 0.32 | 0.66 ± 0.50 | 0.77 ± 0.37 | 0.26 ± 0.25 | 0.84 ± 0.55 |
| CV% | 181.3 | 83.9 | 74.9 | 48.6 | 96.0 | 65.6 |

**Human oral study**

| | 35 mg Fosamax (oral, n=16) | 17.5 mg alendronate/low GIPET I (oral, n=16) | 17.5 mg alendronate/high GIPET I (oral, n=16) |
|---|---|---|---|
| % Excreted | 0.3 ± 0.1 | 1.6 ± 1.7 | 1.5 ± 0.6 |
| CV % | 33.6 | 106.8 | 40.5 |
| Relative F (%) | — | 630.9 ± 600.9 | 644.9 ± 383.7 |
| CV % | — | 95.3 | 59.5 |

*Abbreviations*: ID, intra-duodenal; IJ, intra-jejunal.

subsequent human studies. In each study, the bioavailability of the drug is increased when administered in the GIPET matrix compared to that observed when the control formulations were administered. There is also a decrease in the variability of absorption in both the preclinical and clinical trials with increasing amounts of GIPET in the formulation.

In the human oral study, urinary excretion data indicate that GIPET resulted in a 5-fold increase in the oral bioavailability of alendronate formulations over the reference product. This result is noteworthy as there is a large improvement in bioavailability over the current formulation, which may allow for an expansion of the indications for bisphosphonate tablets to those therapeutic areas that are currently only treated by intravenous infusion. The use of enteric-coated tablets eliminates gastric and esophageal issues with these compounds.

## Low Molecular Weight Heparin/GIPET Feasibility and Clinical Studies

Low molecular weight heparin (LMWH) is used as prophylactic anti-coagulant treatment to prevent deep vein thrombosis or pulmonary embolism following hip or knee replacement surgery, and must be given by subcutaneous injection due to its low oral bioavailability (8). The percentage relative bioavailability of doses of 45,000 IU parnaparin with various amounts of GIPET I, in both dog and human intubation studies, are shown in Figure 1. Bioavailability of up to approximately 10% and 20%

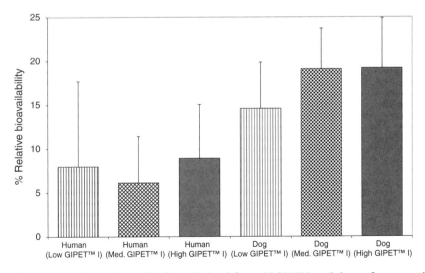

**Figure 1** Relative bioavailability obtained for a 45,000 IU oral dose of parnaparin with various doses of GIPET™ I (low, medium, high) in both human and dog intubation studies. The figures are calculated with respect to the AUC of anti-FactorXa following a subcutaneous dose (3,200 IU) of parnaparin.

was observed in human and dogs respectively in these intubation studies. The dog feasibility model gave a reasonable approximation of the percent bioavailability that could be obtained in humans, as well as providing information for formulation selection. The variability of response decreased in both human and dog models with increasing amounts of GIPET.

Mean data for the anti-FactorXa assay over time in a human oral tablet study are depicted in Figure 2 and the oral data are summarized in Table 2. The relative oral bioavailability of 45,000 IU and 90,000 IU parnaparin with GIPET I, versus the subcutaneous route, were 3.9% and 7.6% respectively in humans. With the higher dose tablet, therapeutic levels of anti-FactorXa activity were seen in all subjects and the responses were sustained in most subjects over a time course comparable to that achieved following subcutaneous delivery.

## Desmopressin/GIPET Feasibility and Clinical Studies

Desmopressin is a peptide that is used as an antidiuretic agent for treatment of vasopressin-sensitive diabetes insipidus, polyuria, and polydypsia. The oral bioavailability for the commercial oral product is low, and in many cases is not able to be calculated due to blood levels remaining below the limit of detection

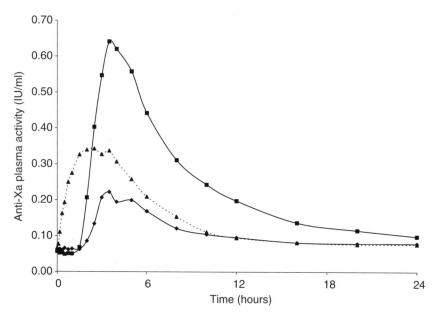

**Figure 2** Plasma profile of anti-FactorXa activity from the oral delivery of LMWH-GIPET I in humans. ■, 90,000 IU parnaparin/high-dose GIPET I; ♦, 45,000 IU parnaparin/low-dose GIPET I; ▲, (dashed) SC reference, 3,200 IU parnaparin. $N$ = 14–16 subjects.

**Table 2**   Human Oral Bioavailability Data: parnaparin-GIPET I

| Pharmacokinetic parameters | 45,000 IU parnaparin/low-dose GIPET I tablets (PO) | 90,000 IU parnaparin/ high-dose GIPET I tablets (PO) | 3,200 IU parnaparin reference subcutaneous |
|---|---|---|---|
| Oral bioavailability (%) | 3.9 ± 3.5 | 7.6 ± 4.8 | N/A |
| Coefficient of variation (%) | 89.1 | 62.9 | N/A |
| Number of responders with levels >0.1 IU/mL (%) | 60 (9/15) | 100 (14/14) | 100 (16/16) |
| Number of responders with levels >0.1 IU/mL for >6 hours (%) | 13 (2/15) | 71 (10/14) | 81 (13/16) |
| Total duration >0.1 IU/mL (hr) | 2.6 ± 3.6 | 10.6 ± 5.4 | 7.1 ± 1.3 |

of the assay. In addition, the compound exhibits considerable intra-subject variability. There is a direct correlation between the amount of drug absorbed and the ultimate pharmacodynamic response. Consequently, an oral formulation with the higher bioavailability may lead to better efficacy and an associated high level of compliance. Desmopressin was formulated into a GIPET II capsule and administered orally to dogs in both an enteric coated and non–enteric-coated form and compared to 100 µg Minirin® tablet (Ferring Pharmaceuticals, New York) and the resultant profiles are depicted in Figure 3.

There was an 11-fold increase in area under the plasma profile curve (AUC) in the case of the uncoated capsule and a 21-fold increase in the AUC in the case of the enteric coated capsule when compared to that observed for the Minirin tablet. These data support the need for the optimum presentation of the drug and permeation enhancer in vitro at the site of absorption.

When desmopressin was administered orally to 18 human subjects, a similar trend to that shown in dogs was observed. These data are summarized in Figure 4 and Table 3.

There was a 10-fold improvement in bioavailability for the GIPET formulation as compared to the currently marketed Minirin tablet. More importantly, the coefficient of variation (CV) of the AUC dropped from more than 240%, to less than 90% with this technology. The coefficient of variation for the GIPET II capsule was similar to that observed for the parenteral product.

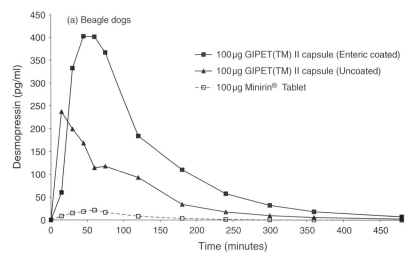

**Figure 3** Plasma profile from the oral delivery of desmopressin in dogs. ■, Desmopressin-GIPET II (100 μg, PO enteric coated capsule); □, desmopressin, Minirin®, (100 μg, PO tablet); ▲, desmopressin-GIPET II (100 μg, PO uncoated capsule). $N = 6$.

## SAFETY SUMMARY

The absorption-promoting excipients of GIPET are approved food additives in both the United States and Europe and numerous safety reviews have been reported (9–11). GIPET I and II systems have been tested orally in rats, dogs and humans to establish their safety profiles and efficacy. To date, more than 300 volunteers have been administered GIPET formulations in 18 Phase I studies on seven APIs. These studies include both single- and repeat-dosing regimes and there have been no reported adverse effects of concern. Intestinal epithelium recovery studies performed in humans indicate that the absorption-promoting effects of GIPET are transient and complete in less than one hour (data not shown).

## TECHNOLOGY POSITION/COMPETITIVE ADVANTAGE

There have been many attempts to promote the oral absorption of poorly absorbable BCS Class III drugs in the past. Many of these approaches have failed due to the inability of the technology to deliver therapeutic levels of API over a sustained period, the need for large amounts of material for product development, and safety issues regarding the long term safety of the enhancer. Additional obstacles have included the lack of reliable and predictive in vitro animal model(s) and the inability to develop practical and reproducible solid oral formulations that can be manufactured on a large

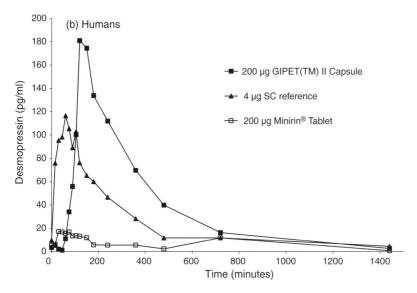

**Figure 4**  Plasma profile from the oral delivery of desmopressin in humans. ■, Desmopressin-GIPET II (200 μg, PO capsule); □, desmopressin, Minirin, (200 μg, PO tablet); ▲, desmopressin (4 μg, SC reference). $N = 18$.

scale. The development of a successful oral formulation of a poorly absorbed drug implies that there is access to the appropriate intestinal region for absorption for a sufficient period of time, and that intact soluble drug is released in a reproducible way so as to improve drug permeability across the gastrointestinal tract membranes.

Merrion has made considerable progress with the GIPET platform in overcoming these obstacles in order to deliver a marketable product. A preclinical feasibility GIPET model has been developed to predict performance of particular API/GIPET combinations in humans and therefore

**Table 3**  Human Oral Bioavailability Data: Desmopressin/GIPET II

|  | 4 μg Desmopressin (SC) $n = 18$ | 200 μg Minirin tablet (PO) $n = 18$ | 200 μg Desmopressin/ GIPET II capsule (PO) $n = 18$ |
|---|---|---|---|
| $AUC_{last}$ | 539.29 ± 517.05 | 159.19 ± 382.96 | 840.58 ± 729.38 |
| (CV %) | (95.88 %) | (240.56 %) | (86.77 %) |
| Relative bioavailability | N/A | 0.18 ± 0.22 | 2.38 ± 2.97 |
| (CV %) | | (122.16 %) | (124.63 %) |

*Abbreviations*: $AUC_{last}$, area under the curve; CV%, coefficient of variation.

aid the advancement of the drug into the clinical phases of drug development. The data presented here show that the GIPET feasibility model can be reflective of subsequent human clinical trials, thereby providing a useful screening tool for a particular API. The feasibility model is an inexpensive, rapid, minimally invasive technique for advancing the oral formulation of poorly absorbed drugs with GIPET into the clinic. Furthermore only a minimal amount of API is required for initial feasibility studies. The model is designed to mimic the enteric-coated co-release of API/GIPET in the intestine, an important factor in enabling the model to be reflective of results in later stage development. The GRAS nature of the excipients used gives GIPET™ a favorable safety profile and permits repeated dosing to subjects. GIPET also provides access to an appropriate region of the intestine by enteric coating of the formulation and reproducible dissolution of the drug and enhancer in vitro. In addition, the GIPET platform provides solid dose formulations which are reproducible and can be scaled-up using conventional equipment available in most pharmaceutical companies.

## FUTURE DIRECTIONS

GIPET III is an extension of the permeation enhancement technology platforms that exist as GIPET I and II. GIPET III consists of novel branched, cyclic, and straight chain fatty acids, also formulated in enteric coated tablets and/or capsules and is currently under investigation.

## REFERENCES

1. Amidon G, Lennernas H, Shah VP, et al. A theoretical basis for a biopharmaceutic drug classification: the correlation of in vitro drug product dissolution and in vitro bioavailability. Pharm Res 1995; 12(3):413–20.
2. Sawada T, Ogawa T, Tomita M, et al. Role of paracellular pathway in non-electrolyte permeation across rat colon epithelium enhanced by sodium caprate and sodium caprylate. Pharm Res 1991; 8(11):1365–71.
3. Anderberg EK, Lindmark T, Artursson P. Sodium caprate elicits dilatations in human intestinal tight junctions and enhances drug absorption by the paracellular route. Pharm Res 1993; 10(6):857–64.
4. Braydon D, Creed E, O'Connell A, et al. Heparin absorption across the intestine: effects of sodium N-[8-(2-hydroxybenzoyl)amino]caprylate in rat in situ intestinal instillations and in Caco-2 monolayers. Pharm Res 1997; 14(12): 1772–9.
5. Physicians' Desk Reference. 59th ed. Montvale, NJ: Thompson PDR; 2005: 2049–57.
6. Cramer JA, Amonkar MM, Mayur M, et al. Compliance and persistence with bisphosphonate dosing regimens among women with postmenopausal osteoporosis. Curr Med Res Opin 2005; 21(9):1453–60.

7.  Gordon DH. Efficacy and safety of intravenous bisphosphonates for patients with breast cancer metastatic to bone: a review of randomized, double-blind, phase III trials. Clin Breast Cancer 2005; 6(2):125–31.

8.  Merli G. Anticoagulants in the treatment of deep vein thrombosis. Am J Med 2005; 118(Suppl. 8A):13S–20S.

9.  Hera, 2002. Hera Targeted Risk Assessment of Fatty Acid Salts. June 2002.

10. JECFA. 29th Report of the Joint FAO/WHO Expert Committee on Food Additives. WHO Technical Report Series No. 733, 1986.

11. SCF. Extracts from First Report on Chemically Defined Flavoring Substances, 1995.

# 23

# The Micropump® Technology

Kenneth Lundstrom, Catherine Castan, Florence Guimberteau,
Roger Kravtzoff, and Rémi Meyrueix

*Flamel Technologies, Vénisieux, France*

## INTRODUCTION

The oral route of delivery is the most desirable route for administration of drugs intended to exert a systemic effect due to patient acceptance, convenience, and relatively simple manufacturing processes (1). However, there are some challenges in using this route, as often the requirements for systemic activity of a drug are dependent on various biopharmaceutical factors. The ideal time over which drug should be released from a dosage form extends over 24 h in relation to a relatively short gastro-intestinal transit time of between 4 and 5 hours and in some cases up to between 8 and 10 hours and which may have an impact on bioavailability. In addition, it is important to control the rate of dissolution of a drug in relation to the short residence time of a delivery system in the stomach and small intestine and highly variable and unpredictable gastric emptying rates when attempting to achieve efficient and effective oral drug therapy.

The major barriers to achieve efficient oral drug delivery are based on physiological, physicochemical, and enzymatic considerations. In the first instance drug molecules have to penetrate the aqueous mucous layer that lines the gastrointestinal tract (GIT) and which acts as a filter for molecules of molecular weights of between 600 and 800 Da prior to their reaching the epithelial layer of the intestinal mucosa (2). Although microvilli in the GIT increase the surface area for absorption by at least two orders of magnitude, the presence of digestive enzymes hampers the absorption of proteins (3). Furthermore physiological conditions such as pH, the texture and permeability of the gastrointestinal membranes, and the presence of proteolytic enzymes influence dramatically on drug absorption (4). Physicochemical factors that affect oral drug delivery include poor solubility and permeability in the GIT fluids and membranes and that are affected by the particle size, associated charge and hydrophobicity of drug compounds (5). Protein degradation due to the acidic environment of the stomach represents the chemical barrier to drug absorption whereas secreted and nonsecreted enzymes represent the biochemical barrier in the GIT fluids (6). Enzymatic barriers are characterized by the presence of large amounts of enzymes that are specific to different regions of the GIT (6).

A number of approaches have been used to improve oral drug delivery and include chemical modification of proteins and peptides to increase their stability and bioavailability and that have been achieved by glycosylation (7), pegylation (8), and crosslinking (9) of the molecules.

The ultimate goal following oral drug delivery is to achieve plasma concentration profiles of a drug (or in some cases of active metabolites) with optimal bioavailability, i.e., the greatest extent of absorption as represented by the area under the concentration time curve (AUC), and in which the plasma concentration remains higher than the minimum effective concentration (MEC) of the molecule over an extended period of time $T_{>MEC}$. Ideally $T_{>MEC}$ should be longer than 24 hours. To achieve an optimal $T_{>MEC}$ and bioavailability and is difficult and has several challenges as summarized herein.

## Bioavailability

The bioavailability of drugs may be limited by several factors including but not limited to poor solubility in the GIT fluids, low permeability through the epithelial membranes of the GIT, a narrow absorption window in the GIT, and/or rapid chemical or enzymatic degradation within the GIT.

The poor solubility of many drugs is a consequence of the degree of hydrophobicity of the molecule and/or a high enthalpy of crystallization. The solubility of poorly soluble drugs can be improved by formulating the poorly soluble or insoluble drug with solubility enhancers such as polyethylene glycol (PEG) (8), by use of amorphous phases that have a lower free energy (10), or by use of drug nanocrystals that increase the surface to volume ratio of the molecule (11).

Enzymatic inhibitors have also been used to slow the rate of degradation of a drug in the GIT and ensure that the drugs are available in a suitable form for absorption for a longer period of time (3). In this context, enzyme inhibitors such as pancreatic enzyme inhibitor (12), camostat mesylate (13), and aprotinin (14) have been used. Another approach is to encapsulate therapeutic protein/peptide molecules in nanoparticles, which will ensure protection against enzymatic degradation due to the presence of a polymeric coating (15).

In the case of small molecule drugs, chemical degradation is frequently accelerated in the low pH or acidic environment of the stomach and efficient inhibition of such degradation is achieved by use of enteric coating materials that are deposited at the surface of tablets, capsules and microparticles (16). The enteric coating material is usually a polyacid polymer that is insoluble and impermeable at acidic pH and that ionizes and becomes water soluble at the alkali pH conditions that prevail in the small intestine.

The use of permeation enhancers to enhance bioavailability results in improved membrane fluidity, decreased viscosity, and facilitates trans-membrane transport. Typical permeation enhancers include chelators, fatty acids, bile salts, and mucoadhesive materials such as anionic polymers and cationic chitosan (17). Multifunctional polymers may inhibit enzymes in addition to enhancing membrane permeability (18) and the most promising polymers used in this context are thiolated polymers (thiomers) (19) which are the focus of Chapter 15 in this book. To improve the bioavailablity of poorly absorbed drugs, liposomal carriers have been developed and applied (20). Although liposome-based delivery seems promising the relatively low stability of conventional liposomal drug delivery systems has restricted their use. The use of soy lecithin/cholesterol coating materials has resulted in the development of a mucoadhesive liposomal delivery system (21). Furthermore transport carriers or "delivery agents" such as protenoid microspheres have been designed to interact with a drug of choice in a noncovalent manner, thereby enhancing the passive transcellular transport across GIT membranes (22). Targeting of the colon as a route for systemic drug delivery has received increased attention due to the less hostile environment of colonic region of the GIT. In order to achieve success using this route of delivery, the drug release must be prevented in the upper GIT must occur immediately when the delivery system reaches the proximal colon (23).

Sustained release (SR) of drugs provides a means for the efficient treatment of nocturnal asthma, angina, and arthritis whereas local treatment is more effective for the treatment of ulcerative colitis and colorectal cancer.

## Extension of the MEC Time ($T_{>MEC}$)

The extension of the time over which the plasma concentration of a drug is greater the MEC for that drug is an essential design feature of oral dosage forms. The plasma concentration profile of a drug reflects a combination of the rate of absorption from the GIT in addition to, distribution and elimination rates and mechanisms.

An increase of the time $T_{>MEC}$ can be achieved by either increasing the time over which absorption occurs or lengthening the elimination half-life of the drug, the latter of which requires chemical modification in order to decrease drug clearance. In the case of proteins, chemical modification is generally achieved by pegylation of the protein, however chemical modification is not always desirable or even possible.

The goal of any SR dosage form is essentially to increase the time over which absorption of a drug can be achieved following administration. It is common for the drug in such systems to be encapsulated in such a way that the drug is release in the lumen over an extended period of time. However, it is important to recognize that prolonging the release of drug from a dosage form is not sufficient to extend the time over which absorption can take place. In many cases, drug absorption is limited to the upper part of the GIT usually the duodenum and/or jejunum. The absorption time ($T_a$) is thus limited to the time a solubilized drug is present at the site of absorption. In other words in order to increase $T_a$ it is necessary to extend the time over which drug is released from a dosage form in addition to increasing the time that the solubilized drug is retained at the site of absorption. In this respect, attempting to increase $T_a$ to 24 hours in relation to a relatively short GIT transit time of 4–5 hours poses a serious challenge.

The focus of this monograph is the Micropump® technology that has been developed for oral drug delivery. Examples of various drug targets and the use of the Micropump technology for the SR of antiviral, antihyperglycemic, and cardiovascular drugs are described in this monograph.

## THE MICROPUMP TECHNOLOGY

The Micropump technology has been developed for the oral delivery of one or more drug components simultaneously (24). The emphasis in the design of the Micropump has been to ensure that the technology allows for the extension of $T_a$ in the upper part of the GIT while maintaining optimal bioavailability. The technology has been applied to the delivery of a number of drugs including aspirin, acyclovir and metformin.

The Micropump technology is based on microparticles that range in the size between 200 and 800 µm (Fig. 1). Each microparticle used in the technology is individually coated and serves as a drug reservoir. The core of the particle contains the active ingredient, which can be present as crystals, granules, or a layered core. The core structure is surrounded by a coating, which is applied to the particles to control drug diffusion in either pH dependent or independent manner as required. The coating materials impart mechanical properties, such as film integrity and compressibility to the particles, and a typical dose of a drug contains from 5,000 to 50,000 particles.

Two versions of the Micropump technology have been developed. Micropump I is designed to produce a continuous SR profile of drug that commences as the technology reaches the stomach. Micropump II is designed as a delayed release technology that releases drug at a precise location in the small intestine and which minimizes the inter- and intra-subject variations in the plasma concentration profile that occur due to

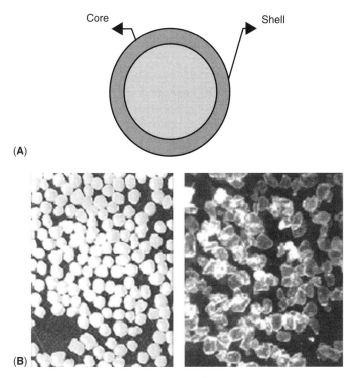

**Figure 1** Preparation of Micropump® microparticles. Granulates of acyclovir (*left*) and Genvir™ coating after 22-hour dissolution (*right*) (× 20).

variations in gastric emptying times. The Micropump technology is particularly useful for delivering drugs that exhibit site-specific absorption in the upper part of the small intestine or require an extended time of absorption. The technology allows for excellent dose-proportionality without any change in the formulation and is readily applied to developing combinations of drugs with different release profiles, reduced intra- and inter-variability and controlled release of poorly (0.01 mg/L) as well as highly (500 g/L) soluble drugs. Due to the high drug loading capacity of the technology Micropump can be applied to both low (4 mg) and high dose (1000 mg) drugs.

## ORAL THERAPEUTICS

The Micropump technology has been applied to the delivery of a number of different drugs via the oral route of administration. Some examples of these applications are presented for antiviral, antihyperglycemic, and cardiovascular drugs.

## Antiviral Drugs

Acyclovir is a commonly used antiviral drug that has been used frequently for the treatment of recurrent genital herpes (RGH). However, the episodic treatment of RGH with acyclovir requires the use of a recommended dosing regimen of 200 mg acyclovir (Zovirax®) five times a day which is a dosing regimen that is inconvenient for the patient. Acyclovir is a sparingly soluble drug and its solubility decreases from 10 mg/mL in solutions of pH 1.6–3.5 mg/mL in solutions of pH > 4.0. Furthermore, the absorption of acyclovir occurs in the upper part of the small intestine and the absolute bioavailability of the immediate release (IR) formulation is in the region of only 20–30% (25). The Micropump technology was applied to acyclovir by granulation of acyclovir crystals to produce granules with a narrow particle-size distribution with an average diameter of 400 µm. Following production each of the granules was coated individually using a thin polymeric Micropump film coating, taking care to avoid the formation of aggregates. On completion of the coating of each granule the coated particles were filled into hard shell capsules (Fig. 1). The resultant product, Genvir™, is able to provide the SR of acyclovir in vitro and the thickness of the coating can be modified so as to release 80% of the dose within 12–15 hours with a resultant pH independent permeation constant (Fig. 2).

The bioavailability of acyclovir from Genvir was compared to that from Zovirax in a randomized Phase I crossover study. The pharmacokinetic and bioavailability parameters of acyclovir were examined following administration of a single dose of Genvir 600 mg or 3 Zovirax 200 mg ablets to 48 healthy volunteers, following a meal. Blood samples were taken until 48 hours post-administration and analyzed using a validated HPLC method with gancyclovir as an internal standard (Fig. 3). The resultant increase in

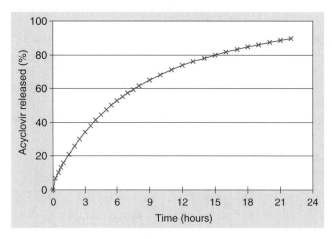

**Figure 2**  Dissolution profile for Genvir™ 600 mg.

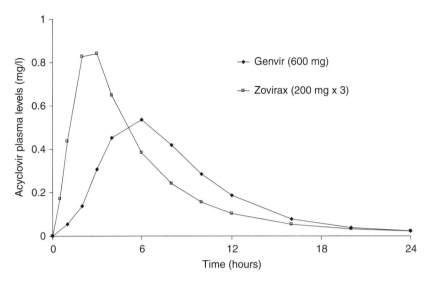

**Figure 3** Mean acyclovir plasma levels (fed) following administration of Genvir (600 mg) and Zovirax (3 ×200 mg).

$T_{max}$ value for Genvir indicates that a prolonged absorption time for the acyclovir was achieved (Table 1). Deconvolution analysis revealed that the absorption time of acyclovir, which in this study was 3.5 hours for Zovirax, was extended beyond 9 hours when using the Micropump technology. In addition, the plasma concentration profile following administration of Genvir remained above the plasma concentration observed following administration of Zovirax for between 5 and 24 hours post dose. The total amount of drug that reached the systemic circulation was statistically equivalent at 20% according to statistical analysis (90% confidence interval). In a Phase III multicenter, multinational, double-blind European trial, Genvir (600 mg dosed twice a day) was compared to Zovirax (200 mg, 5 times a day) in 424 immunocompetent RGH patients. No serious adverse events were observed with either drug treatment. Data analysis revealed that, 53.6% of the patients treated with Genvir were healed, whereas only 45.7% of the patients treated with Zovirax were cured ($p$ = 0.106, 95% CI).

**Table 1** Bioavailability Parameters for Genvir and Zovirax

| Treatment | $C_{max}$ (mg/L) | $T_{max}$ (hr) | $AUC_{tot}$ (mg/L hr) |
|---|---|---|---|
| Genvir (600 mg) | 0.62 | 5.06 | 5.23 |
| Zovirax (200 mg × 3) | 0.98 | 2.27 | 5.95 |
| | F relative Genvir/Zovirax = 86% | | |

Therefore it can be concluded that Genvir proved to be safe alternate for treatment of episodic RGH and was at least equally effective as Zovirax with the advantage of a more convenient twice a day dosage regimen.

## Antihyperglycemic Drugs

Metformin is an oral antihyperglycemic drug used for the treatment of non-insulin-dependent diabetes. In its IR form the drug is administered two to three times daily. Metformin is a highly soluble drug with a solubility of 330 mg/mL. The solubility of metformin is independent of pH and the drug can form large-sized crystals. The Micropump film-coating technology was applied directly to crystals of between 200 and 500 μm in size by spray coating in a fluidized bed drier. Metformin® XL provides SR of metformin over a 6–8 hours period. A Phase I clinical trial comparing Metformin XL to the IR product, Glucophage® was conducted in 12 healthy volunteers. The bioaviliability of 1000 mg Metformin XL was compared to that of two 500 mg Glucophage tablets. As was observed for Genvir the SR Metformin XL formulation had an increased $T_{max}$ value, which gives a clear indication of the extended absorption time from this product (Table 2). Deconvolution analysis of the plasma concentration profiles revealed that the time of absorption of metformin, which was equal to 6 hours for the IR formulation, was extended up to 12 hours for the SR Metformin XL formulation. In addition, the plasma concentration of metformin following administration of Metformin XL remained above the plasma concentration following administration of the IR dosage form for between 6 and 24 hours post dosing. The total amount of drug that reached the systemic circulation was equivalent for both formulations.

## Cardiovascular Drugs

The Micropump technology has recently been applied to the area of cardiovascular diseases. The FDA approved once-a-day Coreg CR™ (carvedilol phosphate) extended release capsule for the treatment of three key cardiovascular conditions such as hypertension, post-myocardial infarction and mild and severe heart failure in 2006. The Micropump technology allows

**Table 2** Bioavailability Parameters for Metformin XL and Glucophage

| Treatment | $C_{max}$ (mg/L) | $T_{max}$ (hr) | $AUC_{tot}$ (mg/L hr) |
|---|---|---|---|
| Metformin XL (1000 mg) | 0.99 | 7.30 | 9.62 |
| Glucophage (500 mg × 2) | 1.23 | 3.70 | 10.22 |
| F relative Metformin XL/Glucophage = 94% | | | |

Coreg CR™ to be dosed once daily in contrast to twice daily administration of the immediate-release product Coreg™ (carvedilol) tablets.

## CONCLUSIONS

The Micropump technology provides a means of modifying drug release profiles for existing drugs. It has been demonstrated that the Micropump formulation of the poorly soluble antiviral drug acyclovir, used for treatment of RGH is able to produce a SR profile, which can significantly modify the dosing regimen and establish a better safety profile and improved patient convenience. The absorption time of Genvir-based acyclovir was significantly increased while the bioavailability remained unchanged. In contrast to acyclovir, metformin is a highly soluble compound and it was demonstrated that the Micropump technology could be efficiently applied to this compound to produce a SR formulation, Metformin XL. Furthermore the absorption time of the drug was increased significantly when compared to that of the reference product, Glucophage. Overall, the technology presents a highly promising approach for the improved and sustained delivery of drugs that are absorbed primarily from the upper part of the GIT.

## ACKNOWLEDGMENTS

The contributions of Philippe Caisse, Frédéric Dargelas, Anne-Sophie Daviaud-Venet, Corinne Vialas, and Rémi Waché at Flamel Technologies are acknowledged. We are also thankful to Dr. Rafael Jorda (Flamel Technologies) for his critical comments to the manuscript.

## REFERENCES

1. Mustata G, Dinh SM. Approaches to oral drug delivery for challenging molecules. Critical Rev Ther Drug Carrier Syst 2006; 23:111–35.
2. Calcagno AM, Siahaan T. Physiological, biochemical and chemical barriers to oral drug delivery. In Wang B, Siahaan TJ, Soltero RA, eds. Drug Delivery: Principles and Applications. New York: Wiley, 2005: 15–28.
3. Carino GP, Mathiowitz E. Oral insulin delivery. Adv Drug Deliv Rev 1999; 35: 249–57.
4. Horer D, Dressman JB. Influence of physicochemical properties on dissulotion of drugs in the gastrointestinal tract. Adv Drug Deliv Rev 2001; 46:75–87.
5. Lipinski CA. Drug-like properties and the causes of poor solubility and poor permeability. J Pharmacol Toxicol Methods 2000; 44:235–49.
6. Mahato RI, Narang AS, Thoma L, Miller DD. Emerging trends in oral delivery of peptide and protein drugs. Crit Rev Ther Drug Carrier Syst 2003; 20:153–214.
7. Davis BG, Robinson MA. Drug delivery systems based on sugar-macro-molecule conjugates. Curr Opin Drug Discov Deliv 2005; 5:279–88.

8. Kodera Y, Matsushima A, Hiroto M, et al. Pegylation of proteins and bio-active substances for medical and technical applications. Progr Polymer Sci 1998; 23:1233–71.

9. Prokop A, Kozlov E, Newman GW, Newman MJ. Water-based nano-particulate polymeric system for protein delivery: permeability control and vaccine application. Biotechnol Bioeng 2002; 78:459–66.

10. Law D, Schmitt EA, Marsh KC, et al. Ritonavir-PEG 8000 amorphous solid dispersions: in vitro and in vivo evaluations. J Pharm Sci 2004; 93:563–70.

11. Keck CM, Muller RH. Drug nanocrystals of poorly soluble drugs produced by high pressure homogenisation. Eur J Pharm Biopharm 2006; 62:3–16.

12. Laskowski M Jr, Haessler HA, Miech RP, Penasky RJ, Lskowski M. Effect of trypsin inhibitor on passage of insulin across the intestinal barrier. Science 1958; 7:1115–6.

13. Tozaki H, Emi Y, Horisaka E, Fujita T, Yamamoto A, Muranishi S. Degradation of insulin and calcitonin and their protection by various protease inhibitors in rat caecal contents: implications in peptide delivery to the colon. J Pharm Pharmacol 1997; 49:164–8.

14. Yamamoto A, Taniguchi T, Rikyuu K, et al. Effects of various protease inhibitors on the intestinal absorption and degradation of insulin in rats. Pharm Res 1994; 11:1496–500.

15. Florence AT. The oral absorption of micro- and nanoparticles: neither exceptional nor unusual. Pharm Res 1997; 14:259–66.

16. Calvor A, Muller BW. Production of microparticles by high-pressure homog-enization. Pharm Dev Technol 1998; 3:297–305.

17. Aungst BJ. Intestinal Permeation enhancers. J Pharm Sci 2000; 89:429–42.

18. Bernkop-Schnurch A, Walker G. Multifunctional matrices for oral peptide delivery. Crit Rev Ther Drug Carrier Syst 2001; 18:459–501.

19. Bernkop-Schnurch A, Hoffer MH, Kafedjiiski K. Thiomers for oral delivery of hydrophilic macromolecular drugs. Expert Opin Drug Deliv 2004; 1:87–95.

20. Stuchlik M, Zak S. Lipid-based vehicle for oral drug delivery. Biomed Papers 2001; 145:17–26.

21. Wu Z-H, Ping Q-N, Wei Y, Lai J-M. Hypoglycemic efficacy of chitosan-coated insulin liposomes after oral administration in mice. Acta Pharmacol Sin 2004; 25:966–72.

22. Steiner SRR. Delivery systems for pharmacological agents encapsulated with protenoids. US Patent 4,925,673, 1990.

23. Van den Moorer G. Colon drug delivery. Expert Opin Drug Deliv 2006; 3: 111–25.

24. Autant P, Selles J-P, Soula G. 1996 Patent FR 2 725 623.

25. de Miranda P, Blum MR. Pharmacokinetics of acyclovir after intravenous and oral administration. J Antimicrob Chemother 1983; 12(Suppl. B):29–37.

# A Novel Microparticle Technology for Tailored Drug Release in the Gastrointestinal Tract

Richard A. Kendall, Emma L. McConnell, Sudaxshina Murdan, and Abdul W. Basit

*The School of Pharmacy, University of London, London, U.K.*

## INTRODUCTION

Conventional solid oral modified release dosage forms that use polymers to alter the time and/or site at which drug release occurs often result in variable and poor in vivo performance in humans. The variability can be attributed, in part, to the large size of normal dosage forms such as tablets, capsules, pellets or granules and the biopharmaceutic interaction of these dosage forms within the gastrointestinal tract (GIT). The human GIT is a physiologically heterogeneous environment and factors such as pH (1), fluid volume (2), and transit times (3) will impact on dosage form behavior. For example, the onset of drug release from enteric coated formulations is unpredictable due to delayed gastric emptying, particularly when dosing occurs after food (4), and the fact that such products may take up to 2 hours to disintegrate in the small intestine (5,6). In addition, modified release dosage forms designed for colon targeting have been found intact in the feces (7,8).

To overcome the aforementioned limitations, a platform microparticle technology has been developed which controls drug release more effectively than conventional formulations due to an increased surface area to volume ratio of the technology. Furthermore, the size and density of the microparticles facilitates their suspension in the liquid contents of the stomach promoting rapid and reproducible gastric emptying and that can overcome the variability in pharmacokinetics that is usually observed following administration of larger preparations.

## HISTORICAL DEVELOPMENT

Over the last 20 years, research into methods of fabrication of modified release microparticles, particularly those based on acrylic polymers, has focused on the use of spray drying and emulsification/solvent evaporation techniques. The use of spray drying for acrylic enteric polymers results in aggregated particles, which must be tableted to achieve control of drug release in acidic conditions. The applicability of emulsification/solvent evaporation methods, on the other hand, is limited by the need for homogenization, control of temperature, and the use of International Conference on Harmonisation (ICH) class II or III solvents in the manufacturing process. Furthermore, microparticles produced using the emulsification/solvent evaporation method fail to control drug release adequately at acidic pH and are often > 500 μm in diameter, a size that has shown variable gastrointestinal transit times similar to that observed for larger pellet and tablet dosage forms (9).

A patented and novel yet simple modified emulsification/solvent evaporation method for the fabrication of delayed and extended release microparticles has been developed. A conventional propeller is used to stir and produce a stable emulsion of a polymer/drug solution in an immiscible liquid paraffin/surfactant phase. The evaporation of solvent (ethanol in the vast majority of applications) proceeds at room temperature and results in the formation of spherical, monodisperse, unaggregated microparticles of diameters of < 50 μm, which are collected by filtration and cleaned of surface liquid paraffin.

## IN VITRO MICROPARTICLE CHARACTERIZATION AND EVALUATION OF DRUG RELEASE

The manufacturing method has been applied to a number of modified release polymers and polymer blends including, e.g., acrylic polymers such as Eudragit L55, L, S, RS, and cellulosic polymers such as cellulose acetate phthalate and ethylcellulose. A summary of the manufacturing and physical attributes of microparticles containing prednisolone 16.7% w/w (5 parts polymer:1 part drug) and prepared using Eudragit L that has a dissolution threshold of pH 6 for delivery to the upper small intestine and Eudragit S that has a dissolution threshold of pH 7 for delivery to the lower small intestine is listed in Table 1. The morphology of the prednisolone loaded Eudragit L and S microparticles as observed using scanning electron microscopy is shown in Figure 1.

**Table 1**  Summary of Manufacturing and Physical Properties of
Prednisolone-Loaded Eudragit L and S Microparticles

|  | Eudragit L microparticles | Eudragit S microparticles |
|---|---|---|
| Yield (%) | 96.4 | 97.1 |
| Encapsulation efficiency (%) | 86.4 | 90.0 |
| Size $dv_{(0.5)}$ (μm) | 31.3 | 50.1 |
| Monodispersity (span) | 0.68 | 0.61 |
| Density (g/cm$^3$) | 1.26 | 1.22 |
| Hausner ratio | 1.16 | 1.15 |
| Flow | Good | Good |

*Source*: From Ref. 10.

The potential for Eudragit L and S microparticles to deliver prednisolone, specifically to the upper and lower small intestine, respectively,
was demonstrated by the use of a pH-change dissolution method (USP
apparatus II, paddle rotation speed 100 rpm, fluid volume 900 mL). The pH
was varied from 1.2 to 6.8 for the assessment of the Eudragit L microparticles and from 1.2 to 7.4 for the Eudragit S microparticles at polymer:
drug loading ratios of 2.5:1 to 30:1. At all drug loadings, prednisolone
release was well controlled and found to be within the pharmacopoeial
limits of < 10% after 2 hours exposure at acidic pH. Furthermore the release
of prednisolone was complete within 5 minutes of the pH change. The
rapidity at which drug release above the threshold pH of the acrylic polymers occurred is primarily due to the large surface area to volume ratio of
the microparticles which is further enhanced by their ease of suspension in
the dissolution media, a factor that can be attributed to a favorable combination of particle size and density (Table 1). In addition, as no crystalline

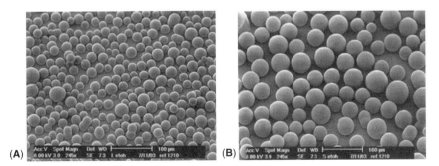

**Figure 1**  Scanning electron micrograph images of (**A**) prednisolone-loaded
Eudragit L microparticles and (**B**) prednisolone-loaded Eudragit S microparticles.

drug was detected by X-ray powder diffraction, it is thought that prednisolone is entrapped within the microparticles as an amorphous material which would also account for the rapid release and dissolution observed above the threshold pH of dissolution of the Eudragit polymers.

The microparticle technology has also been applied to drugs with different physicochemical properties and the in vitro dissolution profiles of Eudragit S microparticles in which prednisolone, budesonide, and bendroflumethiazide were incorporated at 5:1 drug loading are depicted in Figure 2.

The versatility of the technology is further demonstrated by the inclusion of water-insoluble polymers such as Eudragit RS or ethylcellulose into the system to achieve an extended release profile. The in vitro release profiles of prednisolone from microparticles manufactured using 1:1 blends of Eudragit S/ethylcellulose N7 and Eudragit S/Eudragit RS microparticles (pH 1.2–7.4) are shown in Figure 3. The release profiles depicted in Figure 3 show different sustained release patterns, which may be of therapeutic benefit in treatment of the inflammatory bowel diseases which affect large areas of the mucosa of the distal small intestine and colon.

## IN VIVO DRUG ABSORPTION STUDIES

Prednisolone absorption in rats following oral administration by gavage of Eudragit L and S microparticles was evaluated and compared to absorption of micronized prednisolone administered as a suspension. The time to maximum plasma concentration ($T_{max}$) was faster for the Eudragit L microparticles ($45 \pm 15\,min$) than the micronized suspension ($102 \pm 45\,min$), which was attributed to prednisolone being released rapidly from the microparticles in a highly soluble form close to the absorption site of prednisolone in the

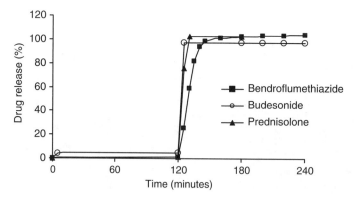

**Figure 2**   In vitro dissolution profiles (pH change) of bendroflumethiazide, budesonide, and prednisolone from Eudragit S microparticles (5:1 drug loading).

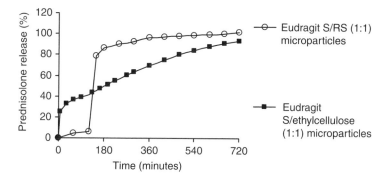

**Figure 3**   Prednisolone release from microparticles manufactured from 1:1 blends of Eudragit S/ethylcellulose N7 and Eudragit S/RS.

upper small intestine (12). The plasma concentration versus time profiles generated following administration of the prednisolone suspension and Eudragit L microparticles are shown in Figure 4 and provide in vivo proof of concept that the "enteric" microparticles are able to overcome the lag time that is usually observed prior to release of drug in the lumen of the small intestine following administration of conventional enteric coated products (5,6).

The relative bioavailability of prednisolone was found to be lower from the Eudragit S microparticles compared to Eudragit L microparticles and the control suspension (Fig. 4). The Eudragit S microparticles do not appear to deliver drug specifically to the ileo-colonic region of the rat and the $T_{max}$ of $72 \pm 24$ min suggests that the microparticles would be located

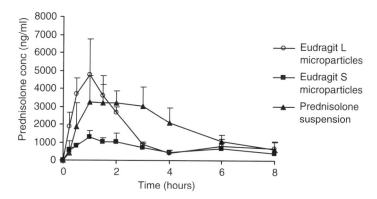

**Figure 4**   Plasma concentration versus time profiles of prednisolone following administration of Eudragit L and S microparticles and a micronized prednisolone suspension.

in the mid-small intestine at this time. The sustained absorption of prednisolone from the Eudragit S microparticles is probably due to release of prednisolone from close to the surface of the microparticles and the efficient absorption in the proximal small bowel and faster release but diminished absorption in the distal small bowel (11,12). The lack of fluid distally and the pH in the rat may have been problematic for this system (13). These findings highlight the need to evaluate pH-sensitive microparticles in a more relevant model and preferably man. A pharmacoscintigraphic study is planned in human volunteers, which is anticipated to unambiguously demonstrate the improved gastrointestinal transit and control of drug release from the Eudragit L and S microparticles.

## COMPETITIVE ADVANTAGE AND CONCLUSIONS

A universal method has been developed that is suitable for the fabrication of tailored release microparticles for drug delivery to the GIT. The method described herein overcomes the limitations of control of drug release that has been described for pH-sensitive microparticles produced by other methods, and furthermore does not require careful control of temperature or homogenization during manufacture and uses the relatively nontoxic solvent ethanol. These factors will facilitate scale-up of the production process for the manufacture of microparticles. The method produces monodisperse microparticles of diameter of $\leq 50\,\mu m$, which may result in improved GIT transit compared to that observed for conventional modified release dosage forms. Specific applications of this technology include the oral delivery of poorly soluble and basic actives which are known to precipitate in the lumen of the small intestine resulting in poor and variable bioavailability. Furthermore, the microparticles may be of particular benefit to pediatric patients, a patient sub-population for whom, currently, no modified release formulations are available, thereby allowing ease and flexibility of dosing and the possibility for taste masking, as well as control of drug release.

## REFERENCES

1. Evans DF, Pye G, Bramley R, Clark AG, Dyson TJ, Hardcastle JD. Measurement of gastrointestinal pH profiles in normal ambulant human subjects. Gut 1988; 29:1035–41.
2. Gotch F, Nadell J, Edelman IS. Gastrointestinal water and electrolytes. IV. The equilibration of deuterium oxide (D20) in gastrointestinal contents and the proportion of total body water (T.B.W.) in the gastrointestinal tract. J Clin Invest 1957; 36:289–96.
3. Davis SS, Hardy JG, Fara JW. Transit of pharmaceutical dosage forms through the small intestine. Gut 1986; 27:886–92.

4. Davis SS, Hardy JG, Taylor MJ, Stockwell A, Whalley DR, Wilson CG. The in-vivo evaluation of an osmotic device (Osmet) using gamma scintigraphy. J Pharm Pharmacol 1984; 36:740–2.
5. Hardy JG, Evans DF, Zaki I, Clark AG, Tønnesen HH, Gamst ON. Evaluation of an enteric coated naproxen tablet using gamma scintigraphy and pH monitoring. Int J Pharm 1987; 37:245–50.
6. Cole ET, Scott RA, Connor AL, et al. Enteric coated HPMC capsules designed to achieve intestinal targeting. Int J Pharm 2002; 231:83–95.
7. Tuleu C, Basit AW, Waddington WA, Ell PJ, Newton JM. Colonic delivery of 4-aminosalicylic acid using amylose-ethylcellulose-coated hydroxypropylmethyl-cellulose capsules. Aliment Pharmacol Ther 2002; 16:1771–9.
8. Ibekwe VC, Liu F, Fadda HM, et al. An investigation into the in vivo performance variability of pH responsive polymers for ileo-colonic drug delivery using gamma scintigraphy in humans. J Pharm Sci 2006; 95:2760–6.
9. Clarke GM, Newton JM, Short MD. Gastrointestinal transit of pellets of differing size and density. Int J Pharm 1993; 100:81–92.
10. Carr RL. Evaluating flow properties of solids. Chem Eng 1965; 72:163–8.
11. Kararli TT. Comparison of the gastrointestinal anatomy, physiology, and biochemistry of humans and commonly used laboratory animals. Biopharm Drug Dispos 1995; 16:351–80.
12. Nakayama A, Eguchi O, Hatakeyama M, Saitoh H, Takada M. Different absorption behaviors among steroid hormones due to possible interaction with P-glycoprotein in the rat small intestine. Biol Pharm Bull 1999; 22:535–8.
13. McConnell EL, Basit AW, Murdan S. Measurements of the gastrointestinal pH, fluid and lymphoid tissue, and implications for in-vivo experiments. J Pharm Pharmacol 2008; 60:63–70.

# 25

# Lipid Nanoparticles (SLN, NLC, LDC) for the Enhancement of Oral Absorption

Cornelia M. Keck, Aiman H. Hommoss, and Rainer H. Müller

*Department of Pharmaceutical Technology, Biopharmaceutics, and Nutricosmetics, The Free University of Berlin, Berlin, Germany*

## INTRODUCTION

Small-sized particulate carriers (microparticles and nanoparticles) are under investigation to enhance oral drug absorption and/or to modulate blood concentration profiles for optimized therapy by controlling drug release from such particles. A further potential benefit of development includes increased retention of formulations in the gastrointestinal tract (GIT). This in turn provides a longer time for drug absorption to occur and is especially useful in the case of active pharmaceutical ingredients (API) that have a narrow absorption window. A slower passage through the absorption window may enhance the bioavailability of an API. One approach to further increase the bioavailability is the combination of mucoadhesive polymers with particulates, which can be achieved by coating and/or stabilizing the particles with mucoadhesive layers such as polyacrylates or chitosan (1,2).

In a pharmaceutical context microparticles by definition are between 1 and 1000 µm (1 mm) in size and therefore include small pellets, polymeric microparticles and micronized drug powders. The reduction in particle size imparts special properties to the particles and with decreasing particle size adhesion to surfaces/membranes increases (3,4). In addition, API release from particles and the velocity of API dissolution increases with decreasing particle size due to an increased surface area. This is the principle of a formulation approach used for micronized Class II drugs or poorly water soluble actives of the biopharmaceutical classification system (BCS). Pellets and micronized powders have been commercially available for many decades. However, the success of using polymeric microparticles for oral delivery has been quite limited.

Decreasing particle size from the micro- to the nano-dimension imparts additional properties to materials as a result of changes to the physicochemical properties of materials. The use of nanotechnology permits the design and fabrication of new products with specific attributes. In pharmaceutical technology, this has been exploited by moving from micronized powders to nanonized powders thereby producing nanocrystals of API. Consequently an increase in the dissolution velocity $dc/dt$ occurs due to the increase in surface area $A$ on application of the Noyes-Whitney equation. Furthermore, saturation solubility increases, leading to steeper concentration gradients between the gut lumen and the systemic circulation (4,5). The increased saturation solubility $c_s$ further increases the dissolution velocity. The first patents describing the technologies for the production of drug nanocrystals were filed at the beginning of the nineties (6–10). Rapamune (Wyeth) was the first commercially available pharmaceutical nanocrystal product and was launched in 2000. Subsequently four additional products have been launched and these are Emend® (Merck), Tricor (Abbott), Triglide (Sciele Pharma Inc.) and Megace ES (Par Pharmaceuticals). A detailed description of the technology and the special product properties can be found in the literature (11). Nanocrystals are a smart formulation technology for poorly soluble API and for which micronization does not provide sufficient advantage as these compounds exhibit extremely low solubility and dissolution velocities (11).

Nanocrystal technology is applicable to many BCS Class II drugs. However, for some molecules the presence of lipids is of further benefit due to increased absorption and greater bioavailability. It is well known that lipophilic vitamins such as vitamin A and E are better absorbed from the GIT in the presence of lipids. Therefore even in case of a diet, low calorie salads should be prepared with some oil in order to promote the absorption of these vitamins. Drug-loaded lipid nanoparticles provide an interesting alternative to drug nanocrystals in situations in which API nanocrystals do not result in adequate bioavailability and where lipids are known to promote the absorption of the respective API. In addition lipid nanoparticles provide flexibility in modulating drug release since the lipid is the release-controlling matrix material. API nanocrystals are free of any matrix material, as they are 100% API. Therefore the rate of release is a function of the dissolution velocity which in turn is a function of dissolution pressure and crystal size. Dissolution can only be controlled to a limited extent by the particle size and the related surface area. Therefore lipid nanoparticles are also of interest for their potential to control the release of API (Fig. 1).

This chapter provides a theoretical background for absorption enhancement by lipids and introduces three types of lipid nanoparticles with a solid matrix. Furthermore the incorporation of lipophilic in addition to hydrophilic drugs is discussed.

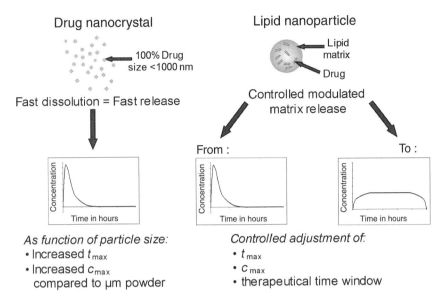

**Figure 1** Difference in effect between APIs formulated as a nanocrystal or as lipid particle matrix system with controlled-release capabilities.

## LIPID ABSORPTION ENHANCING EFFECT

The effect of the molecular structure of lipids on absorption (12–17) using different drugs, such as danazol (18) and halofantrine (19), has been investigated and it is preferable to use glycerides with longer fatty acid chains (chain length C18) (19). In addition to achieve the maximal effect, the API should be closely associated with the lipid, which means it should be dissolved or at least dispersed in the lipid phase. Therefore administration of API and lipid separately obviously reduces the absorption enhancing effect of the lipid. Following the intake of microscopic droplets of oil such as in vinaigrette salad dressing the oil will be dispersed further during the digestion process. Relatively large oil droplets ranging from a few hundred μm up to 1 mm are dispersed by surface active agents in the gut or more specifically be the bile salts. Absorption is enhanced with a decrease in the size of the oil droplets. An example of the effect of the degree of oil dispersion on resultant bioavailability is provided by the first generation cyclosporine product, Sandimmune (Novartis previously Sandoz). Cyclosporine is dissolved in corn oil and consequently the bioavailability is highly dependent on the presence or absence of bile salts. High concentrations of bile salts result in more effective dispersion of the oil and subsequently bioavailability is high. Conversely a lack of bile salts results in a dramatic decrease in bioavailability (20–23). Depending on the status of the patient, the bioavailability of cyclosporine from the Sandimmune product varied between 20% and 60% (23). Therefore to achieve an increase in oral absorption the API should be closely associated with the lipid, ideally it must be dissolved in the lipid, which should be as finely dispersed as possible.

Both prerequisites for optimal absorption enhancement can be realized when using lipid nanoparticles. With a mean particle size of typically between 200 and 300 nm the lipid is extremely finely dispersed and distinctly below droplet sizes for digested oils which is typically a few micrometers in size (24). In addition, the lipophilic API is dissolved or more correctly molecularly dispersed in the particle matrix.

The basic mechanism of absorption enhancement that is valid for oil droplets and lipid nanoparticles within a solid particle matrix (25) is depicted in Figure 2.

Lipid nanoparticles are degraded in a similar manner to liquid lipid droplets, by the enzymes in the gut (26). Lipid nanoparticles are initially dispersed in the gut and subsequently lipase and the co-lipase molecules anchor themselves onto the particle surface. Triglycerides are enzymatically modified to form surface active diglycerides and in particular, monoglycerides. The monoglycerides form micelles on the particle surface and during micelle formation molecularly dispersed drug is solubilized in the micelles. Bile salts then interact with the lipid micelles leading to the formation of mixed micelles that mediate lipid absorption and associated API present. Therefore the API is absorbed together with the lipid. This process

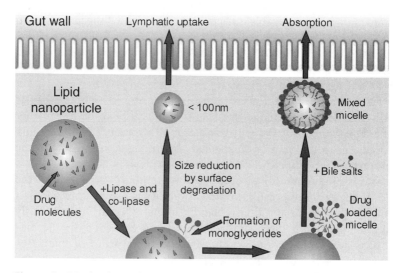

**Figure 2** Mechanism of absorption enhancement by ultrafine dispersed lipids as either a nanoemulsion, or solid nanoparticles in the gut.

is termed the "Trojan horse effect" (25,27). Furthermore lymphatic uptake of small lipid nanoparticles is also possible and has been reported (28).

## SOLID LIPID NANOPARTICLES, NANOSTRUCTURED LIPID CARRIERS, AND LIPID-DRUG CONJUGATE

The first generation of lipid nanoparticles, the so-called "solid lipid nano-particles" (SLNs) were developed in the early 1990s. SLN can be derived from o/w emulsions by exchanging the liquid lipid (oil) for a lipid that is solid at body temperatures. SLN have specific characteristics and are pre-pared from a single solid lipid such as tristearin, Compritol, or waxes such as beeswax or carnauba wax.

At the time of development of SLN, two parallel developments of different production technologies were evident. High pressure homoge-nization (HPH) developed by Müller et al. and Lucks and Müller (29,30) and a microemulsion method developed by Gasco (31). During the past decade additional production methods for SLN have been developed and are described in detail elsewhere (32).

Industrially the most feasible production technology for SLN is HPH. Briefly, the lipid is melted at approximately $5°-10°C$ above its melting point after which the API is dissolved in the molten lipid and the mixture is then dispersed in a hot surfactant solution maintained at an identical temperature with high speed stirring. The resultant coarse pre-emulsion is then passed through a high pressure homogenizer in a process that is identical to the homogenization of milk. Homogenization is performed with a temperature controlled homogenizer and a hot nanoemulsion is formed. Subsequent cooling leads to the re-crystallization of the lipid and the oil droplets solidify and form solid lipid nanoparticles. Figure 3 depicts an atomic force microscopy (AFM) picture of an SLN. The production process is the same for all three particle types and only the lipids used for the particle production are varied.

There are limitations in the use of SLN such as for example the drug loading capacity. In particular when using highly purified lipids such as tristearin the SLN forms a relatively perfect lipid matrix upon cooling (34) and has only a limited number of imperfections for the accommodation of API. Therefore, with increasing perfection of the lipid particle matrix or crystallinity there is a danger of expulsion of the API from the SLNs, leading to formation of crystals of the API in the aqueous phase of the emulsion. The loading capacity can be improved by using of the second generation of lipid nanoparticles or nanostructured lipid carriers (NLCs) in which the formation of a perfect lipid crystal is avoided by the use of blends of spatially different lipids in the particle production process. In contrast to SLNs being made from a single solid lipid, the NLCs are produced from blends of solid lipids with a liquid lipid (oil). The resultant

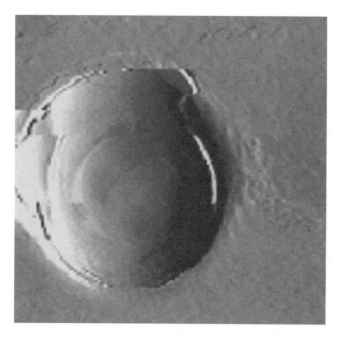

**Figure 3** AFM picture of an SLN showing a single particle. *Abbreviations*: AFM, atomic force microscopy; SLN, solid lipid nanoparticles. *Source*: From Ref. 33.

blends are still solid at body temperature; however, glycerides possessing fatty acid chains that are different in the length can be seen as "mixed" glycerides which are not able to form a perfect crystal lattice. These particles contain a high number of imperfections in which the API can be accommodated thereby promoting a higher drug loading. The "perfectness" of the NLC system is the "imperfectness" of the resultant crystal lattice. Figure 4 provides a schematic representation of the differences between the three lipid particle types.

SLNs and NLCs are preferentially suitable for the incorporation of lipophilic API since the lipophilic matrix is best able to dissolve molecules similar in chemical nature. However, hydrophilic API can be incorporated into SLN and NLC but must be solubilized prior to incorporation. Solubilization is achieved by use of the solubilization effect of surface active monoglycerides or alternatively the use of other w/o surfactants in particular those with a low hydrophilic/lipophilic balance (HLB) values. In addition, surfactant mixtures may be added to the lipid melt to effect solubilization of API. However the loading capacity for hydrophilic molecules is limited and therefore it is only feasible to incorporate high potency API such as erythropoietin (EPO) which has recommended daily doses in the range of approximately 10–30 μg.

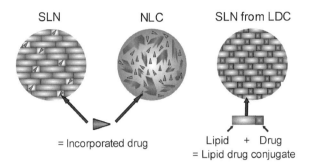

**Figure 4** Structure of SLN made from a single solid lipid (*left*) with almost perfect crystalline structure limiting the drug loading, NLC made from blend of solid lipid and liquid lipid with many imperfections (*middle*) and lipid-drug conjugate (LDC) nanoparticles from conjugates of API with a lipid (*right*). Loading with lipophilic drugs (*triangles*) is highest for NLC. LDC are ideal carriers for hydrophilic actives (*squares in LDC*). *Abbreviations*: LDC, lipid-drug conjugate; NLC, nonostructured lipid carriers; SLN, solid lipid nanoparticles.

Lysozyme as a model peptide was successfully incorporated into SLN (35,36) at a loading capacity of only 500 µg/g of lipid. This load is considered sufficient for incorporation of a highly potent API. Loading of hydrophilic drugs into lipid nanoparticles has been achieved by the development of the lipid-drug conjugate (LDC) nanoparticles and a schematic of these systems is also depicted in Figure 4. The water soluble API is transferred to a poorly water soluble lipophilic compound by conjugating it with lipid by simple salt formation or by covalent linkage (37,38). An example of such a system is exemplified by diminazene diaceturate (38). Most of the lipid conjugates melt at between 50°C and 100°C. Therefore, the conjugate can be processed to form lipid nanoparticles using the same process as that used for the preparation of SLN except that instead of the solid lipid the conjugate is used in the production process. The conjugate is melted, dispersed in a hot surfactant solution and subsequently the resultant emulsion is homogenized. Depending on the molecular weight ratio of lipid and API in the conjugate, loadings of up to between 30% and 40% w/w hydrophilic API are possible.

## FORMULATIONS WITH LIPOPHILIC DRUGS

Cyclosporine was selected as a model candidate for the formulation of SLN for oral administration. The first commercial cyclosporine product, Sandimmune has variable oral bioavailability. A second generation product, cyclosporine microemulsion Sandimmune Optoral/Neoral has distinctly lower variability in bioavailability but has an undesired peak plasma concentration of over 1000 ng/mL that has been implicated in nephrotoxicity (23,39). In an attempt to combine the low advantages of the low variability and low peak plasma concentrations of the "old" and the "new" commercial cyclosporine formulations cyclosporine-loaded SLN were developed.

Cyclosporine SLN were prepared using the lipid, Imwitor 900 at a particle concentration in the SLN suspension of 10%. The SLN were stabilized with 2.5% Tagat S and 0.5% sodium cholate. Sodium cholate was being selected for use since bile salts promote cyclosporine absorption. Oral bioavailability was studied in vivo using a pig model (40). The SLN were administered as a suspension via a gastric catheter. Administration of a suspension was considered appropriate in order to avoid any dosage form effects on absorption such as disintegration and dissolution from a tablet formulation. The Sandimmune microemulsion was used as the reference and a cyclosporine drug nanocrystal suspension was prepared and administered as a second reference.

The plasma profiles generated following administration of the aforementioned formulations are depicted in Figure 5. A typical plasma profile was obtained following administration of the Sandimmune microemulsion with a peak plasma concentration occurring at 2 hours and the plasma concentration being in the therapeutic window up to approximately

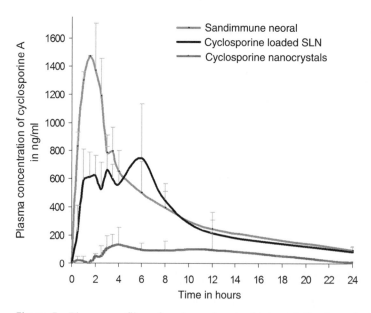

**Figure 5** Plasma profiles of cyclosporine A obtained following administration of Sandimmune microemulsion, cyclosporine loaded solid lipid nanoparticles and cyclosporine drug nanocrystals.

12 hours. Cyclosporine SLN achieved a similar plasma concentration in the therapeutic window as the microemulsion, showed also similar low variation in bioavailability, but avoided the undesired peak plasma concentration. Surprisingly the drug nanocrystal formulation exhibited an extremely low bioavailability.

The lipid nanoparticles proved to be effective for the enhancement of oral absorption and the plasma profile can be modulated due to prolonged release of API from the lipid nanoparticles. The drug nanocrystal formulation was not sufficiently bioavailable for reasons not discussed here despite the fact that for certain drugs lipid nanoparticles are a superior formulation approach.

Further examples relating to the advantages, properties, performance and possible applications of SLN and NLC have been published (32,35,40–45). The in vivo performance of fenofibrate loaded SLN in comparison to other fenofibrate formulations including fenofibrate nano- and microsuspensions with different excipients such as hydroxyl ethyl-cellulose in which lipid nanoparticles showed similar bioavailability and pharmacokinetics data when compared to the nanocrystal formulation have been reported and these data are summarized in Table 1 (45). It is therefore possible to use lipid nanoparticles as a competitive product to the nano-crystal-based Tricor (Abbott) that has a similar plasma profile but avoids intellectual property issues relating to the nanocrystals.

Lipid nanoparticles can also be used to formulate nutraceuticals (46). Fish oils are used in nutraceutical products because of their content of $\omega$-3 and $\omega$-6 unsaturated fatty acids and their beneficial effects in the modulation of fluidity and function of cell membranes, modulation of the inflammatory response, and because they have been shown to be of benefit in treating cardiovascular diseases, Alzheimer's disease, depression, and

**Table 1**  In Vivo Pharmacokinetic Parameters of Fenofibrate Nanocrystals versus Fenofibrate Lipid Nanoparticles

| Formulation | DissoCubes® | SLN | Micro-suspension + Sirupus Simplex | Micro-suspension + HEC |
|---|---|---|---|---|
| $AUC_{0-22hr}$ | $2239.4 \pm 533.0$ | $2170.3 \pm 874.7$ | $1148.0 \pm 717.9$ | $1745.5 \pm 512.5$ |
| $AUC_{0-8hr}$ | $1273.3 \pm 171.0$ | $1163.0 \pm 341.0$ | $340.3 \pm 161.5$ | $628.6 \pm 140.1$ |
| $AUC_{0-inf}$ | $2417.3 \pm 627.3$ | $2438.2 \pm 1024.2$ | $1301.9 \pm 834.4$ | $1906.6 \pm 468.8$ |
| $C_{max}$ | $222.7 \pm 21.9$ | $200.7 \pm 29.9$ | $96.9 \pm 62.4$ | $137.7 \pm 43.4$ |
| $T_{max}$ | $1.5 \pm 0.3$ | $2.3 \pm 1.2$ | $7.2 \pm 3.0$ | $7.3 \pm 3.1$ |
| $MRT_{0-22h}$ | $6.9 \pm 0.9$ | $7.2 \pm 0.9$ | $9.2 \pm 1.2$ | $9.1 \pm 0.3$ |

*Source*: From Ref. 45.

cancer (47–53). NLC in which fish oil represented the liquid lipid in the formulation have been produced. The fish oil was blended with the high melting lipid, Dynasan 118. This allowed 80% (w/w) oil to be incorporated in the particle matrix whilst retaining a melting point for the blend above the body temperature (54). Encapsulation of the fish oil into NLC reduced the unpleasant odor, and to facilitate the oral administration of the fish oil, NLC were transformed into pellets. The pellet excipient mixture was wetted with an aqueous NLC suspension and the plastic mass obtained was then extruded. If desired, the pellets can be coated with an enteric polymer to enable targeted release in the intestine, thereby further minimizing the unpleasant taste associated with regurgitation (55).

## FORMULATION OF HYDROPHILIC DRUGS

As outlined previously the incorporation of hydrophilic drugs into SLN is only possible by use of the solubilization effects of either surface active monoglycerides that are present in the lipid, or alternatively by addition of surfactants such as Span (Fig. 6). Drug loading is usually limited and the effects of processing conditions such as elevated temperature and high pressure of the homogenization process must be considered. In particular, the effects of the lipid environment on API conformation and related activity of the API must be evaluated. Lysozyme was extracted from SLN and its activity checked by using the *Micrococcus lysolydeikticus* assay and it was determined that the lysozyme retained most of its activity (90.5–95.2%) (36).

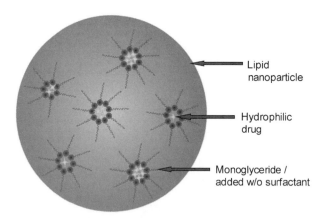

**Figure 6**   Solubilization of a hydrophilic API in lipophilic SLN mediated by use of surface active agents. *Abbreviation*: SLN, solid lipid nanoparticles.

When using HPH or alternatively the microemulsion method for lipid nanoparticle production, the API to be incorporated must be dissolved in the lipid blend or a hot lipid microemulsion, respectively. The solubility of hydrophilic molecules in lipid media is generally low and a higher loading may be achieved by modification of the production method and application of an emulsion-diffusion process. This relatively simple process entails selection of an organic solvent in which both the lipid and hydrophilic API have sufficiently high solubility. Organic liquids are preferred if they have some degree of miscibility with water. Examples of suitable solvents include isobutyric acid (IBA) and isovaleric acid (IVA) (56,57). At the commencement of the process the aqueous and organic solvents are saturated with each other following which the organic phase is dispersed in the water phase. The dispersion results in the formation of an o/w emulsion and the results of saturation ensure that a thermodynamic equilibrium is maintained. The o/w emulsion is then diluted with water and consequently the solvent partitions into the large volume of the water phase due to its solubility in the water resulting in the precipitation of lipid thereby encapsulating the hydrophilic API. A load of 0.92% w/w of insulin was achieved with this method of manufacture of lipid particles (56). Interestingly, following extraction of insulin from the lipid nanoparticles and testing its in vivo activity versus unprocessed bovine insulin, the extracted insulin showed identical activity in vivo and blood glucose levels were reduced to the same extent and for the same duration (57).

Furthermore the insulin that was incorporated into the SLN was protected to a large extent from enzymatic degradation by enzymes present in the water phase. This finding suggests that insulin-loaded lipid nanoparticles may be suitable for the development of an oral insulin product.

There is always the potential for hydrophilic actives to partition between the organic and the water phase when forming the o/w emulsion. Consequently there is a certain loss of the API to the aqueous phase. Despite the potential loss entrapment efficiencies of 80% are possible (56). The loss of API to the aqueous phase appears to be acceptable when considering the potential therapeutic benefits of an oral insulin formulation. A certain loss of API can also be accommodated when considering that recombinant human insulin is available in sufficient quantities.

## FINAL ORAL DOSAGE FORMS

For oral drug delivery the preferred dosage form should be solid such as either a tablet or a capsule. For the production of tablets, lipid nanoparticle suspensions can be used as a granulation fluid if a wet granulation process is considered to be appropriate. In order to achieve success it is preferred that a relatively high particle concentration is used with as little water as possible. Lipid nanoparticle suspensions can also be used as wetting agents for an excipient mass in the production of pellets (Fig. 7).

The first production of pellets from lipid nanoparticle suspensions was described about 10 years ago (58,59). In order for such dosages forms to perform adequately and to benefit from the special properties of SLN it is necessary to ensure that the lipid nanoparticles are released in a non-aggregated, finely dispersed form. Control of the rate of release of the nanoparticles from solid dosage forms can be achieved by evaluation of particle size. A simple approach for success involves the production of pellets using only water soluble excipients such as lactose (58,59). Following dissolution of the excipients the remaining lipid nanoparticles can be analyzed by laser diffractometry.

Alternative formulations include powders for reconstitution (e.g., sachets) or the use of an aqueous suspension itself. In the latter case the suspensions need to exhibit an appropriate physical stability over the shelf life of the product, which is in general 3 years. In case this cannot be achieved for whatever reasons, a lyophilized or spray-dried product can be produced and be reconstituted to yield a suspension for use within 2–4 weeks.

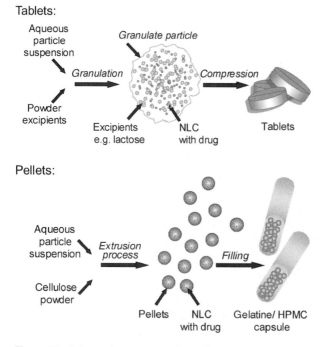

**Figure 7**   Schematic representation of the manufacture of tablets and pellet filled capsules from aqueous lipid nanoparticle suspensions.

Another approach is to produce a highly viscous NLC cream that is then packaged in tubes. Dosing can be performed via the length of an extruded string or alternatively via use of a medicine measure. One approach that was used for fish oil loaded lipid nanoparticles was the production of a paste and dispersing it in soft drinks. For nutraceutical supplements this formulation is acceptable and practical.

## INDUSTRIAL PRODUCTION OF DRUG-LOADED LIPID NANOPARTICLE SUSPENSIONS

The production of lipid nanoparticle suspensions is in principle relatively easy. However, there is a general tendency in industry to outsource the production of such "intermediate" products. The first dermal cosmetic NLC products have been launched. Cosmetic companies can buy API-loaded lipid nanoparticles as ready-made particle concentrates for use in the production of finished products. For example the company Dr. Rimpler GmbH (www.rimpler.de) manufactures such particles under the PharmaSol license as a final product and pharmaceutical companies may purchase drug-loaded concentrated lipid nanoparticle suspensions from Dr. Rimpler GmbH. As excipients they would necessarily undergo the normal internal quality control after which they could be processed further to form oral dosage forms. Dr. Rimpler GmbH is also approved for the production of dermal pharmaceutical products. In conclusion, pharmaceutical companies can outsource the complete production of a pharmaceutical product including having it packaged.

## LIPID NANOPARTICLE PRODUCTS ON THE MARKET

The time-to-market is usually much shorter for cosmetic products than for pharmaceutical products and therefore some formulation technologies and carrier systems were first used in the cosmetic field prior to the pharmaceutical arena. An example in which this is true is evidenced by the use of liposomes in the second half of the 1980s (60–62). Liposomal products appeared on the cosmetic market in 1986 in the form of the product Capture™ (Dior) and was first used in the pharmaceutical field market around 1990 in a product Alveofact® (Boehringer–Ingelheim) (63). The success of this product revealed that liposomal formulations that were stable could be made. Dr. Rimpler GmbH introduced the first two NLC products in Europe in Munich in October 2005, and these were Nanorepair Q10 cream and serum. A third product, Nanovital day cream, was launched in June 2006. The market introduction by Amore Pacific of the first three products in Asia took place in Seoul in September 2006 and the products were SuperVital cream, serum and eye cream. The products were tested with regard to physical stability of the particles, chemical stability of actives and also regarding skin tolerability and cosmetic efficiency. The success of these products will pave the way for pharmaceutical products in the near future.

## CONCLUSION AND PERSPECTIVES

The lipid nanoparticle systems SLN, NLC, and LDC are new carrier technologies that provide new options for oral drug delivery. The simplicity of the technology is what makes it attractive to use as these systems are more likely to enter the market and benefit patients. Large scale production is an essential prerequisite for market introduction and manufacturability on this scale has been established. A further advantage is that a wide range of excipients that have an acceptable regulatory status for oral use are available. All excipients and surfactants/stabilizers used in tablet and capsule technology can be considered thereby reducing regulatory hurdles. It should be noted that this delivery system is of main interest for API that require the use of medium or low doses and doses of 400 mg cannot be formulated into a single tablet since in addition to the API, appropriate quantities of lipid and tablet forming excipients would be necessary.

In vivo data are available and prove the efficiency of lipid based systems in general and in particular data using lipid nanoparticles indicate the value of these technologies. It is expected that the in vivo data will facilitate the development of this technology to create products for patient use.

## REFERENCES

1. Cano-Cebrian MJ, Zornoza T, Granero L, Polache A, et al. Intestinal absorption enhancement via the paracellular route by fatty acids, chitosans and others: a target for drug delivery. Curr Drug Deliv 2005; 2(1):9–22.
2. Chopra S, Mahdi S, Kaur J, et al. Advances and potential applications of chitosan derivatives as mucoadhesive biomaterials in modern drug delivery. J Pharm Pharmacol 2006; 58(8):1021–32.
3. Kulvanich P, Stewart PJ. The effect of particle size and concentration on the adhesive characteristics of a model drug-carrier interactive system. J Pharm Pharmacol 1987; 39(9):673–8.
4. Müller RH. Nanosuspensionen—eine neue Formulierung für schwerlösliche Arzneistoffe. In Müller RH, Hildebrand, GE, eds. Pharmazeutische Technologie: Moderne Arzneiformen. Stuttgart: Wissenschaftliche Verlagsgesellschaft, 1998: 393–400.
5. Möschwitzer J, Müller RH. Drug nanocrystals—the universal formulation approach for poorly soluble drugs. In: Thassu D, Deleers M, Pathak Y, eds. Nanoparticulate Drug Delivery Systems: Recent Trends and Emerging Technologies. Informa Healthcare, 2007. Adv Drug Deliv Rev 59(6):419–26.
6. Liversidge GG, Cundy KC, Bishop JF, Czekai DA. Surface modified drug nanoparticles, in United States Patent 5,145,684. 1992, Sterling Drug Inc. (New York, NY): USA.

7. List M, Sucker H. Pharmaceutical colloidal hydrosols for injection, in GB Patent 2200048. 1988, Sandoz LTD. CH: GB.
8. Sucker H, Gassmann P. Improvements in pharmaceutical compositions, in GB Patent 2269536A. 1994, Sandoz LTD. CH: GB.
9. Violante MR, Fischer HW. Method for making uniformly-sized particles from insoluble compounds, in United States Patent 4,997,454. 1991, The University of Rochester: USA.
10. Müller RH, Becker R, Kruss B, Peters K. Pharmaceutical nanosuspensions for medicament administration as systems with increased saturation solubility and rate of solution. in United States Patent 5,858,410. 1999: USA.
11. Müller RH, Junghanns JU. Drug nanocrystals/nanosuspensions for the delivery of poorly soluble drugs. In: Torchilin VP, ed. Nanoparticulates as Drug Carriers. London: Imperial College Press, 2006: 307–28.
12. Humberstone AJ, Porter CJ, Charman WN. A physicochemical basis for the effect of food on the absolute oral bioavailability of halofantrine. J Pharm Sci 1996; 85(5):525–9.
13. Porter CJ, Charman WN. In vitro assessment of oral lipid based formulations. Adv Drug Deliv Rev 2001; 50 (Suppl. 1):S127–47.
14. Kossena GA, Boyd BJ, Porter CJ, et al. Separation and characterization of the colloidal phases produced on digestion of common formulation lipids and assessment of their impact on the apparent solubility of selected poorly water-soluble drugs. J Pharm Sci 2003; 92(3):634–48.
15. Sek L, Porter CJ, Charman WN. Characterisation and quantification of medium chain and long chain triglycerides and their in vitro digestion products, by HPTLC coupled with in situ densitometric analysis. J Pharmaceut Biomed 2001; 25(3–4):651–61.
16. Sek L, Porter CJ, Kaukonen AM, et al. Evaluation of the in-vitro digestion profiles of long and medium chain glycerides and the phase behaviour of their lipolytic products. J Pharm Pharmacol 2002; 54(1):29–41.
17. Vine DF, et al. Effect of dietary fatty acids on the intestinal permeability of marker drug compounds in excised rat jejunum. J Pharm Pharmacol 2002; 54(6):809–19.
18. Charman WN, Rogge MC, Boddy AW, et al. Effect of food and a mono-glyceride emulsion formulation on danazol bioavailability. J Clin Pharmacol 1993; 33(4):381–6.
19. Caliph SM, Charman WN, Porter CJ. Effect of short-, medium-, and long-chain fatty acid-based vehicles on the absolute oral bioavailability and intestinal lymphatic transport of halofantrine and assessment of mass balance in lymph-cannulated and non-cannulated rats. J Pharm Sci 2000; 89(8):1073–84.
20. Reymond JP. In vitro/in vivo Modelle zur Absorption von Ciclosporin A. Dissertation, 1986.
21. Reymond JP, Sucker H, Vonderscher J. In vivo model for ciclosporin intestinal absorption in lipid vehicles. Pharm Res 1988; 5(10):677–9.
22. Reymond JP, Sucker H. In vitro model for ciclosporin intestinal absorption in lipid vehicles. Pharm Res 1988; 5(10):673–6.
23. Meinzer A, Müller E, Vonderscher J. Perorale Microemulsionsformulierung— Sandimmun Optoral®/Neoral®. In: Müller RH, Hildebrand, GE, eds.

Pharmazeutische Technologie: Moderne Arzneiformen. Stuttgart: Wissenschaftliche Verlagsgesellschaft, 1998: 169–77.

24. Armand M, Borel P, Pasquier B, et al. Physicochemical characteristics of emulsions during fat digestion in human stomach and duodenum. Am J Physiol 1996; 271(1 Pt 1):G172–83.
25. Muller RH, Keck CM. Challenges and solutions for the delivery of biotech drugs—a review of drug nanocrystal technology and lipid nanoparticles. J Biotechnol 2004; 113(1–3):151–70.
26. Olbrich C, Muller RH. Enzymatic degradation of SLN-effect of surfactant and surfactant mixtures. Int J Pharm 1999; 180(1):31–9.
27. Virgil, The Aeneid. appr. 29-19 AC.
28. Cavalli R, Bargoni A, Podio V, et al. Duodenal administration of solid lipid nanoparticles loaded with different percentages of tobramycin. J Pharm Sci 2003; 92(5):1085–94.
29. Müller RH, Mehnert W, Lucks JS, et al. Solid lipid nanoparticles (SLN)—an alternative colloidal carrier system for controlled drug delivery. Eur J Pharm Biopharm 1995; 41(1):62–9.
30. Lucks JS, Müller RH. Medication vehicles made of solid lipid particle (solid lipid nanospheres—SLN), in EP0000605497. 1996, Medac: EP.
31. Gasco MR. Method for producing solid lipid microspheres having a narrow size distribution, in US Patent US 5,250, 236. 1993: USA.
32. Müller RH, Souto EB, Göppert T, et al. Production of biofunctionalized solid lipid nanoparticles (SLN) for site-specific drug delivery. In: Kumar C, ed. Nanotechnologies for the Life Science. Weinheim: Wiley-VCH Verlag GmbH, 2007: 287–303.
33. Dingler A. Feste Lipid-Nanopartikel als kolloidale Wirkstoffträgersysteme zur dermalen Applikation. PhD thesis, 1998.
34. Bunjes H, Westesen K, Koch MHJ. Crystallization tendency and polymorphic transitions in triglyceride nanoparticles. Inte J Pharm 1996; 129:59–73.
35. Almeida AJ, Souto E. Solid lipid nanoparticles as a drug delivery system for peptides and proteins. Adv Drug Deliv Rev 2007; 59(6): 478–90.
36. Almeida AJ, Runge S, Müller RH. Peptide-loaded solid lipid nanoparticles (SLN): influence of production parameters. Int J Pharm 1997; 149(2): 255–65.
37. Müller RH, Olbrich C. Arzneistoffträger zur kontrollierten Wirkstoffapplikation hergestellt aus Lipidmatrix-Arzneistoff-Konjugaten (LAK-Partikel), in EPN 0001176984. 2007, PharmaSol GmbH.
38. Olbrich C, Gebner A, Kayser O, et al. Lipid-drug conjugate (LDC) nanoparticles as novel carrier system for the hydrophilic antitrypanosomal drug Diminazenediaceturate. J Drug Target 2002; 10(5):387–96.
39. Penkler LJ, Muller RH, Runge SA, Ravelli V. Pharmaceutical cyclosporin formulation with improved biopharmaceutical properties, improved physical quality and greater stability, and method for producing said formulation. in United States Patent 6,551,619. 2003, Pharmatec International S.R.L.: USA.
40. Muller RH, et al. Oral bioavailability of cyclosporine: solid lipid nanoparticles (SLN) versus drug nanocrystals. Int J Pharm 2006; 317(1):82–9.

41. He J, Hou SX, Feng JF, et al. Effect of particle size on oral absorption of silymarin-loaded solid lipid nanoparticles. Zhongguo Zhong Yao Za Zhi 2005; 30(21):1651–3.
42. Uner M. Preparation, characterization and physico-chemical properties of solid lipid nanoparticles (SLN) and nanostructured lipid carriers (NLC): their benefits as colloidal drug carrier systems. Pharmazie 2006, 61(5):375–86.
43. Pedersen N, Hansen S, Heydenreich AV, et al. Solid lipid nanoparticles can effectively bind DNA, streptavidin and biotinylated ligands. Eur J Pharm Biopharm 2006; 62(2):155–62.
44. Hu FQ, Wu MZH, Yuan H, et al. A novel preparation of solid lipid nanoparticles with cyclosporin A for prolonged drug release. Pharmazie 2004; 59(9):683–5.
45. Hanafy A, Spann-Langguth H, Vergnault G, et al. Pharmacokinetic evaluation of oral fenofibrate nanosuspensions and SLN in comparison to conventional suspensions of micronized drug. Adv Drug Deliv Rev 2007; 59(6):419–26.
46. Muchow M, Despatova N, Schmitz E, et al. Nanostructured lipid carriers (NLC) containing fish oil as food supplement. In: 5th World Meeting on Pharmaceutics, Biopharmaceutics and Pharmaceutical Technology. 27th–30th March 2006. Geneva.
47. Daubresse JC, Sternon J. Omega-3 fatty acids and cardiovascular diseases. Rev Med Brux 2006; 27(1):43–8.
48. Engler MM, Engler MB. Omega-3 fatty acids: role in cardiovascular health and disease. J Cardiovasc Nurs 2006; 21(1):17–24, quiz 25–6.
49. Vahedi K, Atlan P, Joly F, et al. A 3-month double-blind randomised study comparing an olive oil—with a soyabean oil-based intravenous lipid emulsion in home parenteral nutrition patients. Br J Nutr 2005; 94(6):909–16.
50. n-3 Fatty Acids: Recommendations for Therapeutics and Prevention. Proceedings of a symposium, New York, New York, USA, May 21, 2005. Am J Clin Nutr, 2006. 83(Suppl. 6):1451S–1538S.
51. Black HS, Rhodes LE. The potential of omega-3 fatty acids in the prevention of non-melanoma skin cancer. Cancer Detect Prev 2006; 30(3):224–32.
52. Bougnoux P, Menanteau J. Dietary fatty acids and experimental carcinogenesis. Bull Cancer 2005; 92(7):685–96.
53. Hannon K. Have a daily dose of Omega-3. US News World Rep 2005; 139(24): 54–5.
54. Muchow M, Schmitz E, Despatova N, et al. Omega-3 fatty acid-loaded lipid nanoparticles as oral food supplement. In: AAPS Annual Meeting and Exposition. 5th–10th November 2005. Nashville.
55. Muchow M. Nanostructured Lipid Carrier (NLC) for Oral Administration. PhD thesis 2008 (in preparation).
56. Trotta M, Cavalli R, Carlotti ME, et al. Solid lipid micro-particles carrying insulin formed by solvent-in-water emulsion-diffusion technique. Int J Pharm 2005; 288(2):281–8.
57. Battaglia L, Trotta M, Gallarate M, et al. Solid lipid nanoparticles formed by solvent-in-water emulsion-diffusion technique: development and influence on insulin stability. J Control Release 2007; 24(7):672–84.
58. Pinto JF, Müller RH. Pellets as carriers of "solid lipid nanoparticles" (SLN) for oral administration of drugs. Eur J Pharm Biopharm 1996; 42:35.

59. Pinto JF, Müller RH. Pellets as carriers of solid lipid nanoparticles (SLN) for oral administration of drugs. Die Pharmazie 1999; 54:506–9.
60. Bangham AD, Haydon DA. Ultrastructure of membranes: biomolecular organization. Brit Med Bull 1968; 24(2):124–6.
61. Diederichs JE, Müller RH. Liposome in Kosmetika und Arzeimitteln. Die Pharmazeutische Industrie 1994; 56(3):267–75.
62. Müller RH. Solid lipid nanoparticles, nanosuspensions and liposomes for pharmaceutical and cosmetic applications. In Diederichs JE, Müller RH, eds. Future Strategies for Drug Delivery with Particulate Systems. Boca Raton: CRC Press, 1998: 71–2.
63. Baum P. R&D—key to the future. Boehringer Ingelheim GmbH, Corporate Division Communications. 2003, Ulm: Sueddeutsche Verlagsgesellschaft. 58.

*Part IV: Colonic Technologies*

# 26

# Colonic Drug Delivery

Clive G. Wilson

*Strathclyde Institute of Pharmacy and Biomedical Sciences, Glasgow, Scotland, U.K.*

## INTRODUCTION

Targeted delivery of drugs to the colon has been employed to achieve one or more of four objectives. The desired outcomes can be (*i*) sustained delivery to reduce dosing frequency; (*ii*) to delay delivery to the colon to achieve high local concentrations in the treatment of diseases of the distal gut; (*iii*) to delay delivery to a time appropriate to treat acute phases of disease (chronotherapy or chronopharmaceutics) and historically, (*iv*) to deliver to a region that is less hostile metabolically, e.g., to facilitate absorption of acid and enzymatically labile materials, especially peptides. Further commercial benefits are the extension of patent protection and the ability to promote new claims centered on the provision of patient benefits such as increased effectiveness and the optimization of dosing frequency.

If a colonic system functioned perfectly it would not release drug in the upper and mid-gastrointestinal tract, but open at the beginning of the large bowel where conditions are more favorable for drug dispersion and absorption. More distally, low dispersive forces restrict spread of the formulation. The significant feature of the colon as far as drug delivery is concerned is that the colon is folded but is devoid of villi and microvilli so the effective surface area is much less than the small intestine. The mucus thickness increases moving from proximal to distal colon and the net effect is to reduce permeability. The colon is also a moist rather than a wet environment as the healthy colon reabsorbs 99% of swallowed and secreted fluids, ending with a resident aqueous volume estimated to be between 20 mL and 40 mL. Various estimates derived from fitting regional permeability coefficients using sequential compartment models for drugs in suspension estimate a typical reduction of 10- to

100-fold moving from jejunum to colon. This is a primarily a reflection of reduced absorptive capacity in respect of surface area. There is some debate about the contribution of P-glycoprotein (P-gp) mediated efflux to the reduced flux with a modeling approach assuming that P-gp is expressed maximally in the colon as in a model of the colon (1) whereas direct measurements of segmental capacity suggests a more complex profile. In these experiments, P-gp–mediated efflux is seen to be increasing as the drug moves from duodenum to ileum followed by a decrease in the colon to levels seen in the duodenum (2). In addition the bacterial content may cause significant loss by degradation of the active moiety. In order to appreciate the problems and possibilities of utilizing colonic absorption, the physiological and anatomical aspects need to be considered.

## FUNCTIONS OF THE COLON: THE IMPACT ON DRUG DELIVERY

The large intestine is principally responsible for conservation of water and electrolytes, particularly sodium chloride whose removal facilitates the formation of a solid stool. The structure is easily discriminated from that of the small intestine as the lumen is larger and less convoluted, particularly when it is full of gas. The major regions of the colon are illustrated in Figure 1. The transverse colon is folded in front of the ascending and descending arms. The splenic flexure will generally prevent exposure to the transverse colon following rectal administration. Consolidation occurs from the middle of the ascending colon into a mass, which gradually becomes more homogenous and viscous. By the time the lumenal contents have reached the descending colon, the mass is too solid to allow drug dispersion from a delayed release formulation.

Current studies indicate that the distal transverse colon functions as a conduit, driving material into the descending and sigmoid colon for storage. Studies conducted in patients to measure the relative residence times of materials at steady state shows that the contents are divided two-third into the ascending or right colon and one-third in the descending colon (3). This difference is exaggerated in left-sided colitis to 9:1 which may explain why management is difficult in active disease (4). The change in distribution in left sided colitis is caused by the greater availability of water.

The interior surface differs from that of small intestine by having less surface area [no villi], the presence of plecal folds and movement is sluggish and largely propulsive. The plecal folds are important in drug delivery and are illustrated in Figure 2. The structure and inhomogeneity of the contents causes a separation according to particle size: consolidation starts with lumps of debris pushed ahead of the finer particulates in the liquid phase. In drug delivery this behavior results in the separation of microparticulates and matrix systems; the finer particulates may be trapped in the folds and their retention increased.

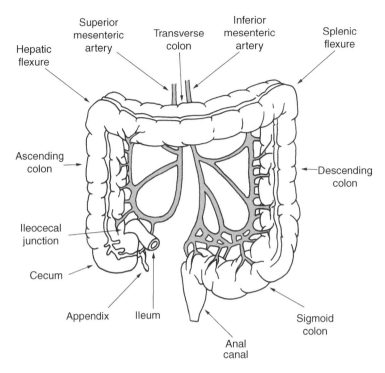

**Figure 1** Main features of the colon. *Source*: Adapted from Ref. 9.

## TRIGGERS FOR DRUG DELIVERY

Previous studies utilizing the technique of scintigraphy have shown that small intestinal transit times in man are relatively consistent, irrespective of the nature of the dosage form (particulate or monolith). Small intestinal transit is usually determined to be between 3 and 4 hours (emptying from the stomach—arrival at the ileocecal junction) although shorter transit times are not unusual, particularly in individuals who regularly engage in high intensity sport.

The emptying from the stomach may however be unpredictable, since it is dependent on the timing of the housekeeper sequence in the fasted state and physical properties when fed. This leads to marked differences in the time of exposure of a formulation under acidic conditions (pH 1.5–2.5) in the fasted state. In the fed state, using the FDA light meal, the pH rises at the beginning of the meal to between 4 and 5, falling to around pH 2 after 1 hour. Protein content is the trigger for acid secretion through central and local action, stimulating a flow of between 2 and 4 mL hydrochloric per minute. The low calorie meal does have one useful attribute: it switches most healthy subjects into the same state and reduces variability in the cohort with regard to gastric emptying of larger formulations.

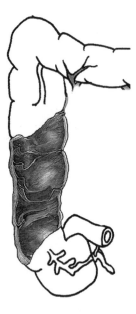

**Figure 2**   Ascending colon showing plecal folds of the mucosal wall.

The entry in the duodenum provides a sharp pH rise and this change can be used to trigger the onset of dissolution of acidic polymers used as coatings or matrices. Thickness of the coating then provides the basis for a process allowing initiation of release at an appropriate point in the intestine. Effectively, both type of polymer and coat thickness are the controlling variables. Early attempts to modify the point of release as far as the colon by thickening the coat were successful and used to facilitate cecal targeting of drugs such as 5-ASA. There are however, a further two triggers which are available: direct bacterial metabolism of the prodrug, which provides the opportunity for reductive and glycosidic cleavage, and release of the active from the formulation following the degradation of suitable polymers by bacterial fermentation.

## ROLE OF CECAL FERMENTATION

The cecal bacteria in the right side of the colon largely control the characteristics of the lumen. Complex carbohydrates are fermented by the bacteria to small chain fatty acids and carbon dioxide, the gas traveling to the transverse colon and being expelled (mostly) through the lungs. The average bacterial load of the colon has been estimated at just over 200 g (equivalent to approximately 35 g dry weight). Water available for dissolution is maximal in the ascending colon, and 1.5 to 2 liters enter from the terminal small intestine each day. The amount of water present varies, being maximal in the period 4 to

8 hours after ingestion of a meal. In the morning, the colon is often empty, and any material remaining in the ascending colon is slowly cleared. In the upright position, the gas produced by fermentation travels to the transverse colon and may limit access of the contents to water. It would be expected that the low water–high gas environment of the transverse colon limit dissolution of materials; it also limits ingress of water into impermeable devices.

In the descending colon, devices may become impacted into the 300 g of fecal contents. The surrounding material limits diffusion and provides a nonabsorbing reservoir. Unless the contents are cleared therefore, there will be no absorption in this region.

From these comments, it is seen that targeted delivery to the large bowel should be directed toward the proximal colon. The ascending colon provides some water for dissolution and contents at the base of the colon will be stirred by the arrivals of additional fluids from gut as meals and accompanying secretions. Figure 3 summarizes the main characteristics of the colon with regard to luminal environments. Transit times are derived from scintigraphic measurements.

## DISEASE AND THE COLONIC ENVIRONMENT

As in all parts drug formulation development, the impact of the disease process is sometimes forgotten by the pharmaceutical scientist, with the outcome that performance is not optimal (5). The three important changes produced by disease are changes in motility, changes in permeability, and changes in intestinal secretion.

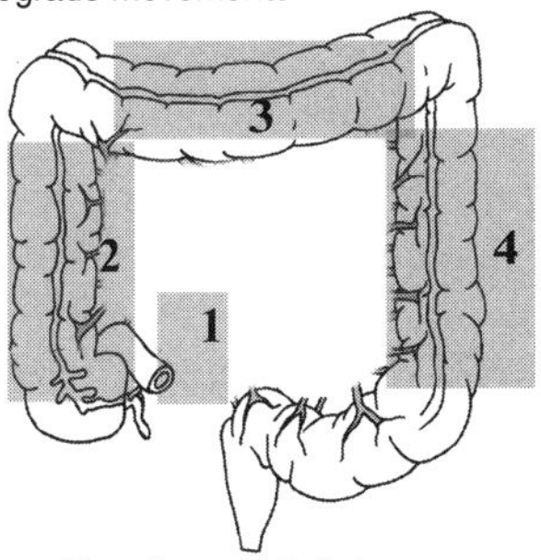

3. Transverse colon: periodically filled with gas. pH 6–8 residence time 0.2 to 4 h, dependent on presence of stool dispersion inhibited by forward propulsive waves by retrograde movements

2. Ascending colon-cecal region periodically filled with liquid, moving in concert with gastric emptying residence time 3–5 h pH 5–8, dependent on fermentation. Stirred by movement of material across ileoce-cal valve: 7–10 litres per day

4. Descending and sigmoid colon periodically filled with feces residence time 5 h to 72 h dependent on bowel habit

1. Ileocecal junction. pH 6–8.4 periodic high dispersive forces propulsion linked to gastric emptying stagnation common, causing bunching of swallowed label

**Figure 3** Physiological features of the colon relevant to modified-release dosage forms.

An observation by Fallingborg et al. that inflammatory bowel disease was associated with an extremely low pH promised a method of targeting drug more specifically to the diseased colon (6). Using radiotelemetry, Fallingborg reported pH as low as 2.8–3.4 and an increased lactate in the stools as a result of gut vessel edema, suggesting an opportunity for a reverse enteric coat system which would release when pH was below 4.5. Unfortunately, a later study by Press and colleagues suggests that most patients do not show such a dramatic change. Nevertheless, even a small change in pH would alter the active transport of vitamins and other important nutrients in the gut. In addition, it is well established that permeability changes are marked in this disease and urinary recovery of a poorly absorbed orally administered marker such as 51Cr-EDTA is increased more twenty-fold in patients with ulcerative colitis (7).

All the specific approaches to colon targeting rely on the concept that enzymes produced by colonic microflora provide the trigger for specific delivery of fermentable coatings, anti-inflammatory azo-bond drugs and other prodrugs to the cecum. An old observation by Carette and colleagues (8) should temper undue enthusiasm. Carette and coworkers demonstrated that in patients with active Crohn's disease, the metabolic activity of digestive flora (assessed on the activity of fecal glycosidases) was decreased. Azo-reductase activity in feces of 14 patients with active Crohn's disease was 20% of that healthy subjects and similarly, beta-D-glucosidase and beta-D-glucuronidase activities in fecal homogenates incubated under anaerobic conditions were also decreased in patients. These data probably reflect large bowel hypermotility and the associated diarrhea, leading to lower bacterial mass in the colon and might contribute to the therapeutic failure of targeting mechanisms in active ileocolic and colic Crohn's disease.

## ORAL ROUTE: ROLE OF EXCIPIENTS AND COATINGS

Since it is virtually impossible to treat the ascending colon via the rectum, oral treatment is the only reliable method of delivery. Colonic delivery via the oral route requires control of four factors: time of release, site of release, extent of dispersion, and modification of low flux across the absorptive epithelium (9). Certain components provide specific mechanisms by which colonic targeting may be achieved: generally they can be grouped as follows:

### Specific

By definition, these must take account of the only nonmammalian cue: the colonic bacteria. The mechanisms are as follows:

1. biodegradable polymers which will release after cecal metabolism of polysaccharide by glucuronidase or glycosidase action (soluble fiber);
2. azo-reduction of polymers containing bonds which can be cleaved by reductive scission.

## Nonspecific

The other group of trigger mechanisms are fairly nonspecific, at least in terms of relying on the bacteria triggers, and may avoid premature release in the upper gastrointestinal tract by

1. a combination of enteric coating and conventional time-dependent barrier coat dissolution;
2. swelling systems which may eject [e.g., Pulsincap (10)] or burst;
3. eroding systems (e.g., Egalet);
4. those using slowed transit due to trapping in plecal folds (e.g., pellet dosage forms) to release the majority of the drug when trapped in the ascending colon.

## CONCLUDING COMMENTS

The examples in the chapters that follow show how the delayed release technologies achieve a measure of modulated delivery in the terminal small bowel and through the proximal large bowel. It should be emphasized that the primary purpose of modified systems is often more related to adjustment of release rate to take account of solubility differences of the drug in the gastric and the intestinal environments; the delayed delivery to facilitate prophylaxis whist sleeping and thirdly, the extension of release to permit once-per-day dosing. Only rarely is true colon-targeting for the topical management of distal gastrointestinal disease an objective to the formulator, in part because the environment is inconvenient to mimic and second, there are few tools which can be conveniently applied to the investigation outside of specialist laboratories.

## REFERENCES

1. Tubic M, Wagner D, Spahn-Langguth H, Bolger MB, Langguth P. In silico modelling of non-linear drug absorption for the P-gp substrate talinolol and of consequences for the resulting pharmacodynamic effect. Pharm Res 2006; 23: 1712–20.
2. Valenzuela B, Nacher A, Ruiz-Carretero P, Martin-Villodre A, Lopez-Carballo G, Barettino D. Profile of p-glycoprotein distribution in the rat and its possible influence on the salbutamol intestinal absorption process. J Pharm Sci 2004; 93:1641–8.

3.  Hebden JM, Gilchrist PJ, Spiller RC, et al. Dispersion, transit, water content and ascending colon volumes in subjects treated with lactulose and codeine scintigraphic and M.R.I assessment. Neurogastroenterol Motility 1996; 175:8.
4.  Hebden JM, Blackshaw E, Perkins AC, Wilson CG, Spiller RC. Limited exposure of the healthy distal colon to orally dosed formulation is further exaggerated in active left-sided ulcerative colitis. Aliment Pharmacol Therap 2000; 14:155–61.
5.  Barrow L, Spiller RC, Wilson CG. Pathological influences on colonic motility: implications for drug delivery. Adv Drug Del Rev 1991; 7:201–18.
6.  Fallingborg J, Christensen LA, Jacobsen BA, Rasmussen SN. Very low intra-luminal colonic pH in patients with active ulcerative colitis. Dig Dis Sci 1993; 38:1989–93.
7.  Arslan G, Atasever T, Cindoruk M, Yildirim IS. [$^{51}$Cr]-EDTA colonic per-meability and therapy response in patients with ulcerative colitis. Nucl Med Comm 2001; 22(9):997–1001.
8.  Carrette O, Favier C, Mizon C, et al. Bacterial enzymes used for colon-specific drug delivery are decreased in active Crohn's disease. Dig Dis Sci 1995; 40: 2641–6.
9.  Washington N, Washington C, Wilson CG. Colon and rectal delivery. In: Physiological Pharmaceutics: Barriers to Drug Absorption. London: Taylor & Francis 2001.
10. Wilson CG, Bakhshaee M, Stevens HE, et al. Evaluation of a gastro-resistant pulsed release delivery system (Pulsincap) in humans. J Drug Deliv 1997; 4: 201–6.

# 27

# Biopolymers and Colonic Delivery

### Clive G. Wilson
*Strathclyde Institute of Pharmacy and Biomedical Sciences,
Glasgow, Scotland, U.K.*

### Gour Mukherji
*Jubilant Organosys Ltd., Noida, India*

### Hardik K. Shah
*Biovail Technologies (Ireland) Ltd., Dublin, Ireland*

## INTRODUCTION

Conventional controlled-release products for oral administration normally lack any unique property which would facilitate drug targeting to a specific location in the gastrointestinal tract. In view of the time course of gastrointestinal transit, any slow release system having a drug release-time profile extending beyond 6 to 8 hours is likely to be present in the colon for release of a high proportion of the drug payload. If the formulation has the appropriate dissolution control, the colon capable of absorbing the drug and the half-life sufficient to achieve therapeutic concentrations, the plasma concentrations can be maintained for longer following each dose. Biopolymers are mainly plant-based polysaccharides, which are digestible by the bacterial enzymes and are almost untouched by enzymes secreted by the gut wall. As a consequence such materials, particularly those which have pronounced swelling properties, have been frequently employed in the formulation of controlled drug release products and are especially valuable as the basis for colonic drug delivery systems.

As unmodified purified materials, biopolymers are often not suitable as single component excipients as the polymers may dissolve in water or may not form impermeable matrices which limits their usage as single component excipients. There is therefore a risk of release of some of the drug in the upper gastrointestinal tract. To ensure minimal drug release in the stomach and proximal small intestine, the product may be enteric coated or mixed with other synthetic polymers.

The mode of drug release from colon targeted biopolymer systems can include one or more of the following mechanisms:

1.  Diffusion
2.  Polymer erosion
3.  Microbial degradation
4.  Enzymatic degradation (mammalian and/or bacterial)

In addition, drug solubility and specific formulations of polymer mixes, play important roles in determining the extent of drug delivery and release in the colon. The breadth of possibilities by combination of selected grades of polymer is impressive and impossible to cover in a single chapter; however, some generalizations may be made. Two broad categories of biopolymers have been employed for formulating into colonic systems: (*i*) biodegradable and (*ii*) nonbiodegradable polymers.

## BIODEGRADABLE SWELLING POLYMERS

The colonic microflora secretes a number of enzymes which are capable of hydrolytic cleavage of glycosidic bonds. These include β-D-glucosidase, β-D-galactosidase, amylase, pectinase, xylanase, α-D-xylosidase, and dextranases. In addition there are scission reactions catalyzed azo-reductases secreted by the anaerobes but these are more generally used in a prodrug approach (e.g., olsalazide, balsalazide, etc.).

The biodegradable polymers are generally hydrophilic in nature and may have limited swelling characteristics in acidic pH. However, these polymers swell in the more neutral pH of the colon. Although the rate of drug release is governed to a limited extent by physical factors such as diffusion and drug solubility, the major mechanism of drug release is by matrix erosion produced by enzymatic or microbial interaction with the polymers.

The biodegradable polysaccharides can be employed (*i*) in the formulation matrix, or (*ii*) as a coat, alone and in combination. Many of these polysaccharides have limited release control properties due to high water solubility. Hence, they are employed in formulations in two ways: (*i*) combination with synthetic nonbiodegradable polymers or (*ii*) synthetic modification such that solubility is decreased without compromising on their specific degradation in the human colon. The modification is normally acheived by introduction of groups by: (*i*) covalent linkages (irreversible complexation) or (*ii*) by ionic linkages (reversible complexation).

## Guar Gum

Guar gum is a galactomannan polysaccharide [β-1,4 D-mannose, α-1,6 D-galactose] having (1→4) linkages. It has a side-branching unit of monomeric D-galactopyranose joined at alternate mannose unit by (1→6) linkage. It has low water solubility but hydrates and swells in cold water forming viscous colloidal dispersions or sols. The rigidity of guar gum can be conferred by cross-linking. Rubinstein and Gliko-Kabir (1) reported cross-linking of guar gum with borax to enhance its drug retaining capacity. The gum is susceptible to bacterial galactomannases present in the large intestine and the viscosity of a guar gum solution incubated with a homogenate of faeces was shown to reduce by 75% over 40 minutes (2).

Wong and colleagues (3) reported the evaluation of the dissolution of dexamethasone and budesonide from guar gum-based matrix tablets using USP Apparatus III. The presence of low grade hydroxymethyl propylcellulose (HPMC) (Methocel E3) or higher grade HPMC (Methocel E50 LV) in dexamethasone formulations altered the rate of the matrix degradation.

Krishnaiah et al. (4) described a scintigraphic study using technetium-99m-diethylenetriaminepentaacetic acid ($^{99m}$Tc-DTPA) as tracer incorporated into tablets to follow the transit and dissolution. Scintiscans revealed that some tracer was released in stomach and small intestine but the bulk of the tracer present in the tablet mass was delivered to the colon. Tugcu-Demiroz and colleagues describe a guar gum based system which was labeled by the incorporation of barium sulfate and administered to volunteers (5). The point of disintegration was estimated by X-ray imaging and the image of the tablet was seen to become more diffuse after 3 or 4 hours in the colon.

Guar gum is commonly used with other biopolymers. Sinha and Kumria used xanthan gum (XG) and guar gum (GG) as a compression coat with a XG:GG ration of 20:10 and 10:20 ratio to deliver 5-fluorouracil to the colon (6). Further studies followed the gastrointestinal behavior of these mixtures XG:GG (10:20) mixtures by incorporation of $^{99m}$Tc-DTPA into solid dosage forms (7). Following administration to six volunteers, the tablets were found to disintegrate in the ascending colon/hepatic flexure; disintegration of the tablet started between 4 and 6 hours post-dose in all the volunteers with a further spread of tracer into the ascending, transverse, descending, and sigmoid colon.

## Chondroitin Sulfate

Chondroitin sulfate is a soluble mucopolysaccharide consisting of β-1,3 D-glucuronic acid linked to N-acetyl-D-galactosamide (Fig. 1). It is a substrate for the *Bacteroides* sp. in the large intestine. Natural chondroitin sulfate is readily water soluble and may not be able to sustain the release of

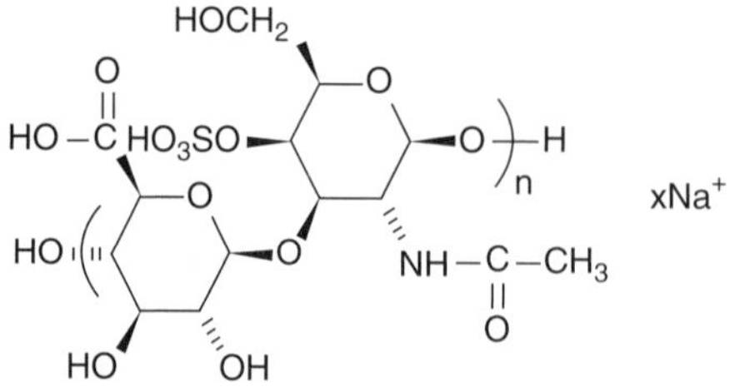

**Figure 1** Chondroitin sulfate.

most drugs from the matrix. Rubinstein and co-workers (8) has reported the use of cross-linked chondroitin sulfate as a carrier for indomethacin specifically for the large bowel. Since natural chondroitin sulfate is readily water soluble, it was cross-linked with 1,12-diaminododecane. The cross-linking reaction was between the carboxyl group in chondroitin and the amino group in diaminododecane, resulting in formation of a dimer of chondroitin sulfate, as shown in Figure 2.

The cross-linked polymer was blended with indomethacin and compressed into tablets. There was enhanced release on incubation with rat cecal contents.

## Pectin

Pectin is a heterogeneous polysaccharide composed mainly of galacturonic acid and its methyl ester. In human nutrition, it is one of the most important sources of dietary fiber and is a constituent of fruit and vegetable cell walls. It is composed mainly of long linear chains α-1,4 D-galacturonic acid (smooth regions, partially esterified with methanol) and "hairy regions" complexed with 1,2 L-rhamnose with D-galactose and L-arabinose side chains (9). It remains intact in stomach and small intestine but is degraded by colonic bacterial enzymes, which appear to work in concert (10). Pectins with high degree of methoxylation can be employed for colonic drug delivery; however, the material is poorly compactable on its own with a high degree of fragmentation, some elastic but little plastic deformation (11). Mura and colleagues overcame these limitations in the formulation of a theophylline matrix tablet by combination of the pectin with a hydrophilic direct compression agent (Emdex) and coated the tablets with Eudragit S100. At high concentrations of Emdex, the tablets increased in hardness but dissolution rate increased suggesting that the Emdex acts as a channeling agent through the gel (12).

ChS–CONH–(CH$_2$)$_{12}$–NHCO–ChS

**Figure 2** Dimer of chrondroitin sulfate. *Abbreviation*: ChS, chrondroitin sulfate.

Pectins with low degree of methoxylation can be cross-linked with a carefully controlled amount of a divalent cation typically calcium (13). In common with many other polymers, calcium or zinc stabilises pectin and other linear, polysaccharides by bridging across the molecules in a conformation often referred to an "eggbox" (Fig. 3). This prevents chain repulsion. Calcium appears to have the ideal elemental dimensions for this type of interaction which occurs in plant walls. If the pectin is heavily methoxylated, this interaction cannot occur (11).

Sriamornsak et al. (14) coated theophylline pellets with calcium pectinate and reported a pH-dependent in-vitro release in 4 hours. The particle size and release rate were reduced with increasing calcium chloride concentration in the treating solution. Muhiddinov and others described the preparation of low methoxy pectin microcapsules from citrus or apple pectin enclosing an oil core (15). The source of the pectin confers properties of flexibility and thus controls the size of the emulsion drops, which appear to be formed by electrostatic attraction of the negatively charged pectin with the positively charged oil dispersion.

Dupuis and colleagues described the use of zinc pectinate beads for the colonic delivery of ketoprofen and reported similar performance when compared to calcium pectinate in hard capsules, but significant differences when the same pellets were compared encapsulated in enteric hard capsules (16). Dissolution of the zinc pectinate beads was noticeably slowed compared to calcium pectinate, which the authors suggest might be more appropriate for colonic delivery of the drug.

Pectin is a poor film former and other polymers, including HPMC, chitosan, and ethylcellulose are often used in combination. Wakerly and colleagues coated paracetamol tablets using a combination of pectin and ethylcellulose, in the form of an aqueous dispersion (17). Based upon

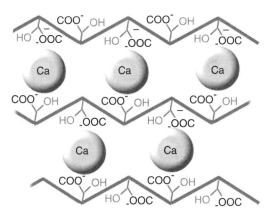

**Figure 3** Eggbox structure of a linear polysaccharide stabilized by calcium cross-linking. Note that zinc will substitute as an alternative cation.

in vitro dissolution, it was concluded that such a system can be used for colonic drug delivery.

Pectins with low degree of methoxylation can also undergo amidation of carboxylic acid groups. Munjeri and colleagues reported entrapment of indomethacin and sulfamethoxazole inside amidated pectin, gelled in the presence of calcium (18). The drug containing core was coated by a chitosan poly-electrolyte complex to obtain desired control in drug release in simulated intestinal media.

Adkin carried out scintigraphic studies to ascertain the behavior of formulations for colonic drug delivery systems containing biodegradable polymers in the matrix and coated with Eudragit L. (19). Two calcium pectinate (CaP) matrix formulations were developed as potential colon targeting systems. One formulation contained calcium pectinate and pectin (CaP/P) and was designed to rapidly disintegrate in the ascending colon. The second formulation contained calcium pectinate and guar gum (CaP/GG) and was designed to disintegrate more slowly than (CaP/P), releasing its contents throughout the ascending and transverse colon. Both formulations were enteric coated by spray coating with aqueous dispersion of Eudragit L. Scintigraphic evaluation was carried out in ten healthy volunteers and fermentation confirmed in rats. Complete tablet disintegration for Formulation CaP/GG appeared to be slower than that of CaP/P and the time and the location of complete tablet disintegration was more reproducible with CaP/P compared to CaP/GG.

## Amylose

Amylose is a linear polymer of glucopyranose units ( α-1,4 D-glucose) linked through α-D -(1,4)-linkages (Fig. 4). The molecule usually consists of around 1000–5000 glucose units. In its glassy amorphous form, amylose is resistant to pancreatic amylases but is susceptible to those of bacterial origin. Amylose has the ability to form films through gelation, and can be applied to tablets using conventional technology although the films are fragile. The biopolymer becomes porous on hydration and swells in water. Addition of ethylcellulose produces a polymer mixture suitable for colon targeting (20).

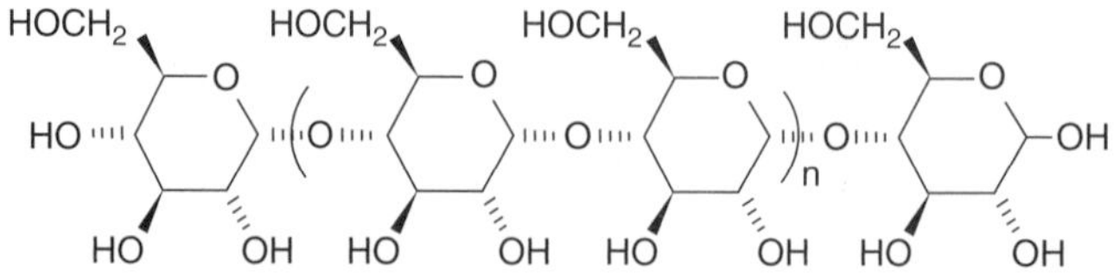

**Figure 4**   Amylose.

Ring and co-workers claimed delayed release compositions comprising an active compound and amorphous amylose and having an outer coating comprising a film forming cellulose or acrylic polymer material (21). The amorphous amylose is glassy amylose and is of particular value for the selective release into the colon. As compared to the other form of amylose, which is rubbery, glassy amylose exists in a glassy state below the glass transition temperature. The film-forming cellulose is preferably ethylcellulose.

In another utilization of amylose, Cartilier and colleagues prepared sustained release tablet containing drug and uncrosslinked substituted amylose (22). Substituted amylose is prepared by the reaction of the hydroxy groups in amylose with a reactive function like an epoxy group. Usual organic substitutents included epoxy, halide, and isocyanate containing groups.

Wilson and Basit (23) prepared the coating mixture containing amorphous-amylose and ethylcellulose (1:1,1:2,1:3) and applied on the single unit tablets containing mesalamine in varied degree of weight gain (2%,4%, and 6%). It was found that these preparations released mesalamine in the simulated colonic condition (fermentation system) because of the possible digestion of amylose by colonic bacterial enzymes. It was concluded that the proportions of amylose and ethylcellulose as well as the thickness of the coating were the key determinants to control the drug release from the system.

## Dextran

Dextran is a polysaccharide consisting of $\alpha$-1,6 D-glucose and $\alpha$-1,3 D-glucose units. Dextran hydrogels are stable when incubated at $37^{\circ}C$ with the small intestinal enzymes amyloglucosidase, invertase and pancreatin (24). However, they are degraded by dextranases, which is a microbial enzyme found in the colon. Hovgaard and Brondsted prepared dextran hydrogels by crosslinking with diisocyanate (25). These hydrogels were characterized by equilibrium degree of swelling and mechanical strength. Release of entrapped hydrocortisone was found to depend on the presence of dextranases in the release medium.

Ahmad and colleagues (26) oxidized dextrans using sodium periodate and coupled the aldehyde product with the alpha-amino group of 5-amino salicylic acid (5-ASA). It was reported that dextrans (MW 20,000) having 93% of degree of oxidation yielded the maximum 5-ASA conjugation (49 mg/100 mg product), which were resistant to dextranase hydrolysis. On the other hand, lower extents of 5-ASA conjugation (around 15 mg/100 mg product) were obtained by using less oxidized dextrans (12%), which were susceptible to dextranase hydrolysis. The authors proposed that the latter group of dextran-5 ASA conjugates could potentially be used to treat the inflammation of the distal ileum and proximal colon.

## Starch

Starch is composed of (*i*) amylose and (*ii*) amylopectin (Fig. 5). The latter is branched with about 10,000 glucose units. Starch is hydrolyzed by several amylolytic enzymes in the gut. The degradation products are mainly composed of oligosaccharides, dextrins and maltose. A colonic drug delivery composition has been prepared using starch capsules to hold the drug and provided with a coating (27). The coating may be a pH-sensitive material, a redox sensitive material, or a material broken down by specific enzymes or bacteria present in the colon.

TARGIT™ is a proprietary starch-based capsule system produced by injection molding. The starch capsule is coated with a 1:1 mix of Eudragits L and S to achieve release at the terminal ileum and ascending colon (28). The starch capsule produced is denser but the manufacturers claim equivalent in terms of disintegration when compared to a gelatin capsule.

## Chitosan

Chitosan is a poly (2-amino-2-deoxy-D-glucopyranose) in which the repeating units are linked by (1–4) β-bonds (Fig. 6). It is biodegradable and nontoxic. It dissolves in acidic pH of the stomach but swells in pH simulating the intestine. Tominaga and colleagues prepared a composite for delivery to the colon comprising an active core, an internal layer of coat comprising chitosan and an external layer, coated on internal layer, containing zein (29). Zein protects the contents by being acid resistant but undergoes proteolysis in the small intestine. Chitosan in the internal layer prevents the elution of the active ingredients in the core in the small intestine. However, in the large intestine the chitosan film breaks due to the combined effect of microorganisms and osmotic pressure.

Raghvan and colleagues (30) reported the use of a bacterially-triggered coating material comprising of chitosan and locust bean gum around a mesalazine core. The authors used an incubation in 2% w/v rat cecal contents in buffer at pH 6.8 as a test in vitro media, and the formulation at a 4:1 (chitosan: locust bean gum) ratio showed almost complete release in 26 hours. This formulation was also shown to be superior compared to the 1:1 mixture in a clinical evaluation in nine volunteers with a five-fold

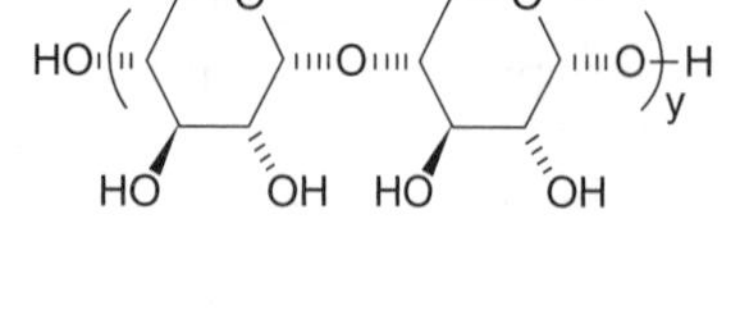

**Figure 5**  Starch.

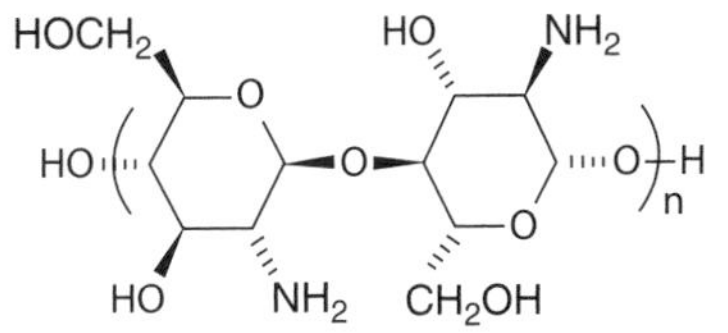

**Figure 6**  Chitosan.

increase in 5-ASA bioavailability. Tozaki and colleagues (31) used enteric-coated chitosan capsules containing 5-amino salicylic acid, which accelerated the healing of trinitrobenzene sulphonic acid-induced colitis in rats and which was significantly more effective than a suspension of the drug in carmellose.

Wilson and Mukherji (32) described a polyelectrolyte complex composed of chitosan and poly-acrylic acid (PAA). PAA was dispersed in absolute ethanol and mixed with chitosan solution in acetic acid. The interaction yielded insoluble precipitates as a result of electrostatic interaction between oppositely charged species. After drying, it was found that the complex had about 20-fold (w/w) degree of swelling. The water retention property suggested its potential to deliver a drug to the dry environment of the colon. Electrostatically-interacted PEC forms a nonpermanent network and dissociation will lead to the release of entrapped species. Furthermore, the utilization of biodegradable polymer in colonic delivery might allow the complete release of an active ingredient following digestion by colonic bacterial enzymes.

## Cyclodextrin

Cyclodextrin is a cyclic oligosaccharide consisting of at least six glucopyranose units joined by $\alpha$-(1→4) linkages (Fig. 7). It is produced by a highly selective enzymatic synthesis. The cyclodextrins consist of six, seven, or eight glucose monomers arranged in a doughnut shaped ring, which are denoted $\alpha$-, $\beta$-, or $\gamma$-cyclodextrin, respectively. The specific coupling of the glucose monomers gives the cyclodextrin a rigid, truncated conical molecular structure with a hollow interior of a specific volume. This internal cavity, which is lipophilic, that is attractive to hydrocarbon materials (in aqueous

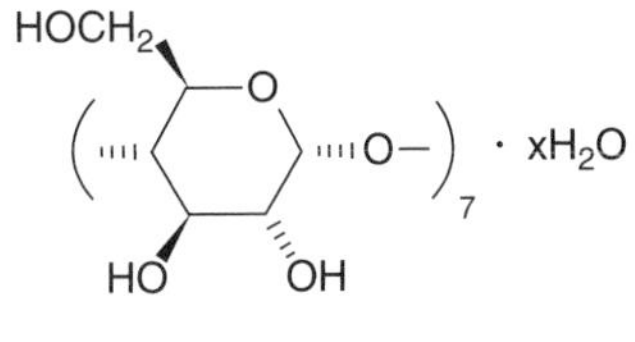

**Figure 7**  Cyclodextrin.

systems is hydrophobic) when compared to the exterior, is a key structural feature of the cyclodextrin, providing the ability to complex molecules including aromatics, alcohols, halides and hydrogen halides, carboxylic acids and their esters (33).

Cyclodextrins are known to be fermented to small saccharides by colonic microflora, whereas they are only slowly hydrolysable in the conditions of the upper gastrointestinal tract. This characteristic, like the other fermentable saccharides may be exploitable for colon specific delivery.

Uekama and colleagues selectively conjugated an anti-inflammatory drug, 4-biphenylylacetic acid (BPAA) onto one of the primary hydroxyl groups of α-, β-, and γ-cyclodextrins through an ester or amide linkage (34). BPAA was found to be released after the ring opening followed by ester hydrolysis, and the activation took place site-specifically in the cecum and colon. Siefke and colleagues reported biodegradable physical mixtures of methacrylic acid copolymers (Eudragit®-RS) and β-cyclodextrins (35).

Zou and colleagues (36) synthesized cyclodextrin–5 ASA conjugates with varying degree of substitution (6–45). It was found that the conjugates having degree of substitution below 30 were more soluble and released a higher amount of 5-ASA in the presence of rat cecal and colonic contents.

## Inulin

Inulin is a naturally occurring glucofructan which can resist hydrolysis and digestion in the upper gastrointestinal tract (Fig. 8). It is fermented by colonic microflora. Inulin, with a high degree of polymerization, was formulated as a biodegradable colon specific coating by suspending it in Eudragit RS films. The films withstood gastric and intestinal fluid but were degraded by fecal degradation medium (37). Later publications from the same group describe further variants in which the inulin was incorporated as the minor component into polymethacrylate aqueous dispersions (38).

Vinyl groups were introduced in inulin chains to form hydrogels, by reacting with glycidyl methacrylate (39). Enzymatic digestibility of the prepared hydrogels was assessed by performing an in-vitro study using an inulinase preparation derived from *Aspergillus niger*. Equilibrium swelling ratio and mechanical strength of the hydrogels were also studied. Based on the mode of swelling it was concluded that inulin-degrading enzymes were able to diffuse into the inulin hydrogel networks causing bulk degradation (40).

Van den Mooter and colleagues (41) studied the in vitro release of model proteins: bovine serum albumin (BSA) and lysozyme from methacrylated inulin hydrogels. The protein release was affected by the loading procedure, loading concentration and also by the molecular weight. The release of BSA was enhanced in the presence of inulinase, which confirmed the biodegrability of the hydrogels in the colonic environment.

n = approx. 35                    **Figure 8**   Inulin.

Akhgari and colleagues (42) studied the drug permeability and swelling properties of the polymethacrylate films (Eudragit RS, Eudragit RL, Eudragit RS-Eudragit RL, Eudragit FS and Eudragit RS-Eudragit S) containing inulin. It was found that the films containing Eudragit RS and Eudragit RL in combination with inulin had better drug permeability in the colonic medium compared to the simulated intestinal medium. It was proposed that this polymer mixture could be a potential coating system to achieve the colon specific delivery.

## NONBIODEGRADABLE SWELLING POLYMERS

Nonbiodegradable polymers are more frequently employed in controlled-release systems rather than in targeted colonic delivery. These polymers are frequently synthetic and undergo dissolution or disintegration in the gastrointestinal tract, without undergoing significant absorption or degradation. They are generally nonspecific carrier systems. Employment of these polymers as carrier matrices for colonic delivery may require a pH or time dependent coat for colon specificity. Hence, products have been commonly formulated containing such polymers in a drug core, followed by application of an enteric polymer coat for controlling drug release in the stomach and the upper intestine.

The solubility characteristics of the active substance can also play an important role. If a drug has high and pH-independent solubility profile, the selection of polymer system for targeted drug delivery, particularly to the colon, is an extremely challenging task. Such matrices tend to release the drug, partially or significantly, in the stomach and the small intestine. Increased application of the polymer may cause incomplete drug release in the colon. Drugs having poor solubility may have intrinsic problems in absorption from the water deficient colon.

Nonbiodegradable swelling polymers do not undergo any cleavage by enzymes or microbes present in the lumen. The prominent examples include the celluloses ethers and the cross-linked polyacrylates. Among the celluloses, there are various grades of HPMC, based upon viscosity, which are commercially marketed under the trade name, Methocel® by Dow. Other cellulose ethers are methyl cellulose, hydroxypropyl cellulose, and carboxymethyl cellulose. The cross-linked polyacrylates of the swelling types include the branded Carbopols® of the oral grade, with suffix 934P, 974P, and 971P, manufactured by BF Goodrich.

Finally, there have been many patents which attempt to exploit azo-reductase activity in the colon. Azo-networks based on an acrylic backbone crosslinked with 4,4'-divinylazobenzene, were prepared and evaluated for drug delivery and muco-adhesive interactions. The data obtained by Kakoulides and others indicated that there is an optimum crosslinking density to allow nonadhesive particles to reach the colon. Within the colonic environment, the azo network degrades to produce a structure capable of developing mucoadhesive interactions with the colonic mucosa (43).

## FURTHER READING

Recently, an excellent review of colon drug delivery has been published by Dr. Van Der Mooter and the reader is referred to this work for additional information (44).

## REFERENCES

1. Rubinstein A, Gliko-Kabir I. Synthesis and swelling dependent enzymatic degradation of borax modified guar gum for colonic delivery purposes. STP Pharma Sci 1995; 5:41–6.
2. Tomlin A, Read NW, Edwards CA, Duerden BI. The degradation of guar gum by a faecal incubation system. Br J Nutr 1986; 55:481–6.
3. Wong D, Larrabee S, Clifford K, Tremblay J, Friend DR. USP dissolution apparatus III (reciprocating cylinder) for screening of guar-based colonic delivery formulations. J Control Release 1997; 47:173–9.

4. Krishnaiah YSR, Satyanarayana S, Prasad YVR, Rao SN. Gamma scintigraphic studies on guar gum matrix tablets for colonic drug delivery in healthy human volunteers. J Control Release 1998; 55:245–52.

5. Tugcu-Demiroz F, Acarturk F, Takka S, Konus-Boyunaga O. In vitro and in vivo evaluation of mesalazine-guar gum matrix tablets for colonic drug delivery. J Drug Target 2004; 12(2):105–12.

6. Sinha VR, Kumria R. Colonic drug delivery of 5-fluorouracil: an in vitro evaluation. Int J Pharm 2003; 249:23–31.

7. Sinha VR, Mittal BR, Kumria K. In vivo evaluation of time and site of disintegration of polysaccharide tablet prepared for colon-specific drug delivery. Int J Pharm 2005; 289:79–85.

8. Rubinstein A, Nakar D, Sintov A. Colonic drug delivery: enhanced release of indomethacin from cross-linked chondroitin matrix in rat cecal content. Pharm Res 1992; 9(2):276–8.

9. Schols HA, Voragen AGJ. Complex pectins: structure elucidation using enzymes. In: Visser J Voragen AGJ, eds. Pectins and Pectinases. Amsterdam, The Netherlands: Elsevier Science, 1996: 3–19.

10. Dongowski G, Lorenz A, Anger H. Degradation of pectins with different degrees of esterification by Bacteroides thetaiotamicron isolated from human gut flora. Appl Environ Microbiol 2000; 66(4):1321–7.

11. Sande SA. Pectin-based oral drug delivery to the colon. Expert Opin Drug Deliv 2005; 2(3):441–50.

12. Mura P, Maestrelli F, Cirri M, Luisa Gonzalez Rodriguez M, Rabasco Alvarez AM. Development of enteric-coated pectin-based matrix tablets for colonic delivery of theophylline. J Drug Target 2003; 11(6):365–71.

13. Ashford M, Fell J, Attwood D, Sharma H, Woodhead P. Studies on pectin formulations for colonic drug delivery. J Control Release 1994; 30:225–32.

14. Sriamornsak P, Prakongpan S, Puttipipatkhachorn S, Kennedy RA. Development of sustained release theophylline pellets coated with calcium pectinate. J Control Release 1997; 47:221–32.

15. Muhiddinov Z, Khalikov D, Speaker T, Fassihi R. Development and characterization of different low methoxy pectin microcapsules by an emulsion–interface reaction technique. J Microencapsulation 2004; 21(7):729–41.

16. Dupuis G, Chambin O, Genelot C, Champion D, Pourcelot Y. Colonic drug delivery: influence of cross linking agent on pectin beadsproperties and role of capsule shell type. Drug Dev Ind Pharm 17 2006; 32(7):847–55.

17. Wakerly Z, Fell JT, Attwood D, Parkins D. Pectin/ethylcellulose film coating formulations for colonic drug delivery. Pharm Res 1996; 13(8):1210–12.

18. Munjeri O, Collett JH, Fell JT. Hydrogel beads based on amidated pectins for colon-specific drug delivery: the role of chitosan in modifying drug release. J Control Release 1997; 46:273–8.

19. Adkin DA, Kenyon CJ, Lerner EI, et al. The use of scintigraphy to provide 'Proof of Concept' for novel polysaccharide preparations designed for colonic drug delivery. Pharm Res 1997; 14(1):103–7.

20. Milojevic S, Newton JM, Cummings JH, et al. Amylose as a coating for drug delivery to the colon: preparation and in vitro evaluation using 5-aminosalicylic acid pellets. J Control Release 1996; 38:75–84.

21. Ring SG, Archer DB, Allwood MC, Newton JM. Delayed release formulations. US Patent 5294448, March 15, 1994.
22. Cartilier L, Moussa I, Chebli C, Buczkowski S. Substituted amylose as a matrix for sustained drug release. US Patent 5879707, March 9, 1999.
23. Wilson PJ, Basit AW. Exploiting gastrointestinal bacteria to target drug to the colon: An in vitro study using amylose coated tablets. Int J Pharm 2005; 300: 89–94.
24. Simonsen L, Hovgaard L, Mortensen PB, Brondsted H. Dextran hydrogels for colon-specific drug delivery 5. Degradation in human intestinal incubation models. Eur J Pharm Sci 1995; 3:329–37.
25. Hovgaard L, Brondsted H. Dextran hydrogels for colon-specific drug delivery. J Control Release 1995; 36:159–66.
26. Ahmad S, Tester RF, Corbett A, Karkalas J. Dextran and 5-aminosalicylic acid (5-ASA) conjugates: synthesis, characterisation and enzymic hydrolysis. Carbohydr Res 2006; 341:2694–701.
27. Watts P. Colonic drug delivery composition. US Patent 6228396, May 8, 2001.
28. Watts P, Smith A. TARGIT technology: coated starch capsules for site-specific drug delivery into the lower gastrointestinal tract. Expert Opin Drug Deliv 2005; 2(1):159–67.
29. Tominaga S, Takizawa T, Yamada M. Large intestinal delivery composite. US Patent 6248362, June 19, 2001.
30. Raghavan CV, Muthulingam C, Amaladoss J, Jenita JL. An in vitro and in vivo investigation into the suitability of bacterially triggered delivery system for colon targeting. Chem Pharm Bull 2002; 50:892–5.
31. Tozaki H, Odoriba T, Okada N, et al. Chitosan capsules for colon-specific drug delivery: enhanced localization of 5-aminosalicylic acid in the large intestine accelerates healing of TNBS-induced colitis in rats. J Control Release 2002; 82: 51–61.
32. Wilson CG, Mukherji G. Glucosamine-polyacrylate inter-polymer complex and applications thereof. Patent: WO 03/067952, 2003.
33. Wood WE, Beaverson NJ. Barrier material comprising a thermoplastic and a compatible cyclodextrin derivative. US Patent 6218013, April 17, 2001.
34. Uekama K, Minami K, Hirayama F. 6(A)-O-[(4-biphenylyl)acetyl]-alpha-, beta- and gamma-cyclodextrins and 6(A)-deoxy-6(A)-[[(4-biphenylyl)acetyl]-amino]-alpha-, beta- and gamma-cyclodextrins: potential prodrugs for colon-specific delivery. Med Chem 1997; 40:2755–61.
35. Siefke V, Weckenmann HP, Bauer KH. β-Cyclodextrin matrix films for colon-specific drug delivery. Proc Int Symp Control Rel Bioact Mater 1993; 20:182.
36. Zou M, Okamoto H, Cheng G, Hao X, Sun J, Cui F, Danjo K. Synthesis and properties of polysaccharide produrgs of 5-aminosalicylic acid as potential colon-specific delivery systems. Eur J Pharm Biopharm 2005; 59:155–60.
37. Vervoort L, Kinget R. In vitro degradation by colonic bacteria of inulin HP incorporated in Eudragit RS films. Int J Pharm 1996; 129(1–2):185–90.
38. Cavalcanti OA, Van den Mooter G, Caramico-Soares I, Kinget R. Polysaccharides as excipients for colon-specific coatings. Permeability and swelling properties of casted films. Drug Dev Ind Pharm 2002; 28(2):157–64.

39. Vervoort L, Van den Mooter G, Augustins P, Bousson R, Toppet S, Kinget R. Inulin hydrogels as carriers for colonic drug targeting: I. Synthesis and characterization of methacrylated inulin and hydrogen formation. Pharm Res 1997; 14(2):1730–37.

40. Vervoort L, Rombaut P, Van den Mooter G, Augustins P, Kinget R. Inulin hydrogels. II. In vitro degradation study. Int J Pharm 1998; 172(1–2):137–45.

41. Van den Mooter G, Vervoort L, Kinget R. Characterisation of methacrylated inulin hydrogels designed for colon targeting: In vitro release of BSA. Pharm Res 2003; 20:303–7.

42. Akhgari A, Farahmand F, Garekani HA, Sadeghi F, Vandamme TF. Permeability and swelling studies of free films containing inulin in combination with different polymethacrylates aimed for colonic drug delivery. Eur J Pharm Sci 2006; 28:307–14.

43. Kakoulides EP, Smart JD, Tsibouklis J. Azocrosslinked poly(acrylic acid) for colonic delivery and adhesion specificity: in vitro degradation and preliminary ex vivo bioadhesion studies. J Control Release 1998; 54:95–109.

44. Van der Mooter G. Colon drug delivery. Expert Opin Drug Deliv 2007; 3(1): 111–25.

# 28

# Enteric Coating for Colonic Delivery

### Hardik K. Shah
*Biovail Technologies (Ireland) Ltd., Dublin, Ireland*

### Gour Mukherji
*Jubilant Organosys Ltd., Noida, India*

### Bianca Brögmann
*Degussa Pharma Polymers GmbH, Darmstadt, Germany*

### Clive G. Wilson
*Strathclyde Institute of Pharmacy and Biomedical Sciences, Glasgow, Scotland, U.K.*

## INTRODUCTION

The most extensive application of a formulation strategy for colonic delivery and generally for controlled release has been the employment of enteric coatings on solid substrates. This is a natural development of conventional coating technologies employed to avoid gastric release thus preventing stability problems such as degradation, or unwanted pharmacological effects including gastric irritation and nausea. The underlying principle in this approach has been the selection of polymers which are insoluble at the lower pH values of the stomach, but which disintegrate and release the drug as the pH increases as the formulation enters the small bowel. The principal discrimination is in the functional use of enteric polymers for delayed release in the mid gut and beyond as compared to a general application for colonic drug delivery. For delayed release, the disintegration and drug release from enteric coated products should be targeted to the proximal small bowel, whilst for colonic delivery release from the enteric coated system should take place closer to the ileo–cecal junction. Since the time of exposure to gastric acid may affect the subsequent release profile further down the tract and gastric emptying is a variable dependent on feeding, idiosyncratic and temporal differences, this is a fairly challenging task.

Early attempts at targeted delivery to the colon utilized those polymers which had previously been used for enteric coating. These dissolved at pH greater than 7 and longer release times were achieved by applying the material at a greater coating thickness. The solid substrate varies and has included tablets, capsules, beads, or microparticles. Subsequent advances in targeted colon delivery has prompted technologists to move to other approaches: e.g., a hybrid strategy employing enteric coating with other excipients or prodrug/coating release approaches based on azo-reductase or glycosidic activity of cecal bacteria. As an illustration of formulation approaches to a particular product, Table 1 gives a brief description of some commercial amino salicylic acid (ASA) products prepared using the current excipients which are available.

## ENTERIC POLYMER MATERIALS

These materials are applied as a coating either dissolved in an organic solvent or as an aqueous dispersion. Traditionally, it has been the practice to restrict enteric polymers dissolving at pH 7 and above for colon targeting. Those dissolving at pH lower than 7 were used in conventional enteric

**Table 1** Different Strategies Adopted in the Marketed 5-ASA Products for Colon Delivery

| Trade name | Molecule | Formulation strategy |
|---|---|---|
| Pentasa® | Mesalazine—250 mg tablets | Ethyl cellulose coated pellets to provide lag time for drug release in the small intestine |
| Asacol® | Mesalazine—400 mg tablets | Tablets coated with methacrylic acid copolymer (EUDRAGIT®-S) to cause drug release at pH ~7 |
| Salofalk® | Mesalazine—250 mg tablets | Tablets coated with EUDRAGIT®-L-100 to release the drug at a pH above 6 |
| Salazopyrin® | Sulfasalazine—500 mg tablets | 5-ASA linked to sulfapyridine through azo-bonds which are cleaved by colonic microflora |
| Dipentum® | Olsalazine sodium— 250 mg capsules and 500 mg tablets | 5-ASA dimer linked through azo-bonds and cleaved by colonic microflora |

*Abbreviation*: ASA, amino salicylic acid.

coating principally to avoid gastric degradation. However, the pH in the small intestine probably remains acidic and a discriminating target to facilitate release in colon is hard to spot. From studies with pH telemetry capsules (1), it has been shown that the pH in the small intestine increases from the duodenum (pH 5.4–6.1) to the ileum (pH 7–8). The colon may have a slightly lower pH than the small intestine (pH 5.5–7), since the acidity of the colon is determined by the availability of fermentable fiber and presence of bacteria (2). Racial differences in the pH and transit times in the colon, probably due to diet, have also been observed.

Selection of enteric polymer dissolving around a pH of 7 is likely to result in drug release in the terminal small bowel. Optimization of coat thickness is essential to ensure drug release in the colon and for the formulation not to escape the entire gastrointestinal tract. The list of enteric polymeric materials commercially available is given in Table 2–4. Adjustments to the thickness of enteric polymer coat will help to extend the choice to those dissolving at pH less than 7. Since in vivo–in vitro correlation is difficult in view of the change of environments, simple predictions are rarely accurate. Employment of imaging techniques, especially scintigraphy of the formulation in the gastrointestinal tract, has been found to be a useful tool in optimizing coat thickness.

## Cellulose Acetate Phthalate

Cellulose acetate phthalate (CAP) is a cellulose derivative in which about half the hydroxyl groups are acetylated, and about a quarter are esterified with one of two acid groups being phthalic acid, where the remaining acid group is free (Fig. 1). It is a hygroscopic, white to off-white, free-flowing powder, granule or flake, with a slight odor of acetic acid. It is insoluble in water, alcohols and chlorinated hydrocarbons, but soluble in acetone

**Table 2**  List of Phthalate-Based Enteric Polymers

| Polymer | Threshold pH | Product name | Manufacturer |
|---|---|---|---|
| Cellulose acetate phthalate | 6.0–6.4 | CAP Aquacoat CPD | Eastman FMC Corp. |
| Hydroxypropyl methylcellulose phthalate-50 | 4.8 | HPMCP 50 HP-50 | Eastman Shin-Etsu |
| Hydroxypropyl methylcellulose phthalate-55 | 5.2 | HPMCP 55 HP-55 | Eastman Shin-Etsu |
| Polyvinylacetate phthalate | 5.0 | Sureteric | Colorcon |

*Abbreviations*: CAP, cellulose acetate phthalate; HPMCP, hydroxypropyl methylcellulose phthalate.

**Table 3**  List of Methacrylic Acid-Based Copolymers

| Polymer | Threshold pH | Brand name | Manufacturer |
|---|---|---|---|
| Methacrylic acid–methyl methacrylate copolymer (1:1) | 6.0 | EUDRAGIT L 100/L 12.5 | Degussa Pharma Polymers GmbH |
| Methacrylic acid–methyl methacrylate copolymer (2:1) | 7.0 | EUDRAGIT S 100/S 12.5 | Degussa Pharma Polymers GmbH |
| Methacrylic acid–methylacrylate– methyl methacrylate copolymer | 7.0 | EUDRAGIT FS 30 D | Degussa Pharma Polymers GmbH |
| Methacrylic acid–ethyl acrylate copolymer (2:1) | 5.5 | EUDRAGITL 100-55/L 30 D-55 Acryl-EZE Eastacryl 30D | Degussa Pharma Polymers GmbH Colorcon Eastman |

and its mixtures with alcohols, ethyl acetate–IPA mixture and aqueous alkali (pH 6). The pseudolatex version (Aquacoat CPD) offers the convenience of aqueous-based processing. The use of CAP to deliver beclamethasone dipropionate has been described by Levine and colleagues, sampling ileostomy content during a single dose protocol. CAP-coating was shown

**Table 4**  Miscellaneous Enteric Polymers

| Polymer | Threshold pH | Product name | Manufacturer |
|---|---|---|---|
| Shellac | 7.0 | – | Zinsser Pangaea Sciences |
| Hydroxypropyl methylcellulose acetate succinate (HPMCAS) | 7.0 | Aqoat AS-HF | Shin-Etsu |
| Poly(methyl vinyl ether/ maleic acid) monoethyl ester | 4.5–5.0 | Gantrez ES-225 | International Speciality Products (ISP) |
| Poly(methyl vinyl ether/ maleic acid) n-butyl ester | 5.4 | Gantrez ES-425 | International Speciality Products (ISP) |

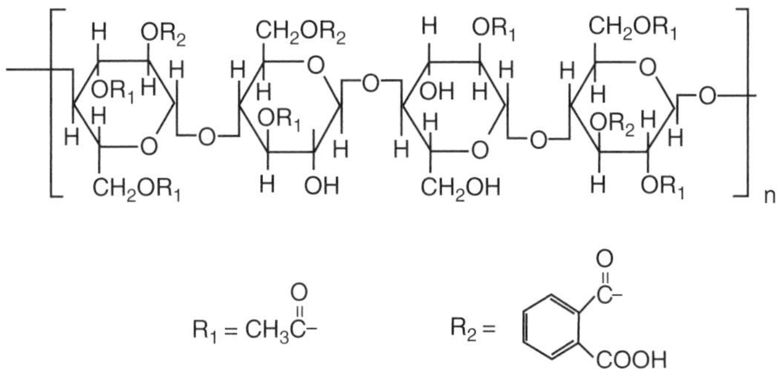

Figure 1 The structure of cellulose acetate phthalate.

to produce a three-fold increase in ileal effluent recovery compared to the uncoated capsules suggesting that such a formulation would be useful in treating ileocolitis (3).

## Polyvinyl Acetate Phthalate

Polyvinyl acetate phthalate (PVAP) is a free flowing white to off-white, essentially amorphous powder and may have a slight odor of acetic acid. It is a reaction product of phthalic anhydride, sodium acetate and a partially hydrolyzed polyvinyl alcohol. It is soluble in methanol and its mixture with methylene chloride, ethanol, and ethanol–water mixture, acetone and its mixtures with alcohols, ethyl acetate-IPA mixture and alkali (pH 5). Sureteric™ powder is a specially blended combination of PVAP, plasticizer, and other ingredients for reconstitution with water to make a totally aqueous coating dispersion of PVAP.

## Hydroxypropyl Methylcellulose Phthalate

Hydroxypropyl methylcellulose phthalate (HPMCP) is a cellulose in which some of the hydroxyl groups are replaced with methyl ether, 2-hydroxypropyl ether or phthalyl ether. It is a white to slightly off-white granular powder or free flowing flake. It is odorless or with a slightly acidic odor and has a barely detectable taste. It is insoluble in water but soluble in alkaline media (pH 4.5) and acetone–water mixture.

HPMCP is a more flexible polymer than CAP and is included in many monographs. Commercially, the available forms are HPMCP-50 (HP-50) and HPMCP-55 (HP-55). The numbers refer to pH ($\times$ 10) of the aqueous buffer solubility. A special type of HPMCP-55 (HP-55S), which is distinguished by its higher molecular weight, higher film strength, and higher resistance to simulated gastric fluid, is also available in the market.

## Shellac

Shellac is a material of natural origin and is now less popular in commercial pharmaceutical applications for enteric coatings. It is a purified resinous secretion of the insect *Laccifer lacca*. It is soluble in aqueous alkali at pH of 7.0 and suited for drug release in the distal small intestine.

## Methacrylic Acid Copolymers

These are anionic copolymers and are very commonly utilized for enteric coating, including applications in colonic delivery. This range of copolymers is principally marketed by Degussa, Pharma Polymers (Darmstadt, Germany) under the brand names, EUDRAGIT®. The enteric grades of EUDRAGIT dissolves at raised pH due to ioniZation of its carboxyl groups forming salts. The most commonly employed methacrylate polymers are EUDRAGIT L and EUDRAGIT S which are copolymers of methacrylic acid and methyl methacrylate and are available as fine solids. Their aqueous solubility depends on the ratio of carboxyl to ester groups, being approximately 1:1 in EUDRAGIT L100 and 1:2 in EUDRAGIT S100 (Fig. 2). This has a direct effect on solubility with regard to pH sensitivity and they dissolve above pH 6 and pH 7, respectively.

EUDRAGIT L100-55 is a copolymer of methacrylic acid and ethyl acrylate, and it dissolves at pH above 5.5. Among the anionic copolymers, it is the only polymer which is available as a 30% aqueous dispersion (EUDRAGIT L30D-55). Others are recommended for use after dissolution in acetone or alcohols.

EUDRAGIT L100, S100 and L100-55 are listed in USP/NF as methacrylic acid copolymer A, B, and C, respectively.

Preferred coating compositions for the colonic drug delivery are often mixtures of EUDRAGIT L100 and EUDRAGIT S100. The most preferable range for the two in a coating composition comprises around 70% to 80% of EUDRAGIT L100 and 20% to 30% of EUDRAGIT S100. Depending upon the pH at the target site in the colon, the coating thickness would be varied accordingly such that as the pH increases, the optimal coating thickness would be decreased. Formulations for colonic delivery containing

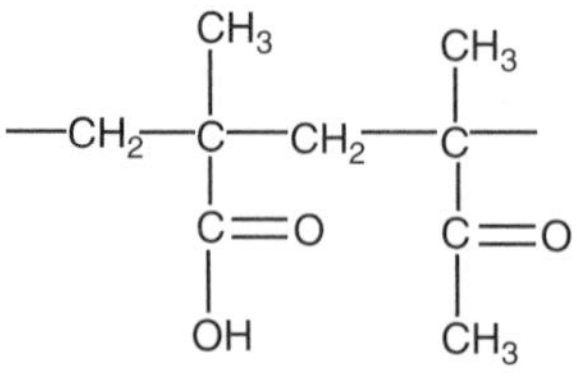

Figure 2   EUDRAGIT® L100/S100.

combination of EUDRAGIT L100 and S100 normally receive a target coating thickness of 80–120 μm.

The approach for using enteric polymers in the coat for colonic drug delivery is based on the assumption that the gastrointestinal pH increases progressively from the small intestine to colon. However, studies have shown that the pH in the distal small intestine is usually around 7.5, while the pH in the proximal colon is closer to 6. Hence, EUDRAGIT L and S containing products have a tendency to release their drug load prior to reaching the colon.

One of the issues in preparing multilayer formulations is the residual organic solvent which may be unacceptable. To overcome the problem of organic phase coating, a copolymer of methacrylic acid, methyl methacrylate, and ethyl acrylate (EUDRAGIT FS) was developed, which dissolves at a similar rate to EUDRAGIT S, however with big advantage of aqueous product processing.

## Hydroxypropyl Methylcellulose Acetate Succinate (HPMCAS)

Hydroxypropyl methylcellulose acetate succinate (HPMCAS) consists of a cellulose backbone to which are attached methyl, hydroxypropyl succinate, and hydroxymethyl acetate groups. The ratio of these side groups affects the extent to which the polymer becomes soluble in the intestine. It dissolves in aqueous buffers of pH 7.

## Polymethyl Vinyl Ether/Maleic Acid Copolymers

International Speciality Products, markets a range of polymethyl vinyl ether copolymers under the brand, Gantrez (Fig. 3). The ES series of Gantrez are available in ethyl (ES-225), n-propyl or n-butyl ester (ES-425) forms and are supplied as a 50% solution in ethanol. They are insoluble in aqueous acidic pH conditions and are suitable for use as enteric materials.

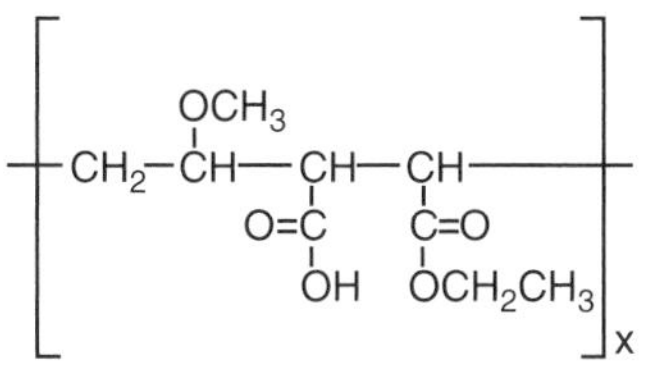

Gantrez ES-225
monoethyl ester of
poly (methyl vinyl ether/maleic acid)
(CAS#: 25087-06-3)

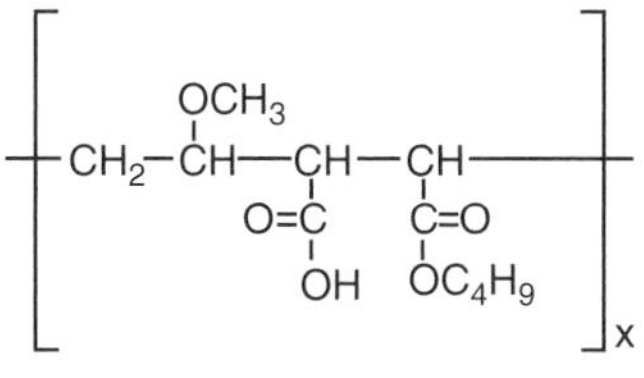

Gantrez ES-425
monobutyl ester of poly (methyl vinyl
ether/maleic acid)
(CAS#: 25119-68-0)

**Figure 3**   Gantrez polymers.

## EXAMPLES OF ENTERIC COATED SYSTEMS FOR COLONIC DELIVERY EUDRACOL

EUDRACOL™ is a drug delivery platform technology, marketed as complementing the two EUDRAMODE and EUDRAPULSE™ technologies by Degussa Pharma Polymers GmbH (Fig. 4). EUDRACOL™ is a multiparticulate, multilayer system that uses aqueous polymethycrylate dispersions in the design of the release profile. The pellets can be produced in conventional process equipment. The final dosage forms can either be capsules or pellets compressed to disintegrating tablets. These technologies are patent-protected and the concepts have been confirmed in proof-of-concept studies.

This concept takes advantage of relatively constant transit time of the small intestine (3–4 hr) and a high pH of the distal small intestine and hence combine pH characteristics of different EUDRAGIT polymers and transit time in the small intestine to develop a reliable multiunit colonic delivery system.

The outer layer is an EUDRAGIT FS 30 D layer that dissolves above pH 7. Since the pH at the ileum and ileocaecal valve is reported to be pH 7–8, it is expected that EUDRAGIT FS 30 D dissolves in that region and can be used to control the site of release of a pellet system previously coated with EUDRAGIT RL and/or RS layer for sustained release in the colon (4).

The pellet core consists either of a nonpareil and a drug-layer coating or of a drug core.

An HPMC capsule coated with EUDRAGIT FS 30 D was investigated in a gamma scintigraphy study, where the capsule passed the stomach without being damaged and shortly before entering the colon, the dissolution was observed to occur (5). Bott and colleagues (6) manufactured caffeine pellets coated with inner EUDRAGIT RL/RS 30 D and outer

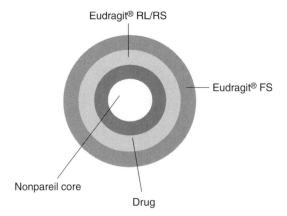

Eudragit® RL/RS

Eudragit® FS

Nonpareil core

Drug

**Figure 4**   The structure of a EUDRACOL™ pellet.

EUDRAGIT FS 30D. Additionally a lactose [$^{13}$C]-ureide was administered to study orocaecal transit time in twelve healthy male volunteers. The coated pellets reached the ileo-cecal region within 4 hours and also prolonged the caffeine release (serum levels) compared to the pellets containing only one coat (EUDRAGIT FS 30 D). The authors proposed that the oral delivery of these systems could be more beneficial to treat the colonic diseases compared to the existing conventional therapies.

Sekigawa and colleagues (7) claim a coated solid dosage form suitable for oral administration having reliable medicament release only in the large intestine. The product was prepared by coating a core containing the active ingredient, first with a chitosan having a specific degree of deacetylation and a specific degree of polymerization, and then top-coating with a specific enteric-soluble polymer, such as hydroxypropyl methylcellulose acetate succinate (Fig. 5). The release of the active ingredient in the large intestine can be more reliable when, prior to coating with chitosan, the core is provided with an enteric undercoating layer.

An oral pharmaceutical preparation for releasing a principal agent in the lower gastrointestinal tract was reported by Yamada and coworkers (8), comprising an active component and a solid organic acid, filled into a hard capsule composed mainly of chitosan, and the surface of the filled capsule coated with an enteric coating film consisting of hydroxypropyl methyl cellulose phthalate, hydroxypropyl methyl cellulose acetate succinate, cellulose acetate phthalate, methacrylate copolymer and shellac.

A controlled release coated bead formulation (9) has been described incorporating a lag phase prior to the release of the drug which is tailored to begin release at the beginning of the large bowel, releasing the active at a predetermined rate to the colon (Fig. 6). It comprises drug layered onto inert seed surrounded by a drug release control membrane, which is a pH-independent or pH-dependent dissolving first membrane (typically, an enteric polymer). The next layer is an acid layer, followed by a release time-controlling compound membrane consisting of a pH-sensitive polymer as an inner layer and an insoluble polymer in the outer layer.

EUDRAGIT S was first used by Dew and colleagues for the targeted delivery of 5-ASA in colitic patients (10). This early paper laid the principle

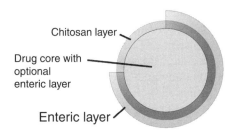

Chitosan layer

Drug core with optional enteric layer

Enteric layer

**Figure 5** Coated dosage form suitable for oral administration. *Source*: Adapted from Ref. 7.

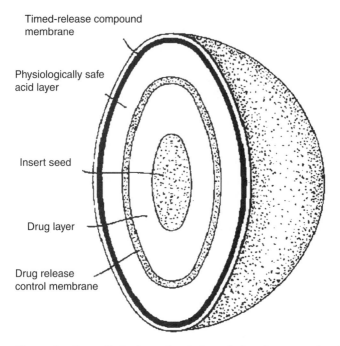

Timed-release compound
membrane

Physiologically safe
acid layer

Insert seed

Drug layer

Drug release
control membrane

**Figure 6** Controlled-release bead formulation incorporating lag phase. *Source*: From Ref. 9.

of utilizing delayed release to achieve better colonic-drug delivery and the workers used x-ray imaging to follow the transit of the formulation. The adoption of gamma scintigraphy to follow gastrointestinal transit in animals was reported in a very early study by our group (11) and our later papers showed gamma scintigraphy could be used to demonstrate targeted delivery to the colon (12). Similar studies were then carried out using gamma scintigraphy by Adkin and colleagues carried out scintigraphic studies to ascertain the behavior of formulations for colonic drug delivery systems containing biodegradable polymers in the matrix and coated with EUDRAGIT L (13).

Ishibashi's group prepared four capsule formulations for colon delivery containing theophylline, each of which had a different in-vitro dissolution lag time (14). The capsules also contained sulfasalazine as a colon arrival marker. A powder mixture consisting of 20 mg of theophylline, 50 mg of sulfasalazine, and 100 mg of succinic acid was filled into a hard gelatin capsule, and the joint of the capsule body and cap was sealed with a small amount of 5% (w/w) ethylcellulose ethanolic solution. Four batches of the sealed capsules were spray-coated with ethanolic solutions containing different amounts of EUDRAGIT E (0, 11, 21, and 33 mg/capsule) to provide a different onset time for drug release. Each batch of the EUDRAGIT-E coated capsules were next coated with a hydrophilic intermediate layer containing hydroxypropyl methylcellulose and acetaminophen, in a hydroxyethanolic solution. Finally, the capsules were coated with hydroxypropyl methylcellulose acetate succinate as the outmost enteric layer. Succinic acid was used as the pH-adjusting agent.

Marvola and coworkers at the University of Helsinki reported a multiple-unit system for drug release in the colon using enteric polymers (15). Film-coated matrix pellets were prepared with enteric polymers as both binders and coating materials. It was found that drug release from the formulations took place in the distal part of the small intestine and the colon if enteric polymers dissolving at pH 7 were used.

Fukui and colleagues reported on the use of enteric coated timed-release press-coated tablets (16). The tablet core contains diltiazem hydrochloride as a model drug, followed by the outer press-coated shell of hydroxypropylcellulose and, finally, an outer-most shell of an enteric polymer. The tablets were found potentially useful for oral site-specific drug delivery including colon targeting.

Gupta et al. utilized a pellet-based colon delivery system for 5-ASA (17) The core was prepared by drug layering on nonpareils followed by coating with an inner layer of a combination of two pH-independent polymers ammonio–methacrylate copolymers (EUDRAGIT RL and RS), and an outer layer of a pH-dependent methacrylic acid copolymer, EUDRAGIT FS.

Akhgari and colleagues (18) prepared the mixture of pH dependent (EUDRAGIT S100 and EUDRAGIT L100) and pH independent (EUDRAGIT RS) polymers following statistical full factorial design. The mixture containing different proportions of these polymers was applied on indomethacin pellets to obtain coating levels of 5%, 10%, and 15%. The in vitro dissolution profiles of all the formulations were obtained and the one containing EUDRAGIT RS: EUDRAGIT S100: EUDRAGIT L100 (20: 64: 16) with 10% coating level gave optimum dissolution profile. The studies revealed that the combination of this polymer-coating system might be suitable to achieve the colonic delivery.

Ibekwe and colleagues (19) compared the dissolution profiles of prednisolone tablets coated with EUDRAGIT S (organic solution), EUDRAGIT S (aqueous dispersion), EUDRAGIT FS (aqueous dispersion) and EUDRAGIT P4135 to obtain a 5% weight gain. EUDRAGIT P4135 was not sufficiently acid-resistant and abandoned fairly early on by the authors. The in vitro release profiles of the coated tablets after a 2-hour exposure to acid were dissimilar for Sorenson phosphate buffer (pH 7.4) compared to a physiological phosphate buffer (Hank's buffer, pH 7.4) and this was found to be due to solubility effects on the polymer rather than the prednisolone. It was suggested that EUDRAGIT FS was more appropriate to achieve the delivery in the ileo-colonic region. In addition, the authors conclude that the dissolution medium should have the ionic composition similar to the intestinal fluid while assessing the performance of the enteric coated dosage forms.

Gao and colleagues (20) utilized EUDRAGIT FS 30D to coat the meloxicam loaded cores at a 15% (w/w) coating level. It was found that the in vitro release of meloxicam was pH dependent. In vivo studies were conducted using pentagastrin-pretreated beagle dogs. This treatment was carried out to maximally stimulate acid secretion as dogs tend to have a higher resting pH than humans. It was demonstrated that the release of the drug was significantly delayed from the coated pellets compared to the non-coated pellets and the authors proposed that this weight gain using EUDRAGIT FS 30D was appropriate to achieve the colonic delivery of meloxicam.

Krogars et al. prepared pH-sensitive matrix pellets for colon-specific drug delivery of ibuprofen (21). Using an extrusion-spheronization pellet-ization technique, EUDRAGIT S and citric acid were the principal for-mulation ingredients of the matrix core, which also contained microcrystalline cellulose. The pellets were enteric coated to achieve a lag time of 15 minutes in pH 7.4 phosphate buffer.

Alvarez-Fuentes and colleagues (22) prepared matrix tablets of theo-phylline containing different properties of hydroxyl ethyl cellulose (HEC) with microcrystalline cellulose (MCC) which were compared to HEC with ethyl cellulose (EC). The matrix tablets were enteric coated with EUDRAGIT S100 with a coating level between 10% and 40%. After per-forming in vitro dissolution studies, it was found that the tablets containing theophylline: MCC:HEC (1:0.3:0.7) with 27% coating level had a lag time of about 260 minutes and released 90% of the drug content within 10 hours. The authors proposed that these coated-tablets could be ideal to target the colon while treating the inflammatory bowel diseases.

## CONCLUDING REMARKS

The use of a pH-based trigger to target the colon is probably insufficient to guarantee reproducible treatment both when the patient has active disease and when in remission, since normal rhythms of distal gastrointestinal tran-sit and reabsorption of secretions are altered in inflammatory disease. In order to avoid premature release in the upper gastrointestinal tract, a combination of acid-resistant barrier coat and time-dependent release has to be employed as conditions in the lumen remain fairly homogenous until the cecum is reached. The small dip in pH caused by bacterial fermen-tation may not be exploitable and other factors including the physical form of the formulation become important determinants of colonic resi-dence time.

## ACKNOWLEDGMENTS

The authors wish to express their gratitude to Dr. Pradip Kumar Ghosh, Jubilant Organosys, India, for having reviewed this chapter and providing valuable information based upon his experience in the use of enteric coating polymers.

## REFERENCES

1. Hardy JG, Evans DF, Zaki I, Clark AG, Tonnenson HH, Gamst ON. Evaluation of an enteric-coated tablet using gamma scintigraphy and pH monitoring. Int J Pharm 1987; 37:245–50.
2. Reddy SM, Sinha VR, Reddy DS. Novel oral colon-specific drug delivery systems for pharmacotherapy of peptide and nonpeptide drugs. Drugs Today 1999; 35:537–80.
3. Levine DS, Raisys VA, Alnardi V. Coating of oral beclamethasone dipropri-onate capsules with cellulose acetate phthalate enhances delivery of topically active antiinflammatory drug to the terminal ileum. Gastroenterology 1987; 94(4):1037–44.
4. Gupta VK, Beckert TE, Price JC. Development of a novel multi-particulate colonic delivery system using multifunctional coatings of aqueous poly-methacrylates. In: Third world meeting (APV/APGI) on Pharmaceutics, Biopharmaceutics and Pharmaceutical Technology, 4–6 April, Berlin, Germany, 2000.
5. Cole ET, Scott RA, Connor AL, et al. Enteric coated HPMC capsules designed to achieve intestinal targeting. Int J Pharm 2002; 231:83–95.
6. Bott C, Rudolph MW, Schneider ARJ, et al. In vivo evaluation of a novel pH- and time-based multiunit colonic drug delivery system. Aliment Pharmacol Ther 2004; 20:347–53.
7. Sekigawa F, Onda Y. Coated solid medicament form having releasability in large intestine. US Patent: 5217720, 1993
8. Yamada A, Wato T, Uchida N, Fujisawa M, Takama S, Inamoto Y. Oral pharmaceutical preparation released in the gastrointestinal tract. US Patent: 5468503, 1995
9. Klokkers-Bethke K, Fischer W. Pharmaceutical preparation to be administered orally with controlled release of active substance and method for manufacture. US Patent: 5472710, 1995
10. Dew MJ, Ryder REJ, Evans N, Rhodes J. Colonic release of 5-aminosalicylic acid from an oral preparation in active ulcerative colitis. Br J Clin Pharmac 1983; 16:185–7.
11. Curt NE, Hardy JG, Wilson CG. The use of the gamma camera to study the gastrointestinal transit of model drug formulations. In: Drug Measurement and Drug Effects in Laboratory Health Science. Karger, Basel, 1980: 147–50.
12. Hardy JG, Wilson CG, Wood E. Drug delivery to the proximal colon. J Pharm Pharmacol 1985; 37:874–7.
13. Adkin DA, Kenyon CJ, EI Lerner, et al. The use of scintigraphy to provide "proof of concept" for novel polysaccharide preparations designed for colonic drug delivery. Pharm Res 1997; 14:103–7.

14.  Ishibashi T, Ikegami K, Kubo H, Kobayashi M, Mizobe M, Yoshina H. Evaluation of colonic absorbability of drugs in dogs using a novel colon-targeted delivery capsule (CTDC). J Control Release 1999; 59:361–76.

15.  Marvola M, Nykänen P, Rautio S, Isonen N, Autere AM. Enteric polymers as binders and coating materials in multiple-unit site-specific drug delivery systems. Eur J Pharm Sci 1999; 7:259–67.

16.  Fukui E, Miyamura N, Uemura K, Kobayash M. Preparation of enteric coated timed-release press-coated tablets and evaluation of their function by in vitro and in vivo tests for colon targeting. Int J Pharm 2000; 204:7–15.

17.  Gupta VK, Beckert TE, Price JC. A novel pH- and time-based multiunit potential colonic drug delivery system. I. Development. Int J Pharm 2001; 213: 83–91.

18.  Akhgari A, Sadeghi F, Garekani HA. Combination of time-dependent and pH-dependent polymethacrylates as a single coating formulation for colonic delivery of indomethacin pellets. Int J Pharm 2006; 320:137–42.

19.  Ibekwe VC, Fadda HM, Parsons GE, Basit AW. A comparative in vitro assessment of the drug release performance of pH-responsive polymers for ileo-colonic delivery. Int J Pharm 2006; 308:52–60.

20.  Gao C, Huang J, Jiao Y, et al. In vitro release and in vivo absorption in beagle dogs of meloxicam from EUDRAGIT FS 30 D-coated pellets. Int J Pharm 2006; 322:104–12.

21.  Krogars K, Heinamaki J, Vesalahti J, Marvola M, Antikainen O, Yliruusi J. Extrusion-spheronization of pH-sensitive polymeric matrix pellets for possible colonic drug delivery. Int J Pharm 2000; 199:187–94.

22.  Alvarez-Fuentes J, Fernández-Arévalo M, González-Rodríguez ML, Cirri M, Mura P. Development of enteric-coated timed-release matrix tablets for colon targeting. J Drug Target 2004; 12:607–12.

# 29

# Programmed Drug Delivery Systems and the Colon

## Clive G. Wilson

*Strathclyde Institute of Pharmacy and Biomedical Sciences, Glasgow, Scotland, U.K.*

## Hardik K. Shah

*Biovail Technologies (Ireland) Ltd., Dublin, Ireland*

## Wang Wang Lee

*AstraZeneca, Macclesfield, U.K.*

## Bianca Brögmann

*Degussa Pharma Polymers GmbH, Darmstadt, Germany*

## Gour Mukherji

*Jubilant Organosys Ltd., Noida, India*

## INTRODUCTION

In many therapeutic applications it would be advantageous to deliver orally-administered drug into the systemic circulation some time after swallowing the formulation. Examples include the treatment of nocturnal asthma and prevention of secondary serious arrhythmias provoked by postural changes following previous severe cardiac ischemia. Many physiological and pathophysiological events have a circadian rhythm which suggests that treatment could be optimized by delivering the drug at the most appropriate time. By delaying the release of the drug until a programmed interval after swallowing, more sophisticated and efficient therapies can be designed.

Enteric coating allows a simple delivery solution to avoiding dissolution of the formulation in the gastric milieu and the presentation of a pulse of drug after a pre-programmed interval. The physicochemical characteristics and thickness of the polymer coat controls release and simple distinctions of pH and time dependent release are not always applicable. Moreover, the formulator still has a relatively narrow window of gastrointestinal transit in which to operate. For some actives, a rapid onset of release may not be appropriate but applying too much retardation will inevitably lead to a slower absorption if the unit delivers past the terminal ileum/ascending colon. The initial approach to overcoming these limitations was to employ zero-order release devices, but this would not allow for slower agitation and altered absorption profiles in the terminal gut. Perhaps other shapes of drug release pattern, with an upswing in release rate with time, might be more effective? This thinking led formulators to consider the generation of more complex release profiles and the term "programmed release" should therefore include a description of the profile as well as the delay. The extent to which in vivo–in vitro correlation can be expected for such systems is questionable as gastrointestinal transit is influenced by daily activity, especially meal timing, and postural changes.

Time-dependent systems have been developed for colon targeted delivery utilizing nonbiodegradable polymers which are more frequently employed as excipients in controlled-release systems. The polymers are usually synthetic in nature and undergo dissolution or disintegration in the gastrointestinal tract, without undergoing significant absorption or degradation. They are generally nonspecific with respect to pH-solubility characteristics and the employment of these polymers as carrier matrices for colonic delivery often utilizes a time-dependent mechanism to provide an initial lag phase of low or no release during transit through the upper gastrointestinal tract. Other physical attributes of the material can be used to achieve targeting include bioadhesion, mechanical strength (i.e., systems which are ruptured during passage from ileum to cecum) and biological properties especially fermentation by bacterial enzymes. The fermentation of biopolymers is a further extension of this concept, but here the coverage is restricted to small molecule fermentation such as lactose. In addition, some of the systems described in the patent literature are based on well-established osmotic core technology. Products have been formulated in a variety of compositions, including incorporation of polymers in a drug core, with an application of an enteric polymer coat for preventing drug release in the stomach. This may provide release in the terminal ileum or if the lag time is sufficient, 3–4 hours, in the colon. In another variation, the outermost nonenteric layer completely replaces the enteric inner layer resulting in a complete time-dependent drug release mechanism.

The mechanisms employed for timed release have been recently summarized in a review of oral pulsed delivery systems (1). Maroni and colleagues separate the oral pulsatile systems into the following types of systems:

- Drug delivery system with rupturable coating layer
- DDS with swellable/erodible layers
- DDS with increasingly permeable coating layers
- Capsule-shaped systems with release-controlling plugs
- Osmotic systems

Film rupture systems work by the development of an internal pressure generated by expansion of the core. Expanding systems include cros-car-mellose (Ac-Di-Sol®) which was found to be most effective as the core material in soft gelatin capsules as opposed to formulation in hard gelatin capsules (2). Ethyl cellulose is often used as the outer-layer as it possesses excellent strength and film-coating properties and can be press-coated at different thicknesses onto drug cores as sides or faces as described by Lin and colleagues (3,4).

The solubility characteristics of the active substance can play an important role. If a drug has high solubility, the selection of the polymer system for targeted drug delivery particularly to the colon, is an extremely challenging task. Such matrices may tend to release the drug prematurely, at least partially, in the stomach and the small intestine. Application of a thicker coat of the polymer may cause incomplete drug release in the colon. In contrast, drugs having poor solubility may have intrinsic problems with regards to absorption from the colon, where the availability of water is less.

Prominent examples of these synthetic materials include the cellulosic ethers and the cross-linked polyacrylates. Among the celluloses, there are grades of hydroxypropyl methylcellulose (HPMC) of various viscosity, which are commercially marketed under the trade name, Methocel® (Dow). Other cellulose ethers include methyl cellulose, hydroxypropyl cellulose and carboxymethyl cellulose. The cross-linked polyacrylates of the swelling types include the branded Carbopols of the oral grade, with suffix 934P, 974P, and 971P, manufactured by BF Goodrich. Polymethacrylates are often employed in nonswelling polymers in modified release products. The poly-methacrylic acids are frequently employed as enteric polymer coats on matrices, while the anionic, cationic and the neutral polymethacrylates have been used in controlled-release products. The most commonly used brands of these polymers are the various EUDRAGIT® products from Degussa Pharma Polymers. The polyethylene oxides are also useful polymers for controlled release, suitable for application in colonic drug delivery.

The following section illustrates some of the technologies that have been commercialized employing nonbiodegradable polymeric systems for colon-specific delivery.

## EXAMPLE TECHNOLOGIES

## CODES

The technology used in CODES™ system comprises a series of polymers which are combined to protect the drug core until the formulation arrives in the colon. CODES, an oral tablet technology, consists of an enteric outer coating, with a cationic polymer coating for retarding release during transit along the small intestine. Once in the colon, lactulose, which is incorporated in the drug core, is degraded by the colonic microflora allowing drug release.

### Colon Targeted Delivery System

This system first described by Shah and coworkers uses lagtime to achieve colon delivery. The system comprises of three parts; an outer enteric coat, an inner semipermeable polymer membrane and a central core comprising of swelling excipients and an active component (5). These parts of the system function to prevent premature release in the upper gastrointestinal tract. The dosage form releases drug consistently in the colon by a time-dependent rupturing mechanism.

The outer enteric coating prevents drug release until the tablet reaches the small intestine. In the small intestine, the enteric coating dissolves allowing gastrointestinal fluids to diffuse through the semipermeable membrane into the core. The core swells until after a period of 4–6 hours, when it bursts the membrane releasing the active component in the colon.

The precision and predictability of release time relies on the functional properties of the semipermeable membrane; in particular the percent elongation of the membrane which increases by between 2.0% and 3.5% during manufacture. This membrane elongation allows the release of the active ingredient 4–6 hours after entering the small intestine, which is consistent with the literature values for the small intestine transit time (SITT). The elongation is achieved using a plasticizer which comprises between 10% and 30% w/w of the membrane. The concentration of the plasticiser determines the percentage elongation.

The enteric coating has a thickness of 100 μm at a weight of about 15% of the core. The polymer used is hydroxypropyl methylcellulose phthalate which dissolves at pH 5.5. The enteric coating is typically formulated with distilled acetylated monoglyceride as the plasticizer. The role of the membrane is to allow water influx but to prevent outward diffusion of the active drug. Several polymers have suitable properties and include ethyl cellulose, cellulose acetate, and polyvinyl chloride. Conventional excipients, dibutyl sebacate, acetylated monoglycerides, and diethyl phthalate, are utilized.

In addition to the active component, the core contains of a swelling agent, e.g., croscarmellose sodium or sodium starch glycolate, and osmotic agent such as mannitol, sucrose or glucose in the percentages of 10–30% and 15–25% w/w, respectively.

The formulation is prepared by conventional methods. The core is prepared by wet granulation and the semipermeable and the enteric coating are applied by suitable air spray systems. In vitro dissolution experiments carried out showed that release occurred after 4–6 hours exposure of the system to phosphate buffer pH 7.5. This release occurred regardless of the time of initial exposure in an acid medium. These data suggests that this system should be applicable for colonic delivery.

## Time-Controlled Ethyl Cellulose System

A novel four compartment system was described by Niwa and colleagues (6) which releases drug in a time-controlled system based on an ethyl cellulose shell. The base of the system is drilled to allow the ingress of water to allow access to a swellable system causing rupture of the system at a rate dependent on the thickness of the cap. Published in vivo data obtained in beagle dog studies investigated cap thicknesses of 39, 63, and 76 μm. Increasing the thickness of the coating shifted showed peak plasma peaks of the marker substance fluorescein from 1.5 to 4 and 7 hours, respectively, suggesting that the thicker coating maybe sufficient to target the colon. Such systems show low pH specificity and thus taking this system with food may cause premature release in the upper gastrointestinal tract (7).

## OROS-CT

The following two examples illustrate the use of osmotic agents to provide colon-targeted delivery. OROS-CT® is a technology developed by Alza Corporation and consists of an enteric coating, a semipermeable membrane, a layer to delay drug release and a core consisting of two compartments. The first compartment contains the active drug in any layer adjacent to an exit passageway and the other is an osmopolymer composition to provide the osmotic push in the system (8).

The enteric coating used does not dissolve, disintegrate or change its structural nature in the stomach. The material consists of phthalates, keratin, formalin-treated protein, oils and anionic polymers. The semipermeable wall consists of selectively permeable polymers that are insoluble in body fluids, nonerodible but permeable to the passage of fluids. These polymers, cellulose acylate and cellulose acetates, form good semipermeable membranes.

The layer below the semipermeable membrane consists of polyethers, polyoxyethylene, and hydroxypropylmethylcellulose depending on the formulation. It delays the release of drug for about 2–4 hours. As the system passes through the small intestine, it absorbs fluid and begins to dispense drug at a controlled rate.

In the core, the osmopolymer swells or expands to push the composition containing the active drug from the delivery system. The osmopolymers are typically hydrophilic polymers including poly(hydroxyalkylmethacrylate), poly(vinylpyrrolidone) and poly(vinylalcohol) or acidic carboxypolymers.

The compartment containing the active drug and the osmopolymer are manufactured either by wet or dry granulation and the dosage form is formed by tablet press. The wall and the delay coat are formed by an air suspension procedure. The enteric coating is applied onto the surface of the delay layer. On the semipermeable membrane, a 6.35-μm orifice is laser drilled through to the core components.

The OROS-CT system has been utilized in the delivery of drugs for the treatment of colitis, ulcerative colitis, Crohn's disease, idiopathic proctitis, and other conditions affecting the colon (8).

## Controlled-Release Drug Delivery Device

The delivery device is an osmotic system with a solid core comprising an active drug, a substantially soluble delay jacket, a semipermeable membrane and an enteric coating. The delay jacket comprises at least one component selected from the group consisting of a binder, an osmotic agent and a lubricant. The semipermeable membrane may have a release orifice as a part of the structure (9).

The enteric coating resists dissolution in gastric fluid and limits drug release in intestinal fluid. The enteric coating usually consists of phthalate based material such as cellulose acetate phthalate, hydroxypropyl methylcellulose phthalate and polyvinyl acetate phthalate. The semipermeable membrane consisting of cellulose acetate, ethyl cellulose and polymethacrylic acid esters which function to maintain physical integrity. To impede the dissolution and release of the active agent as the system travels through the small intestine, a jacket delaying release is included in the formulation.

The solid core comprises an active drug and excipients including osmotic agents, lubricants, binders and suspending agents. The osmotic agent induces a hydrostatic pressure after water enters the core which drives out the active drug in solution or as a suspension. Suitable osmotic agents include salts of organic or inorganic acids.

The delay jacket may be applied to the core using conventional means, e.g., a tablet press or a spray coater. This is followed by the application of the semipermeable membrane using film coating techniques and the enteric coating applied utilizing a conventional perforated pan coating technique.

## TIMECLOCK

The TIMECLOCK delivery device developed by Pozzi and colleagues is a pulsed delivery system based on a coated solid dosage form. The coating which is applied by aqueous dispersion at 75°C, is a hydrophobic-surfactant layer with the addition of a water-soluble polymer to improve adhesion of the coating to the core. The dispersion rehydrates and redisperses once in an aqueous environment in a time proportional to the thickness of the film. The delay in drug release correlates with the thickness of the originally applied layer. Following redispersion, the core is available for dissolution (10).

In vitro studies described by the authors showed that the lag time interval was highly reproducible despite variation of the parameters simulating differing physiological conditions. The authors used the dye, sunset yellow E110, to visualize the behavior of the system in vitro. The dissolution of the dye was always rapid and complete for all the tablets tested. In vivo studies confirmed the high reproducibility of the lag time. In a clinical study conducted using scintigraphy, the effect of food was investigated. After the administration of TIMECLOCK following either a low or a high calorie meal, the mean lag time was 345 and 333 minutes, respectively.

The hydrophobic film redispersion appears not to be influenced by the presence of intestinal digestive enzymes or by the mechanical action of the stomach. The lag time interval can therefore be considered independent of the digestive state. However, the TIMECLOCK releases its core content at a set lag time, regardless of the position of the delivery system in the gastrointestinal tract (10). This is a disadvantage if a positioned site-specific drug delivery is required. Product development work was described by Steed and colleagues (11), which used a hydrophobic enteric-coating to increase the specificity of drug release.

## TARGIT™

West pharmaceutical services developed TARGIT™ technology particularly to deliver the therapeutic agent for the topical treatment of the colonic diseases (12). The technology utilizes starch capsules coated with combination of pH dependent polymers (EUDRAGIT L100:EUDRAGIT S100, 3:1). TARGIT™ capsules were evaluated for the phase I studies in 90 volunteers (fasted state) using gamma scintigraphy (12). The studies revealed that 90% of the TARGIT capsules ($n = 73$) disintegrated within terminal ileum and colon. TARGIT capsules promise the delivery of the active ingredient to the colon supported by extensive clinical studies. In addition, the dissolution of the coating was not affected by the drug formulation, which resulted in a flexible technology allowing the incorporation of different active ingredients.

## EUDRAPULSE™

EUDRAPULSE™ is a multiparticulate, multilayer system that uses aqueous polymethacrylate dispersions in the design of pulsatile release profile with various lag times, marketed as complementing the two EUDRACOL™ and EUDRAMODE™ technologies by Degussa Pharma Polymers GmbH. EUDRACOL has been described in Chapter add place holders "Enteric Coating for Colonic Delivery." The technology is patent protected and the concept has been confirmed in proof-of-concept studies.

The design is based on a core with a combination of drug with organic acids or salts from organic acids, top-coated with EUDRAGIT RL and/or RS polymer dispersion. Alternatively the pellet preparation can be started with a nonpareil core (Fig. 1). The final dosage form can either be a capsule or pellets compressed to disintegrating tablets.

The pulsatile drug delivery is achieved through an ionic interaction of the organic anion and the quarternary ammonium group of the polymethacrylate copolymer, where the chloride is replaced by the respective organic anion, thus leading to different film properties, e.g., permeabilities (13,14). Formulation variations using different organic anions, EUDRAGIT RS/RL ratios and polymer layer lead to a high flexibility with regard to lag time and slope of pulsed release (15).

This drug delivery technology has been applied to the commercial product Dilzem®, where the necessity of a night dosing is required.

### Pulsatile Drug Delivery System

Krögel and Bodmeier (16) have described a capsular drug delivery system where drug release occurred after erosion of plug material in a manner reminiscent of Egalet TM. The capsule consists of insoluble and impermeable poly(propylene). The plug was formed by congealing a melt of polyglycolated glycerides or compressing low viscosity grade HPMC within the capsule body. An anionic surfactant, sodium dodecyl sulfate,

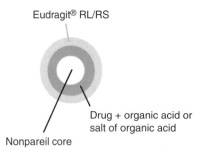

Eudragit® RL/RS

Drug + organic acid or
salt of organic acid

Nonpareil core

**Figure 1** The structure of the EUDRAPULSE pellets.

was added to improve the erodability of the plugs. Release time was affected by the grade of HPMC used to make the plugs, position and thickness of plugs but not the plug hardness. Effervescent agents, disintegrating agents and surfactant were investigated to accelerate drug release from the capsule body where release was less than 40% within 2 hours. It was found that drug release was quicker with increasing concentration of effervescent agents with 20% effervescent agent resulting in complete release within 5 minutes, which was desirable. The addition of the super-disintegrant, Ac-Di-Sol, marginally improved the release, while sodium dodecyl sulfate had no effect.

Problems with premature and irreproducible plug ejection time were also encountered. This was overcome by modifying the opening of the capsule body to be conically shaped. Sometimes the HPMC plug remained as a highly viscous polymer solution at the opening of the capsule body, thus retarding drug release. To overcome this, the researchers further developed a pectin/pectinolytic enzyme-containing plug (17). Both enzyme and substrate is incorporated into the plug where degradation of plug material was not controlled by enzymes present in the gastrointestinal tract but by the enzyme incorporated into the plug. The viscous solution of pectin is completely degraded by the pectinolytic enzyme. Hence, a nonhindered diffusion and release of the content was achieved.

## PORT

PORT developed by Port Systems, LLC consists of a hard-gelatin capsule film coated with celluloses to render it semipermeable, an insoluble plug made of fats, waxes and fatty esters and an osmotic agent within the capsule shell (18). The osmotic agent consists of simple sugars such as lactose, sorbitol, mannitol, and sodium bicarbonate to increase internal pressure on hydration inside the shell. The increased pressure forces the plug to slide out of the shell to release the drug. The lagtime is controlled by the thickness of the capsule film; increasing thickness lengthens the time to reach the required amount of pressure inside the shell to expel the plug. The system tested in humans showed good agreement between lag times for in vitro dissolution and in vivo release of Samarium-153 chloride (19).

## SUMMARY

From these remarks, it is noted that the general construction used for the time-dependent systems is similar. The composition consists of three main layers; an outer enteric coating, a lag phase layer and a core containing the active component. The characteristics of polymers used to form the layers should allow sufficient flexibility to provide gastric protection and low release during intestinal transit allowing delivery to the colon.

## FURTHER READING

The review by Maroni provides an extensive discussion on oral pulsatile devices and should be consulted in addition to this chapter.

## REFERENCES

1. Maroni A, Zema L, Cerea M, Sangalli ME. Oral pulsatile drug delivery systems. Expert Opin Drug Deliv 2005; 2(5):855–71.
2. Sungthongjeen S, Puttipipatkhacorn S, Paeratakul O, Dashevsky A, Bodmeier R. Development of pulsatile release tablets with swelling and rupturable layers. J Control Release 2004; 95(2):147–59.
3. Lin S-Y, Lin K-H, Li MJ. Micronized ethylcellulose used for designing a directly compressed time-controlled disintegration tablet. J Control Release 2001; 70(3):321–8.
4. Lin S-Y, Lin K-H, Li MJ. Compression forces and amount of outer coating layer affecting the time-controlled disintegration of compression-coated tablets prepared by direct compression with micronized ethylcellulose. J Pharm Sci 2001; 90(12):2005–9.
5. Shah H, Railkar AM, Phuapradit W. Colon targeted delivery system. US patent: 6,039,975, 2000.
6. Niwa K, Takaya T, Morimoto T, Takada K, Preparation and evaluation of a time-controlled release capsule made of ethylcellulose for colon delivery of drugs. J Drug Target 1995; 3:83–9.
7. Matsuda KI, Takaya T, Shimoji F, Muraoka M, Yoshikawa M, Takada K. Effect of food intake on the delivery of fluorescein as a model drug in colon delivery capsule after oral to beagle dogs. J Drug Target 1996; 4:59–67.
8. Theeuwes F, Guittard GV, Wong PSL. Delivery of drug to colon by oral dosage form. US patent: 4,904,474, 1990.
9. Savastano L, Carr J, Quadros E, Shah S, Khanna SC. Controlled release drug delivery device. US patent: 5,681,584, 1997.
10. Pozzi F, Furlani P, Gazzaniga A, Davis SS, IR Wilding, The Time Clock system: a new oral dosage form for fast and complete release of drug after a predetermined lag time. J Control Release 1994; 31:99–108.
11. Steed KP, Hooper G, Monti N, Benedetti MS, Fornasini G, Wilding IR. The use of pharmacoscintigraphy to focus the development strategy for a novel 5-ASA colon targeting system ["Time Clock(R)" system]. J Control Release 1997; 49:115–22.
12. Watts P, Smith A. TARGIT™ technology: coated starch capsules for site-specific drug delivery into the lower gastrointestinal tract. Expert Opin Drug Deliv 2005; 2:159–67.
13. Beckert TE, Pogarelli K, Hack I, Peterreit HU. Pulsed drug release with film coatings of EUDRAGIT® RS 30 D, Poster presentation at Controlled Release Society, 1999.

14. Ravishankar H, et al. Factors influencing the pulsatile EUDRAPULSE™ technology, Poster presentation at Control Society, 2005.

15. Narisawa S, Nagata M, Hirakawa Y, Kobayashi M, Yoshino H. acid-induced sigmoidal release system for oral controlled-release pı 2. Permeability enhancement of EUDRAGIT RS coating led by icochemical interactions with organic acid. J Pharm Sci 1996; 85:1!

16. Krogel I, Bodmeier R. Pulsatile drug release from an insoluble ca controlled by an erodible plug. Pharm Res 1998; 15:474–81.

17. Krogel I, Bodmeier R. Evaluation of an enzyme-containing capsu pulsatile drug delivery system. Pharm Res 1999; 16:1424–9.

18. Amidon GL, Crison JR. Method for making a multi-stage drug dı tem. US Patent. US, Port Systems, L.L.C, 1997.

19. Crison, JR, Siersma PR, Amidon GL. A novel programmable o technology for delivering drugs: human feasibility testing using gaı tigraphy. Proc Int Symp Control Rel Bioac Mater 1996; 51–2.

# 30

# Pulsincap™ and Hydrophilic Sandwich Capsules: Innovative Time-Delayed Oral Drug Delivery Technologies

H. N. E. Stevens

*Department of Pharmaceutical Sciences, University of Strathclyde, Glasgow, Scotland*

## INTRODUCTION

Chronopharmaceutical drug delivery (1) discussed the delivery of drugs in accordance with the circadian rhythms of the disease. The identification of a specific time-dependent "trigger" capable of provoking drug release from an oral formulation after a pre-determined time interval represents a significant challenge to the pharmaceutical formulator.

## PULSINCAP™ TECHNOLOGIES

Three variants on a capsule theme have been developed that trace their origins back to PolySystems Ltd, a small Scottish company in the late 1980s. The first concept consisted of a device based on the separation of a plug from an insoluble capsule body which was first described by Rashid (2). This formulation, which was described in the patent literature, comprised a water permeable body (Fig. 1) prepared from a water swellable hydrogel cross-linked polyethylene glycol (PEG) polymer. Depending on their composition, such polymers have the capacity to swell significantly, but in a controlled manner, in aqueous media. A swelling agent (powdered high-swelling polymer) mixed with drug, was filled into the internal cavity of Rashid's molded capsule body and a plug (also of high-swelling polymer) was used to seal the contents into the internal cavity. The rate at which water diffused

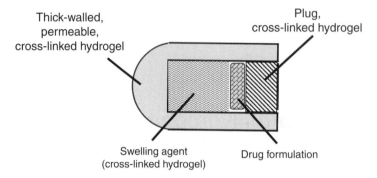

**Figure 1**  Pulsatile hydrogel capsule. *Source*: From Ref. 2.

into the core was controlled by the hydrogel composition and wall thickness of the capsule. The delay period prior to drug release was defined by the time taken for fluid to diffuse through the wall. When fluid came into contact with the capsule contents, the high-swelling polymer absorbed water rapidly, swelled and caused internal pressure to be generated inside the capsule. This pressure caused the plug to be expelled from the neck of the capsule and drug to be released in a pulsatile manner. Optimization of the construction of the components and the chemistry of the hydrogel polymers enabled time-delays to be controlled reproducibly.

A manually prepared prototype formulation with a 5-hour lag time was the subject of a pharmacokinetic study in man designed to release captopril in the colon of the fasted volunteers. Scintigraphic observations confirmed that drug was released from the capsule at the target site, however, pharmacokinetic analysis confirmed that minimal absorption had taken place from the colon (3).

Molding the thermosetting hydrogel polymers required for the capsule body was a very complex process that did not lend itself to industrial scale-up. Further developments of this technology, now more widely referred to as Pulsincap™, were undertaken and improved devices were described in the patent literature (4). Polysystems was acquired by RP Scherer Corporation in 1990 and the Pulsincap technology was then developed by Scherer DDS Ltd. This second generation Pulsincap device was less complex than Rashid's earlier capsule and the hydrogel body of the earlier formulation was now replaced by a gelatin capsule, film-coated with ethyl cellulose to render it impermeable (Fig. 2). The link to hydrogel polymer chemistry was retained and a molded hydrogel plug was used to seal the drug contents into the capsule body. In the presence of fluid, the plug swelled at a controlled rate that was independent of the nature or pH of the medium (5).

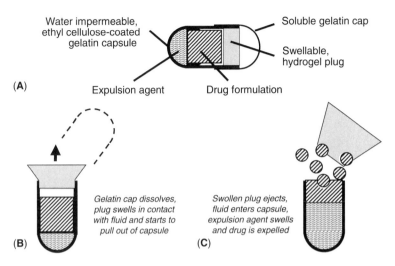

**Figure 2** Pulsincap™ delivery system. *Source*: From Ref. 4.

As it swelled, the plug developed a frustro-conical shape and slowly pulled itself out of the capsule. The length of the plug and its insertion distance into the capsule controlled the pulse time reliably.

This second generation Pulsincap formulation has been studied in numerous human volunteer studies (e.g., (6,7)) and was well tolerated in man (8). In order to effect complete drug release from the capsule following plug ejection, an active expulsion system was employed to rapidly and completely expel the contents from the capsule, as demonstrated with delivery of salbutamol to human volunteers, where the expulsion system low-substituted hydroxypropylcellulose (LH-21®, Shin-Etsu) was employed (9,10).

Due to the fact that the mechanism of action was controlled by the plug sliding out of the capsule, a significant factor for the correct operation of Pulsincap was the tightness of fit of the hydrogel plug in the capsule. If the fit of the plug was too slack it ejected prematurely, whereas when it fitted too tightly, drug was released erratically (11). In order to respect the very tight dimensional specifications demanded for predictable operation, each plug was subjected to three-dimensional measurement using laser gauges. As a result of the cost implication of this requirement, the delivery system was never adopted for large scale human healthcare applications. However, a low volume diagnostic test kit based on Pulsincap releasing nutrient components into a microbial test medium after a 6-hour lag time, was commercialized in 1997 (SprintSalmonella™, Oxoid Ltd, Basingstoke, UK).

More recent studies have been undertaken on a further simplified adaptation of the technology. Now working at Strathclyde University Stevens et al. (12) and Ross et al. (13) eliminated reliance on hydrogel

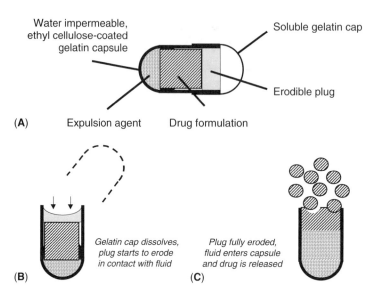

**Figure 3**   Erodible plug time-delayed capsule. *Source*: From Ref. 12.

polymers and developed a Pulsincap formulation that employed a simple erodible compressed tablet in place of the swelling hydrogel plug (Fig. 3). Since the tablet eroded in place, it did not move relative to the capsule body and this factor overcame the need for the precise dimensional tolerances between plug and capsule required by the sliding mechanism of the plug in the earlier Pulsincap formulations.

A range of erodible tablet formulations were studied using ethyl cellulose-coated gelatin capsule bodies. It was shown that controllable time-delayed release of propranolol could be achieved with pulse-time being determined by either plug composition or its thickness. Ross et al. (13) again utilized low-substituted hydroxypropylcellulose (LH-21®, Shin-Etsu) as a swellable expulsion system and achieved release of propranolol over a controllable 2–10 hour range using erodible tablet plugs compressed from mixed lactose and HPMC (Methocel®, DOW) excipients.

Krögel and Bodmeier (14) similarly studied the application of erodible plugs fitted in plastic capsules using formulations based on either compressed tablets or congealed semi-solid materials. Release of chlorpheniramine after time-delays was obtained by manipulating plug composition or weight.

## HYDROPHILIC SANDWICH CAPSULE

In an attempt to develop a simple, time-delayed probe capsule, Stevens et al. (15) devised a manually assembled delivery system based on a

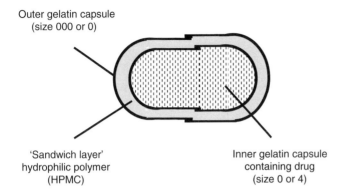

**Figure 4**   The hydrophilic sandwich capsule. *Source*: From Ref. 15.

capsule-within-a capsule, in which the intercapsular space was filled with a layer of hydrophilic polymer (HPMC). This effectively created a "hydrophilic sandwich" (HS) between the two gelatin capsules. When the outer capsule dissolved, the sandwich of HPMC formed a gel barrier layer which provided a time-delay before fluid could enter the inner capsule and cause drug release. The time-delay was controlled by the molecular weight of the polymer and could be further manipulated by the inclusion of a soluble filler, e.g., lactose, in the hydrophilic layer (Fig. 4).

The HS capsule was studied in two configurations, either with an external size 000 capsule and an internal size 0, or a "mini HS," in which the external capsule was size 0 and the internal capsule was size 4. Soutar et al. (16) employed a gastroresistant version of the larger HS capsule in a cohort of 13 volunteers to deliver 500 mg paracetamol to the ileocecal junction/proximal colon. Absorbed drug was monitored using salivary analysis and a mean $T_{max}$ value of 7.9 hours (SD ± 0.96) was observed.

## CONCLUDING REMARKS

Pulsed drug delivery using systems based on Pulsincap technology and derivatives has been demonstrated in the clinic using scintigraphy. Current research is focused on providing a readily adaptable configuration whose release characteristics in vivo can accurately be reflected in compedial in vitro tests. Results so far are extremely encouraging with good concordance in healthy volunteers.

## REFERENCES

1.  Stevens HNE. Chronopharmaceutical drug delivery. J Pharm Pharmacol 1998; 50:S5.
2.  Rashid A. Dispensing device. EP 0 384 642, 1990.

3. Wilding IR, Davis SS, Bakhshaee M, Stevens HNE, Sparrow RA, Brennan J. Gastrointestinal transit and systemic absorption of captopril from a pulsed-release formulation. Pharm Res 1992; 9:654–7.
4. McNeill ME, Rashid A, Stevens HNE. Drug dispensing device. GB patent, 2 230 442, 1993.
5. Binns JS, Bakhshaee M, Miller CJ, Stevens HNE. Application of a pH independent PEG based hydrogel to afford pulsatile delivery. Proc Int Symp Control Rel Bioact Mater 1993; 20:226–7.
6. Bakhshaee M, Binns JS, Stevens HNE, Miller CJ. Pulsatile drug delivery to the colon monitored by gamma scintigraphy. Pharm Res 1992; 9(Suppl):F230.
7. Hebden JM, Wilson CG, Spiller RC, et al. Regional differences in quinine absorption from the undisturbed human colon assessed using a timed release delivery system. Pharm Res 1999; 16:1087–92.
8. Binns JS, Stevens HNE, McEwen J, et al. The tolerability of multiple oral doses of Pulsincap capsules in healthy volunteers. J Control Release 1996; 38:151–8.
9. Stevens HNE, Binns JS, Guy MI. Drug expelled from oral delivery device by gas. International Patent Application WO 95/17173, 1995.
10. Stevens HNE, Rashid A, Bakhshaee M, Binns JS, Miller CJ. Expulsion of material from a delivery device. US patent 5 897 874, 1999.
11. Hegarty M, Atkins G. Controlled release device. International patent application WO 95/10263A1, 1995.
12. Stevens HNE, Rashid A, Bakhshaee M. Drug dispensing device. US patent, 5 474 784, 1995.
13. Ross AC, MacRae RJ, Walther M, Stevens HNE. Chronopharmaceutical drug delivery from a pulsatile capsule device based on programmable erosion. J Pharm Pharmacol 2000; 52:903–9.
14. Krögel I, Bodmeier R. Pulsatile drug release from an insoluble capsule body controlled by an insoluble plug. Pharm Res 1998; 15:474–81.
15. Stevens HNE, Ross AC, Johnson JR. The hydrophilic sandwich (HS) capsule: a convenient time-delayed oral probe device. J Pharm Pharmac 2000; 52:S41.
16. Soutar S, O'Mahony B, Bakhshaee M, et al. Pulsed release of paracetamol from the Hydrophilic Sandwich (HS) capsule. Proc Int Symp Control Rel Bioact Mater 2001; 28:790–1.

# 31

# Targeting the Colon Using COLAL™: A Novel Bacteria-Sensitive Drug Delivery System

**Emma L. McConnell and Abdul W. Basit**

*The School of Pharmacy, University of London, London, U.K.*

## INTRODUCTION

The colon, by virtue of favorable pH and reduced motility, is home to a dense population of micro-organisms [over 400 species (1), numbering $10^{11}$–$10^{12}$ colony forming units per ml of colonic material (2)]. The presence of a resident microflora is a highly specific environmental feature of the colon, contrasting markedly with the sparsely populated upper gastrointestinal tract; this difference can be exploited in order to effect site-specific drug release in the colon (3). The consistently high levels of bacteria in the colon mean that it is much more reliable than the more variable pH (4) or transit time (5) which have been investigated for colonic delivery. Prodrugs, e.g., sulfasalazine, which rely on the action of colonic bacteria to break down an inactive precursor and release the active drug moiety (mesalazine or 5-aminosalicylic acid), have been in use for many years, but are highly drug specific, and there is a need for the development of a more universal system which can be adapted to a variety of drugs for both local and systemic treatment. An amylose based, bacterially triggered system has been developed to fulfil this need.

## DEVELOPMENT OF A UNIVERSAL COLONIC DRUG DELIVERY SYSTEM

The colonic microflora, reliant on undigested polysaccharides as their energy source, are the producers of large quantities of polysaccharidase enzymes. This has led to the identification of polysaccharides as good candidates for colonic drug delivery. A wide variety of polysaccharides, have been shown to be digested by human colonic bacteria (6) but, of these, amylose, one of the main polysaccharides from starch, has shown the most promise and progress for colonic delivery.

In order to effect colon specific release, an amylose based dosage form must first reach the colon intact. Amylose must therefore firstly resist digestion by the endogenous enzymes of the pancreas, and a proportion of amylose termed "resistant starch" is capable of doing this (7). Digestion of resistant starch by colonic bacteria can still occur due to greater efficiency of colonic bacterial enzymes (8). Amylose, in its glassy form, is a form of "resistant starch" and the properties which lend it to colonic drug delivery are summarized in Table 1.

Amylose, due to its tendency to swell in contact with water, cannot be used alone to control drug delivery. Mixing amylose with a water insoluble polymer such as ethyl cellulose, allows intermingling of polymer chains sufficient to cause a reduction in the swelling properties of amylose films (9,10).

## DESCRIPTION OF THE AMYLOSE/ETHYLCELLULOSE TECHNOLOGY

Amylose and ethyl cellulose (as an aqueous suspension) can be mixed and used as a film coat. This technology is versatile and, using conventional fluid bed coating, can be adapted to coat tablets (11), capsules (12) and pellets (9,13,14). Amylose and ethyl cellulose are not completely miscible and the result is a heterogeneous film coating in which the amylose exists interspersed within the polymer. Thus, the film coat is a matrix system, in which the amylose is behaving as a pore forming agent, in that it provides areas within a water insoluble film that are subject to swelling or enzymatic degradation, and drug release will occur by this route (9).

## RESEARCH AND DEVELOPMENT

### In Vitro

Through in vitro investigations, the system of film coating with amylose and ethyl cellulose proved capable of controlling drug release in simulated gastric and small intestinal conditions. Through optimization of variables, primarily

**Table 1**  Properties of Glassy Amylose That Enable Its Use as a Colonic Specific Coating

- Good film forming properties
- Nontoxic
- Resistant to pancreatic enzyme digestion
- Susceptible to fermentation by bacterial enzymes in the colon

coating thickness and amylose/ethyl cellulose ratio, a coating with appropriate controlled-release characteristics could be developed for a variety of drugs; glucose (13), 5-aminosalicylic acid (9), propranolol (14), 4-aminosalicylic acid (12), and prednisolone sodium metasulphobenzoate (15).

After successful retardation of drug release in simulated upper gastrointestinal conditions, it was necessary to establish whether release would occur in the presence of colonic bacteria. This was done in vitro using human fecal material as a model for the colonic contents. Colonic bacteria are mainly anaerobic (2) and the anaerobic environment was provided by batch fermenters, in which inoculums of human fecal material (10% w/v in pH 7.2 buffer media under an atmosphere of nitrogen) were introduced (16) and drug-loaded dosage forms were then added to this. Any amylose present in the film was then available for digestion by the colonic bacteria, and drug release into the fecal media, brought about by permeation through the pores left by amylose, was assessed.

Rapid release of drug into simulated colonic conditions was shown, using several drugs (9,11,13,14). Figure 1 shows the release of 5-aminosalicylic acid into control dissolution systems, and colonic conditions (9). Thus the amylose/ethyl cellulose coating shows the desired formulation characteristics for colonic drug delivery.

Although amylose/ethyl cellulose coatings for pellets or tablets performed well in vitro, the in vivo performance cannot always be predicted. Therefore, these systems were investigated in man, by coupling drug release with gamma scintigraphic methods of following transit. Since glassy amylose is present in many foodstuffs, and ethyl cellulose is generally regarded as safe, the clinical trials did not require preclinical safety data.

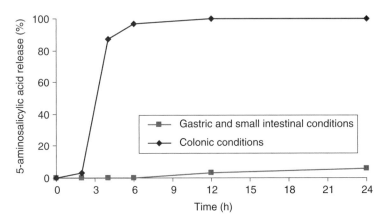

**Figure 1** In vitro release of amylose/ethyl cellulose coated pellets (containing 5-aminosalicylic acid) under simulated gastric and small intestinal conditions, and a simulated colonic environment.

## CLINICAL TRIALS IN HEALTHY VOLUNTEERS

Noninvasive in vivo studies in humans, using [$^{13}$C] glucose pellets, utilized the fact that, upon release in the colon, [$^{13}$C] glucose is fermented by the gut microflora to $CO_2$ and short chain fatty acids, which are absorbed and metabolized, and can be detected as $^{13}CO_2$ in the breath. Ingestion of [$^{13}$C] glucose pellets coated with amylose/ethyl cellulose, followed by breath measurements and gamma scintigraphy, showed that $^{13}CO_2$ excretion in the breath did not occur until the pellets reached the cecum (17). This demonstration of successful in vivo release was further confirmed by studies in which dosage forms coated with amylose/ethyl cellulose (containing 4-aminosalicylic acid, ranitidine or prednisolone sodium meta-sulphobenzoate) were found, by blood testing and gamma scintigraphy, to release drug into the blood corresponding with the entry of the dosage form in the colon (12,15,18). Figure 2 shows the release of ranitidine in one volunteer, which coincided with arrival of the dosage form in the colon.

Successful in vivo results in healthy subjects has led to the development of the amylose/ethyl cellulose formulation concept into COLAL™, which is currently under investigation in further clinical trials, and the technology is subject to a number of patents.

## CLINICAL TRIALS IN DISEASE STATE PATIENTS

The COLAL system is the first universal colonic drug delivery system to progress beyond Phase I trials. The corticosteroid prednisolone sodium metasulfobenzoate has been incorporated into the COLAL system and the

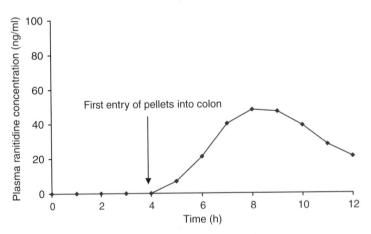

**Figure 2** Correlation between arrival of amylose/ethyl cellulose coated ranitidine pellets in the colon, and the appearance of drug in the blood.

resultant product (COLAL-PRED™) has been assessed in Phase II clinical trials for the treatment of inflammatory bowel disease, primarily ulcerative colitis. In a randomized, double-blind, parallel study, a dose-dependent improvement in disease activity and disease severity of ulcerative colitis was shown with COLAL-PRED. Clinical remission was achieved with a 60-mg dose and, beneficially, systemic exposure to prednisolone was found to be low, with an associated low incidence of side effects, and no depression of adrenal function (19). Positive results here have enabled Phase III clinical trials for moderate to severe ulcerative colitis to begin, and these are currently underway.

## CONCLUSION

Amylose has been combined with ethyl cellulose to produce a novel coating system, known as COLAL, which can be used to coat pellets, tablets and capsules. This coating has been shown in vitro to resist breakdown in the upper gastrointestinal tract but allow drug release in the colon, by bacterial fermentation of the amylose component. The system is versatile and can be used to modify the release of a variety of drugs, making it effectively a universal colonic delivery system. In vivo, the system has been shown to allow drug release, so that it available for local or systemic treatment, in the colon. This patented technology, in the form of for the treatment of ulcerative colitis COLAL-PRED has shown impressive results in Phase II clinical trials, with good clinical efficacy coupled with a decrease in corticosteroid associated side effects. Currently, Phase III trials are underway.

## REFERENCES

1. Finegold SM, Sutter VL, Mathisen GE. Normal indigenous intestinal flora. In: Hentges DJ, ed. Human Intestinal Flora in Health and Disease. New York: Academic Press, 1987: 3–13.
2. Moore WEC, Holdeman LV. Discussion of current bacteriologic investigation of the relationships between intestinal flora, diet and colon cancer. Cancer Res 1975; 35:3418–20.
3. Basit AW. Advances in colonic drug delivery. Drugs 2005; 65:1991–2007.
4. Nugent SG, Kumar D, Rampton DS, Evans DF. Intestinal luminal pH in inflammatory bowel disease: possible determinants and implications for therapy with aminosalicylates and other drugs. Gut 2001; 48:571–7.
5. SS Davis, JG Hardy, JW Fara. Transit of Pharmaceutical Dosage Forms through the small intestine. Gut 1986; 27(8):886–92.
6. Salyers AA, West SHE, Vercellotti JR, Wilkins TD. Fermentation of mucins and plant polysaccharides by anaerobic bacteria from the human colon. Appl Environ Microb 1977; 34:529–33.
7. Englyst HN, Cummings JH. Digestion of the polysaccharides of some cereal foods in the human small intestine. Am J Clin Nutr 1985; 42:778–87.

8.  MacFarlane GT, Englyst HN. Starch utilisation by the human large intestine. Lett Appl Microbiol 1986; 60:195–201.
9.  Milojevic S, Newton JM, Cummings JH, et al. Amylose as a coating for drug delivery to the colon: preparation and in vitro evaluation using 5-aminosalicylic acid pellets. J Control Release 1996; 38:75–84.
10. Leong CW, Newton JM, Basit AW, Podczeck F, Cummings JH, Ring SG. The formation of colonic digestible films of amylose and ethyl cellulose from aqueous dispersions at temperatures below 37°C. Eur J Pharm Biopharm 2002; 54:291–7.
11. Wilson PJ, Basit AW. Exploiting gastrointestinal bacteria to target drugs to the colon: An in vitro study using amylose coated tablets. Int J Pharm 2005; 300: 89–94.
12. Tuleu C, Basit AW, Waddington WA, Ell PJ, Newton JM. Colonic delivery of 4-aminosalicylic acid using amylose-ethyl cellulose-coated hydroxypropylmethylcellulose capsules. Aliment Pharm Ther 2002; 16(10):1771–9.
13. Milojevic S, Newton JM, Cummings JH, et al. Amylose as a coating for drug delivery to the colon: Preparation and in vitro evaluation using glucose pellets. J Control Release 1996; 38:85–94.
14. McConnell EL, Tutas J, Mohammed MAM, Banning D, Basit AW. Colonic drug delivery using amylose films: the role of aqueous ethyl cellulose dispersions in controlling drug release. Cellulose 2007; 14:25–34.
15. Bloor JR, Basit AW, Chatchawalsaisin J, et al. Targeting of ATL-2502 (prednisolone sodium metasulphobenzoate) using COLAL coating. AAPS Pharm Sci 1999; 1(4):S438.
16. Siew LF, Man S-M, Newton JM, Basit AW. Amylose formulations for drug delivery to the colon: a comparison of two fermentation models to assess colonic targeting performance in vitro. Int J Pharm 2004; 273:129–34.
17. Cummings JH, Milojevic S, Harding M, et al. In vivo studies of amylose- and ethyl cellulose-coated [13C] glucose microspheres as a model for drug delivery to the colon. J Control Release 1996; 40:123–31.
18. Basit AW, Podczeck F, Newton JM, Waddington WA, Ell PJ, Lacey LF. The use of formulation technology to assess regional gastrointestinal drug absorption in humans. Eur J Pharm Sci 2004; 21:179–89.
19. Thompson RPH, Bloor JR, Ede RJ, et al. Preserved endogenous cortisol levels during treatment of ulcerative colitis with COLAL-PRED, a novel oral system consistently delivery prednisolone metasulphobenzoate to the colon [abstract]. Gastroenterology 2002; 122(S1):T1207.

# 32

# Development of the Egalet Technology

Daniel Bar-Shalom and Christine Andersen

*Egalet a/s, Vaerlose, Denmark*

Clive G. Wilson and Neena Washington

*Strathclyde Institute of Pharmacy and Biomedical Sciences, Glasgow, Scotland, U.K.*

## INTRODUCTION

The market for controlled and sustained release delivery forms is well established. Apart form the obvious applications for drugs with short half-lives and narrow therapeutic windows, sophisticated delivery systems open up the path for development of drugs with less than ideal physicochemical properties and allow better treatment of diseases which display chrono-biology, e.g., rheumatoid arthritis and asthma.

Currently, the commercially successful solid oral controlled-release technologies are almost exclusively based upon diffusion of water either directly into a matrix or through a membrane to release drug. This systems works well for water soluble drugs, however diffusion of a poorly soluble or nonwater soluble drug through a matrix poses difficulties. Currently only one system exists to meet this challenge, the Oros® osmotic technology from the ALZA Corporation.

This leaves many unmet needs in formulation development, with respect to successful delivery of labile drugs, providing burst or delayed-release characteristics, and allowing combinations of different drugs in one unit. Egalet® technology (1, 2) from Egalet a/s, Denmark is relatively new to the market, but offers distinct advantages over more conventional controlled release dose forms. The primary one is its ability to deliver water-insoluble compounds in a controlled manner as drug release involves the processes of erosion rather than diffusion. An added advantage is that active compounds entrapped in the Egalet matrix are also protected from oxygen and humidity and therefore the technology appears suited for chemically unstable substances and thus may increase shelf-life.

Chronotherapeutics will represent one of the next most significant challenges to the drug delivery sector (3). Chronobiology has long recognized that biological systems alter with days or seasons, taking their cue from the environment, e.g., mating seasons for animals and flowering seasons for plants and that a "body clock" alters the overall homeostatic controls of the body. The magnitude to which this "body clock" affects almost all systems is still quite a new concept and has been shown to affect periodicity and/or amplitude. What is less well recognized is that the disease state of a body will also display a periodicity. The realization that this occurs has led to the development chronotherapeutics, a new branch of therapy. This aims to take maximum advantage of the disease's chronobiology to provide optimum plasma levels of drug resulting in maximum health benefit and minimum side effects to the patient. This can be achieved by a combination of accurately timing both the dosing of the patient and the release of the drug from the delivery system.

The dosage forms which can meet the challenges posed by chronotherapeutics have to cope not only with the huge physiological variations which they will encounter, but they will have to precisely deliver their payload of drug to a specific time window. These parameters will not only vary with the disease state, but also on the physiochemical and pharmacokinetic properties of each individual drug. One important factor for a dosage form to meet these challenges is that it needs to be very flexible and fully customizable (4).

## OVERVIEW OF THE EGALET

The Egalet technology offers two distinct systems, the Constant-Release (2K) system or the Delayed-Release (3K) system (Fig. 1).

The 2K system consists of two components: and impermeable coat and matrix. The drug is distributed evenly throughout the matrix, which is eroded by gut movements and gastrointestinal fluids as it travels through the gut. The 3K form of the Egalet technology consists of an impermeable shell with two lag plugs, enclosing a plug of active drug in the middle of the unit. After the inert plugs have eroded, the drug is released, thus a lagtime occurs. Time of release can then be modulated by the length and composition of the plugs.

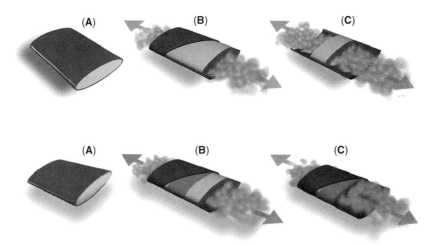

**Figure 1** *Top row*: Release from the 2K system demonstrating heterogeneous erosion and constant release: **(A)** whole Egalet, **(B)** during erosion, and **(C)** almost complete erosion. *Bottom row*: Burst release from a 3K Egalet: **(A)** intact, **(B)** outer inert cores eroding, and **(C)** erosion of central drug-laden core.

## DEVELOPMENT OF THE EGALET TECHNOLOGY

### Manufacture

The Egalet manufacturing process consists of a conventional two color, injection molding. The key components of both the tube and matrix are thermoplastic. The premixed powders, usually in the form of extruded granulates, which are used to form either the active matrix or plug, are fed into the mold. A reciprocating injection-molding process allows sequential molding of the shell and the core contents within the dies.

One issue with controlled-release technologies is that it can be a lengthy and costly process to tailor the dose form to match the required in vivo release profile of the drug. Often only a few different designs are tried in vitro and only the most promising one or two are selected to be tested in humans. The efficient manufacturing process for the Egalet leads to highly accurate dimensions, weight and content. It also allows for flexibility in dosage form design at minimum cost as the fill content and the size and length of the coat can be altered relatively easily. The same active substance can be used in the outer and inner plugs but a different concentration to create a customized release profile.

### Matrix Erosion

The shells are made of cetostearyl alcohol and ethyl cellulose while the matrix of the plugs comprises a mixture of polyethylene glycol (PEG) monostearates and polyethylene oxides. The drug release mechanism is believed to be surface erosion, effected through water diffusion, polymer hydration, disentanglement and dissolution. The matrix is designed to erode when in contact with available water but, at the same time, it is desirable that water does not diffuse into the matrix until the point of release thus avoiding hydrolysis and diffusion and reducing the effects of luminal enzymatic activity. A balance is required where the erosion is as fast as the diffusion of water into the matrix. The diffusion of water into the edges of the matrix producing only a hydrating/dissolving thin layer and leaving a dry core even after 4 hours (5).

The rate of drug release from an Egalet can be altered by adjusting the composition of the PEG carrier within the matrix. One explanation may be that when molten PEG cools and solidifies, it produces a structure that is partly crystalline and partly amorphous containing cracks or fissures. Water will penetrate rapidly through the fissures causing the surface and deeper layers to begin to dissolve simultaneously resulting in gel formation. If PEG-monosterate and PEG are co-melted and then cooled, the PEG/PEG parts will align whereas the monosterate groups will tend to be left on the surface of the particles, rendering the fissures hydrophobic and impassable to water. This results in heterogeneous erosion, because the erosion proceeds layer by layer. This matrix gives a zero-order release profile of drugs in vitro independent of pH but directly dependent upon rate of agitation (6).

## In Vitro Dissolution

The 2K Egalets, tested according to the generic USP dissolution tests (120–150 rpm for 2 hours, 30–50 rpm the rest of time) demonstrated that release in the first 2 hours during high agitation was much higher than in the later period of low agitation. Addition of small amounts (<10%) of cellulose derivatives of the type used for enteric coatings [cellulose acetate phthalate (CAP), hydroxypropylmethyl cellulose phthalate (HPMCA), hydroxypropylmethyl cellulose succinate] were found to slow down the rate of erosion at low pH but not at near-neutral or basic pH. This effect can be used to modify the relative rates of erosion at different agitations if the agitation is associated with a particular pH as, e.g., in the stomach relative to the small intestine.

Different materials, including the drug itself, when added to the matrix can have profound effects on the erosion rates. Water soluble drugs will speed the erosion, whereas water-insoluble ones will slow it, e.g., testosterone base will stop it altogether even at low concentrations. The pKs of the active compounds can also have a significant effect on the erosion. This is, of course, also true for excipients; cellulose derivatives, e.g., add plasticity. Starch, lactose, sucrose, and mannitol are convenient fillers as they normally have little impact on the release other than the solubility effect mentioned above. This can be used to compensate for water-soluble or insoluble drugs or to adjust the rate of erosion.

## CLINICAL EXPERIENCE

The correlation of in vitro to in vivo data been performed using the Egalet 2K constant-release system containing caffeine and samarium oxide in a scintigraphic study (6). The samarium oxide can be activated to $^{153}Sm_2O_3$ upon irradiation which is detected by a gamma camera hence allowing visualization of the behavior of the dose within the gastrointestinal tract.

Caffeine release consisted of three linear phases with constant slopes (Fig. 2) there was an initial burst release followed by 3 hours constant release than 10 hours of decreasing release and constant but slower release.

The potential to use a 2K Egalet for sustained drug delivery has been demonstrated in the development process of a once-daily antihypertensive drug. Two pharmacokinetic studies were carried out; the first to compare the pharmacokinetics of the Egalet formulation and an immediate release (IR) tablet formulation each containing 25 mg of carvedilol (7). In the second study, one 25 mg carvedilol Egalet was compared to twice-daily dosing of 12.5 mg IR tablets (7).

For the first study, the differences in area under the plasma-concentration time curve (AUC) were equivalent with a 90% confidence interval for the Egalet and IR formulations. The $C_{max}$ for carvedilol was statistically lower with the Egalet formulation than the IR formulation

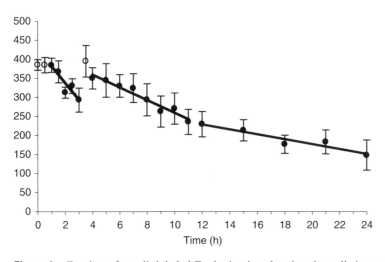

**Figure 2** Erosion of a radiolabeled Egalet in vivo showing three distinct rates which correspond to different areas of the gastrointestinal tract. *Source*: From Ref. 6.

($p < 0.001$). The $T_{max}$ was delayed from 60 minutes with the IR formulation to 180 minutes with the Egalet formulation.

The steady-state plasma concentration time curve for study 2 is shown in Figure 3. The $AUC_{(0-24)}$ for the single 25 mg dose of carvedilol delivered in the Egalet and twice daily 12.5 mg doses of carvedilol delivered in the IR formulation were $312.5 \pm 185.7$ and $303.4 \pm 195.4\,ng \cdot mL^{-1}h^{-1}$, respectively (mean $\pm$ SD). The $AUC_{(0-24)}$ for the Egalet formulation was tested and found to be equivalent to the IR tablets with 90% CI. Hence, it can be concluded that a once-daily 25 mg dose of carvedilol delivered in an Egalet drug delivery system in healthy volunteers provides the same total daily systemic exposure of drug as when administered with twice-daily dosing in a 12.5 mg IR tablet[®].

As with many complex controlled release devices, obtaining a close in vitro/in vivo correlation has proven to be more challenging for the 3K system. In vitro release of Egalet 2-hour system and a 6-hour system was between 90 and 100 minutes and 240–300 minutes, respectively. Initial work with effervescent agents has shown some promise, but a delicate balance is required to ensure that the effervescent agent assists drug release without causing bubbles which block its exit from the tube.

Drug release from the 3K Egalet formulation has been demonstrated in vivo also using the technique of gamma scintigraphy. The radiolabeled core was released when the unit entered the ascending colon. The released radioactivity gives a close approximation to the release and spread of the drug prior to absorption from the large bowel. The radiolabel can be seen to disperse as it passes through the ascending and transverse sections of the colon. Drug absorption usually ceases past the transverse colon due to the lack of water available. Preliminary work using quinine as a model drug demonstrates that the in vivo release of drug from the 3K Egalet is

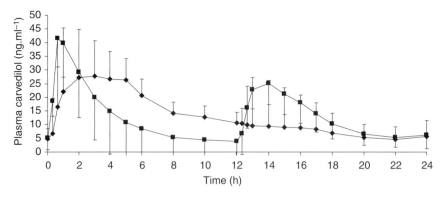

**Figure 3** Plasma concentration-time curves for carvedilol when dosed once daily with a 25-mg Egalet or twice daily with 12.5 mg immediate-release formulation.

consistently slower than the in vitro prediction. This is almost certainly due to the reduced motility and water availability in the distal regions of the gastrointestinal tract. The data from these studies confirm the need for more sophisticated in vitro testing methods which can more closely mimic the in vivo conditions and thus be better predictors of in vivo behavior.

## CONCLUDING REMARKS

The concept of erosion technology for sustained release appears to have a number of advantages over more conventional delivery systems. In summary, these are the ability to

- deliver poorly water-soluble drugs;
- possess zero-order release, the rate of which is dependent on gastrointestinal motility and water availability;
- easily tailor dosage form manufacture to obtain the desired release profile by altering size, width and matrix composition;
- have timed release, which may have great potential in chronotherapeutics.

Although this short description has concentrated on oral drug delivery, there are other possible alternative routes of use. These include utilization as part of another device, which is not necessarily designed for administration of drugs, e.g., insertion into the urinary bladder mounted on the tip of a catheter. Other routes, such as vaginal delivery, may allow this technology to be used to provide controlled release of actives over several days or even weeks as required.

## REFERENCES

1. Bar-Shalom D, Kindt-Larsen T. Controlled release composition US Patent No 5, 213:808.
2. Bar-Shalom D, Kindt-Larsen T. Controlled release composition US Patent No 5, 1993; 213:808.
3. Ura J, Shirachi D, Ferrill M. The chronotherapeutic approach to pharmaceutical treatment. California Pharmacist 1992; 23(9):46–53.
4. Washington N, Wilson CG. Can oral controlled drug delivery meet the challenges posed by chronotherapeutics? Drug Deliv Technol 2006; 6:57–9.
5. Metz H, Bar-Shalom D, Hemmingsen P, Fischer G, Mäder K. EPR and NMR imaging in monitoring the release mechanisms from Egalet® dosage units. Paper presented at the Controlled Release Society, Vienna, Austria, 2006.
6. Marvola J, Kanerva H, Slot L, et al. Neutron activation-based gamma scintigraphy in pharmacokinetic evaluation of and Egalet constant-release system. Int J Pharm 2004; 281:3–10.
7. Data on File. A randomised, steady-state, two-treatment, two-way crossover pharmacokinetic study investigating the relative bioavailabilities of two formulations of carvedilol tablets. Egalet, 2004.

# 33

# Regulatory Aspects in Modified-Release Drug Delivery

**Michael S. Roberts**

*School of Medicine, University of Queensland, Princess Alexandra Hospital, Brisbane, Queensland, Australia*

**Andrew Bartholomaeus**

*Drug Safety Evaluation Branch, Therapeutic Goods Administration, Canberra, ACT, Australia*

**George Wade**

*European Medicines Agency (EMEA), London, U.K.*

**Sultan Ghani**

*Drugs and Health Products, Health Canada, Ottawa, Ontario, Canada*

**Patrick J. Marroum**

*Division of Pharmaceutical Evaluation I, Office of Clinical Pharmacology, Center for Drug Evaluation and Research, Food and Drug Administration, Silver Spring, Maryland, U.S.A.*

## INTRODUCTION

Modified-release products are produced with the goal of delivering medicines that are efficacious, are acceptably safe and have a predictable time course of delivery. In this context, modified release refers to all types of formulations with modified release, including fast (rapid), delay, sustained release, targeted, and controlled-release formulations for the various routes of administration possible. Achieving regulatory approval is an integral part in the development and commercialization of any modified-release product. This overview chapter will emphasize conventional products, recognizing that although approaches differ somewhat between the major regulatory jurisdictions regulatory authorities will require documentation demonstrating that, in common with more standard preparations, such pharmaceutical products meet Good Manufacturing Practices (GMP); quality control specifications; and pharmaceutical product interchangeability (1). In general, such approval requires evidence that the following are well defined:

- As an active drug substance in its properties, manufacture, characterization, control, choice of storage container, and stability
- The drug product in terms of its formulation, manufacturing process, manufacture, excipient control, its control, choice of storage container and stability
- The pharmacokinetics and biopharmaceutics and, possibly, pharmacodynamics of the drug product and/or
- Demonstration of safety and efficacy by clinical trial

The precise nature and form of the evidence does differ greatly between the countries providing regulatory approval. In general, two somewhat different but increasingly convergent strategies are used. The United States has very detailed process driven procedures that are applied in product approval as described in a later chapter by Marroum (2). In contrast, the European Union (EU) provides guidelines for what is seen as the norm for various delivery systems (3). Here, it is possible to depart from the guidance with justification. The Japanese (4) and Canadian (5) systems appear to have a number of aspects in common with the US system. In contrast, the Australian system is somewhat more flexible, largely following, and formally adopting, the European Medicines Agency (EMEA) guidelines (6) but utilizing other sources of guidance or adopting a case by case approach where appropriate. The World Health Organization (WHO) provides effectively an overall harmonizing system. Interestingly, EMEA, WHO, and FDA each have one formulation category referred to as Delayed Release (1). The second is referred to as Prolonged Release by EMEA and as Extended (controlled, prolonged, sustained) Release by WHO and FDA.

In addition, the criteria being applied in regulatory approvals are continually evolving. In general, the criteria are becoming increasingly more drug and target specific. These considerations are of particular importance for modified-release dosage forms as many of these systems are specific in terms of both the active drug and the target site. For instance, topical corticosteroids are applied to exert an effect in the viable epidermis and/or upper dermis. Assessment of efficacy is dependent on defining activity at that site. Plasma concentrations may be useful, but mainly in terms of measuring the safety of topical steroids. Prolonged and significant plasma levels may be indicative of an excessive systemic steroid exposure and may, in some cases, lead to suppression of natural corticosteroid production—which may need to be addressed when the topical steroid is stopped.

In this chapter, we first consider the state of regulatory requirements as they exist in various countries for modified-release products. We then examine some examples of regulatory requirements that are in various evolutionary stages. Much of the emphasis is placed on oral formulations as they represent the bulk (>80%) of the 50 most-sold products in the western world.

## RATIONALE FOR DEVELOPMENT OF MODIFIED-RELEASE FORMULATIONS

In principle, modified release implies some modification of release rate and it may take the form of being faster, prolonged, delayed, controlled, responsive, or targeted. From a regulatory viewpoint, EMEA (7,8,9) proposes that the prolonged release product

- be effective and safe;
- leads to avoidance of high peaks and low troughs in plasma active substance concentration—time profiles;
- leads to less adverse reactions and/or the desirable clinical effect with a lower dose;
- potentially improves patient compliance through a lower frequency of administration.

EMEA (7) further proposes that a delayed release form may: protect the active substance from stomach acid; or the stomach from the active substance; or facilitate local action by release in a defined segment of the intestine.

Further, any dossier submitted in support of a marketing authorization application must provide (7)

- the modified-release device physical form and release mechanism;
- the dosage form description and in vitro and/or in vivo performance;
- active substance content;
- the dosage form clinical relevance, including proposed indications and posology.

In addition, the modified-release formulation administration conditions must be defined in terms of starting, maintaining or modifying dosing, managing acute conditions, co-dosing with an immediate release formulation and in terms of any special patient groups (e.g., elderly, children, patients with renal or hepatic insufficiency). Special consideration also needs to be given to (7)

- situations and modes of use of a combination of modified and immediate release forms "so as to avoid new prescribing problems for the physician and the risk of overdosing (or underdosing) for a significant proportion of the treated patients";

- having other dosages "to guarantee the therapeutic effect in terms of dose adjustment and to preclude harmful effects under normal conditions of use";
- "optimum conditions of use (e.g., not to chew or crush tablets)."

In pharmacokinetic terms, one goal may be to maximize the time a drug is within the therapeutic range over a dosing interval. In order to maximize patient compliance, this interval may be 12 or 24 hours. In principle, the shorter the half-life of a drug, the greater is the fluctuation in plasma concentrations. This can be expressed formally by the equation below. Here, the extent of fluctuation over a dosage interval at steady state, given by $R$, and equal to the ratio of the $C_{max,ss}$ to $C_{min,ss}$, is related to the drug's terminal half-life $t_{0.5}$ and the dosing interval $\tau$:

$$R = \frac{C_{max,ss}}{C_{min,ss}} = \frac{1}{\exp\left[-\frac{0.693\tau}{t_{0.5}}\right]}$$

Hence, if it is desired to dose twice daily for maximal compliance ($\tau = 12\,h$), the values for $R$ would be 64, 8, 3, 2, and 1 for half lives of 2, 4, 8, 12, and 24 hours. Now, if a drug has an elimination half-life of 2 hours and the desired fluctuation ($R$) is $<3$, the desirable half-life (defined by the release from the modified-release dosage form being rate limiting, i.e., absorption rate limited or "flip-flop" kinetics) is $>8$ hours. Accordingly, a modified-release dosage form must have an in vivo rate of release of $>8$ hours to achieve this target. If $R$ was 8, then an in vivo rate of release of $>4$ hours would be sufficient.

## MEDICINES EVALUATION

The regulation of therapeutic goods varies by jurisdiction and in the definition of therapeutic goods. In general, therapeutic goods are comprised of drugs and therapeutic devices, but in the United States, for instance, what is a cosmetic and what is a drug is defined by the proposed use of the product whereas in other jurisdictions, a drug is defined more specifically by its nature, concentration and site of application. Appropriate therapeutic goods regulation should facilitate their safety, quality, and efficacy.

The WHO provides a key global quality framework for drug regulation for its 193 member states (10). It suggests "effective drug regulation promotes and protects public health by ensuring that

- medicines are of the required quality, safety and efficacy;
- health professionals and patients have the necessary information to enable them to use medicines rationally;

- medicines are appropriately manufactured, stored, distributed and dispensed;
- illegal manufacturing and trade are detected and adequately sanctioned;
- promotion and adverting is fair, balanced and aimed at rational drug use;
- access to medicines is not hindered by unjustified regulatory work."

A recent survey (11) has shown that only some 50 drug regulatory agencies across the globe offer their respective information resources via a website to the internet audience. Websites of drug regulatory agencies as defined by WHO are given in Table 1. We now consider guidelines from countries in each geographical region. Table 2 outlines examples of developed and guidelines readily available from a range of countries.

## Africa

The Medicines Control Council of South Africa, established in 1965, has undergone considerable change in its performance and regulatory processes over the past five years. Its pharmaceutical and analytical guideline, for instance, was implemented in July 2007. The components of its guideline (Table 2) include:

| | |
|---|---|
| PART 2A | Pharmaceutical and biological availability |
| PART 3A | Active pharmaceutical ingredient (API) biological medicine primary production lot/batch |
| PART 3B | Formulation |
| PART 3C | Specifications and control procedures for pharmaceutical ingredients |
| PART 3D | Containers and packaging materials |
| PART 3E | Manufacturing procedure |
| PART 3F | Final product specifications and control |
| PART 3G | Stability data of the finished pharmaceutical product |
| PART 3H | Pharmaceutical development |
| PART 3I | Expertise and premises used for the manufacture of a biological medicine. |

Part 2A requires comparative data for a relevant method such as bioavailability, dissolution, disintegration, acid neutralizing capacity, microbial growth inhibition zones, proof of release by membrane diffusion, particle size distribution, blanching test, any other method provided the rationale for submitting the particular method is included. Proof of release by membrane diffusion is used as proof of efficacy for creams, ointments and gels; particle size distribution, by the Anderson sampler or equivalent apparatus, is proposed for inhalation efficacy; and blanching test for topical corticosteroids proof of efficacy in topical dosage forms. It is noted that, for appropriate oral dosage forms, biowaiver (waiver of boavailabilty or bioequivalence studies for biologicals) may be applied for on the basis of either

362 *Roberts et al.*

**Table 1** Drug Regulatory Authority Websites

*Africa*: 4 of 49 countries (8.5%)
  Algeria: http://www.ands.dz/
  Mauritius; http://ncb.intnet.mu/moh/index.htm
  South Africa: http://www.doh.gov.za/about/index.html
  Botswana: http://www.gov.bw/government/ministry_of_health.html (http://
    www.moh.gov.bw/index.php?id = 284) (http://www.moh.gov.bw/fileadmin/
    documents/Policies/registration_guidelines.pdf.)

*The Americas*: 7 of 36 countries (19.5%)
  Canada: http://www.hc-sc.gc.ca/hpb-dgps/therapeut/
  Colombia: http://anticorrupcion.gov.co/invima/
  Costa Rica: http://regcon.netsalud.sa.cr/
  Guatemala: http://www.mspas.gob.gt/default.html
  Mexico: http://www.ssa.gob.mx/unidades/dgcis/
  Peru http://www.minsa.gob.pe/digemid/
  United States of America: http://www.fda.gov/

*The Eastern Mediterranean*: 1 of 22 countries (4.5%)
  Morocco: http://www.sante.gov.ma/ministere/medicament/
    direction_du_médicament.htm

*Europe*: 28 of 51 countries (excluding EMEA) (55.8%)
  Austria: http://www.bmsg.gv.at/
  Belgium: http://www.afigp.fgov.be
  Bulgaria: http://www.bda.bg/
  Czech Republic: http://www.sukl.cz/
  Denmark: http://www.dkma.dk/
  EMEA: http://www.emea.eu.int/
  Estonia: http://www.sam.ee/
  Finland: http://www.nam.fi/
  France: http://agmed.sante.gouv.fr/
  Germany: http://www.bfarm.de/gb_ver/
  Greece: http://www.ypyp.gr/
  Hungary: http://www.ogyi.hu/ENG011.HTM
  Ireland: http://www.imb.ie/
  Israel: http://www.health.gov.il/ (We would categorise this as being in Middle
    East)
  Italy: http://www.sanita.it/farmaci/
  Latvia: http://www.vza.gov.lv/english/default.html
  Lithuania: http://www.vvkt.lt/ENG/default.htm
  Luxembourg: http://www.etat.lu/MS/DPM/fr/fr_index.html
  Netherlands: http://www.cbg-meb.nl/
  United Kingdom: http://www.mca.gov.uk/
  Poland: http://www.il.waw.pl/eng/version.htm
  Portugal: http://www.infarmed.pt/
  Slovakia. http://www.sukl.sk/sukl_en.htm
  Spain: http://www.msc.es/agemed/main.htm
  Sweden: http://www.mpa.se/ie_index.html

(*Continued*)

**Table 1**   Drug Regulatory Authority Websites (*Continued*)

Switzerland: http://www.iks.ch/default_E.asp
Turkey: http://www.iegm.gov.tr/
Norway: http://www.legemiddelverket.no/eng/reg/regulatory.htm
Slovenia: http://www.sigov.si/mz/ur-zdrav/english/index_en.htm

*Southeast Asia*: 3 of 10 countries (30%)
India: http://www.mohfw.nic.in/kk/95/ia/toc.htm
Republic of Korea: http://www.kfda.go.kr/english/index.html
Thailand: http://www.fda.moph.go.th/enginfo.htm

*Western Pacific Region*: 9 of 28 countries (32.1%)
Australia: http://www.tga.gov.au
China: http://www.sda.gov.cn
Japan. http://www.mhlw.go.jp
Malaysia: http://www.bpfk.org/html/index.htm
Mongolia: http://www.pmis.gov.mn/health/Epos_NHP/default.htm
New Zealand: http://www.medsafe.govt.nz/indexie4.htm
Philippines: http://web.doh.gov.ph/BFAD/
Singapore: http://www.hsa.gov.sg/cpa/
Hong Kong SAR: http://www.info.gov.hk/dh/

*Source*: From Ref. 11.

similarity with an existing product or in accordance with the U.S. FDA Biopharmaceutical Classification System (BCS). This guideline defines a modified-release product as

> one for which the drug release characteristics of time course and/or location are chosen to accomplish therapeutic or convenience objectives not offered by conventional dosage forms such as solutions, ointments, or promptly dissolving dosage forms.... Delayed-release and extended-release dosage forms are two types of modified-release dosage forms... *Delayed-release dosage forms*— A delayed-release dosage form is one that releases a drug(s) at a time other than promptly after administration... *Extended-release dosage forms*—An extended-release dosage form is one that allows at least a twofold reduction in dosing frequency or significant increase in patient compliance or therapeutic performance as compared to that presented as a conventional dosage form (e.g., as a solution or a prompt drug-releasing, conventional solid dosage form)... The terms *controlled release, prolonged action,* and *sustained release* are used synonymously with extended release. This document uses the term *extended release* to describe a formulation that does not release active drug substance immediately after oral dosing and that also allows a reduction in dosage frequency. This

(*Text continues on p. 368*)

**Table 2**   Selected Recent Guidelines Relevant to Modified Drug Release
Registration

---

Argentina
- GCP in Clinical Studies: 1997, amended 2005 http://www.anmat.gov.ar/
  Normativa/Normativa/Medicamentos/Disposicion_ANMAT_5330-1997.pdf
- BA/BE: Final Sep 2006, amended Mar 2007 http://www.anmat.gov.ar/
  Normativa/Normativa/Medicamentos/Disposicion_ANMAT_5040-2006.pdf

ASEAN States (ACCSQ)
Pharmaceutical Product Working Group http://www.aseansec.org/14904.htm
- BA/BE: Final Draft, Jul 2004 http://www.bpfk.gov.my/pdfworddownload/drug/
  ASEAN%20GUIDELINES%20FOR.pdf

Australia (TGA)
http://www.tga.gov.au/pmeds/pmeds.htm#guidelines
- BA and BE Guidelines: Apr 2002 http://www.tga.gov.au/docs/pdf/euguide/ewp/
  140198entga.pdf
- Summary of a BA or BE Study: Dec 2002 http://www.tga.gov.au/docs/pdf/
  forms/pmbiosum.pdf
- Australian Regulatory Guidelines for Prescription Medicines, Appendix 15:
  Biopharmaceutic Studies: Jun 2004 http://www.tga.gov.au/pmeds/argpmap15.pdf

Botswana (MOH Drugs Regulatory Unit)
(http://www.moh.gov.bw/index.php?id = 284)
- Guidelines On Drug Registration Applications: March 2000 (http://www.moh.
  gov.bw/fileadmin/documents/Policies/registration_guidelines.pdf.

Brazil (ANVISA)
- Implementation of Relative BA and BE Studies: Apr 2006 http://e-legis.anvisa.
  gov.br/leisref/public/showAct.php?id = 21746
- Pharmaceutical Equivalence/Dissolution: Sep 2004 http://e-legis.anvisa.gov.br/
  leisref/public/showAct.php?id = 15466
- Series of documents in 2003

Canada (HPFB)
http://www.hc-sc.gc.ca/dhp-mps/prodpharma/applic-demande/guide-ld/bio/index_e.
html
- BA/BE—Part A [IR]: 1992
- BA/BE—Part B [MR]: Nov 1996
- BA/BE—Part C [IR, complicated or highly variable PK]: Dec 1992
- CTAs for Comparative Bioavailability Studies: Draft, Oct 2001
- Draft Policy: BE Requirements: Drugs Exhibiting Non-linear Pharmacokinetics,
  Jun 2003
- BE of HVDs/HVDPs: Discussion Paper, Jun 2003
- Removal of Requirement for 15% Random Replicate Samples: Notice, Sep 2003
- BE of Combination Drug Products: Notice, Jun 2004
- Metabolites in Comparative BA Studies: Draft, May 2004

---

*(Continued)*

**Table 2**  Selected Recent Guidelines Relevant to Modified Drug Release
Registration (*Continued*)

- Preparation of Comparative BA Information for Drug Submissions in the CTD Format: Draft, May 2004
- BE in Fed State: Jun 2005
- BE for Long Half-life Drugs: Notice, Jun 2005
- BE for Rapid Onset Drugs: Notice, Jun 2005
- BE for Critical Dose Drugs: May 2006—Critical Dose Drugs are: cyclosporine, digoxin, flecainide, lithium, phenytoin, sirolimus, tacrolimus, theophylline, and warfarin.

Danish Medicines Agency (DKMA)
http://www.dkma.dk/1024/visUKLSArtikel.asp?artikelID = 1586
- Bioequivalence and labelling of medicinal products with regard to generic substitution: Jan 2006 http://www.laegemiddelstyrelsen.dk/1024/visLSArtikel.asp?artikelID = 6410

European Medicines Agency (EMEA)
http://www.emea.europa.eu/sitemap.htm
*Bioavailability/Bioequivalence:* Note for Guidance and associated documents
- Bioavailability/Bioequivalence: Jul 2001 http://www.emea.europa.eu/pdfs/human/ewp/140198en.pdf
- BA/BE for HVDs/HVDPs: Concept Paper, Apr 2006—Draft expected to be released for consultation in Q2/3 2007. http://www.emea.europa.eu/pdfs/human/ewp/14723106en.pdf
- Questions & Answers on the BA and BE Guideline: Jul 2006 http://www.emea.europa.eu/pdfs/human/ewp/4032606en.pdf
- Recommendation on the Need for Revision of NfG on BA/BE: May 2007 http://www.emea.europa.eu/pdfs/human/ewp/20094307en.pdf
- Concept Paper on BCS-based Biowaiver: May 2007 http://www.emea.europa.eu/pdfs/human/ewp/21303507en.pdf

*Modified Release Oral/Transdermals:* Draft 15, Jul 1999
http://www.emea.europa.eu/pdfs/human/ewp/028096en.pdf
Pharmacokinetics—range of documents
Statistical Issues—Biostatistical Methodology & Multiplicity Issues in Clinical Trials
Miscellaneous—range of documents, including:
- Development Pharmaceutics (of modified release dosage forms): Jan 1998 http://www.emea.europa.eu/pdfs/human/qwp/015596en.pdf
- Dry Powder Inhalers: Jun 1998 http://www.emea.europa.eu/pdfs/human/qwp/015896en.pdf

India (CDSCO)
http://cdsco.nic.in/
- Bioavailability/Bioequivalence: Current Draft, Mar 2005 http://cdsco.nic.in/html/BE%20Guidelines%20Draft%20Ver10%20March%2016,%2005.pdf

(*Continued*)

**Table 2**   Selected Recent Guidelines Relevant to Modified Drug Release
Registration (*Continued*)

Japan (NIHS)

http://www.nihs.go.jp/drug/DrugDiv-E.html

- Oral Prolonged Release Dosage Forms: Mar 1988 http://www.nihs.go.jp/drug/
  be-guide(e)/CR-new.pdf
- BE Studies for Generic Products: http://www.nihs.go.jp/drug/be-guide/
  GL061124_BE.pdf; http://www.nihs.go.jp/drug/be-guide/QA061124_BE.pdf
- Guideline for BE Test on Oral Solid Preparation with Different Drug Strengths:
  http://www.nihs.go.jp/drug/be-guide/GL061124_ganryo.pdf; http://www.nihs.
  go.jp/drug/be-guide/QA061124_ganryo_shoho.pdf
- Guideline for BE Test on Oral Solid Preparation for which the Formulation has
  been changed: http://www.nihs.go.jp/drug/be-guide/GL061124_shohou.pdf;
  http://www.nihs.go.jp/drug/be-guide/QA061124_ganryo_shoho.pdf
- Guideline for BE Studies of Generic Products for Topical Use: http://www.nihs.
  go.jp/drug/be-guide/GL061124_hifu.pdf; http://www.nihs.go.jp/drug/be-guide/
  QA061124_hifu.pdf
- Guideline for BE Studies of Adding Dosage Form for Topical Use: new 24 Nov
  2006 http://www.nihs.go.jp/drug/be-guide/GL061124_hifu_zaikei.pdf; http://
  www.nihs.go.jp/drug/be-guide/QA061124_hifu_zaikei.pdf

Mexico

- BA/BE: Final, May 1999 http://www.farmacopea.org.mx/legisla/legal28.asp
- BA/BE Update, Biowaivers: Mar 2000 http://www.salud.gob.mx/unidades/cdi/
  nom/acl177ssa1.html

New Zealand (Medsafe)

http://www.medsafe.govt.nz/Regulatory/guidelines.asp

- Biostudy Reference Products: Jul 2006 http://www.medsafe.govt.nz/Regulatory/
  Guideline/biostudy.asp

Saudi Arabia

http://www.sfda.gov.sa/En/Drug/Topics/Regulations+-+Guidelines.htm

- BE: Draft, May 2005 (297kB PDF)
- Drug Master File Requirements for the Registration of Biosimilars: Draft, Aug
  2007 (105kB PDF)

(South) Korea

http://www.kfda.go.kr/open_content/english/index.html

- Minimum Requirements for BE Test: Dec 2005 http://www.kfda.go.kr/open_-
  content/file/%BF%B5%B9%AE%BB%FD%B9%B0%C7%D0%C0%FB%
  B5%BF%B5%EE%BC%BA%BD%C3%C7%E8%B1%E2%C1%D8.pdf

South Africa (MCC)

http://www.mccza.com/showdocument.asp?Cat = 17 Desc = Guidelines%20-%
  20Human%20Medicines

- Generic Substitution: Final, Dec 2003
- Pharmaceutical and Analytical Guideline: Jul 2006

(*Continued*)

**Table 2** Selected Recent Guidelines Relevant to Modified Drug Release Registration (*Continued*)

- Biostudies: 02 Jul 2007
- Dissolution: 02 Jul 2007, except section 4.1

Switzerland
http://www.swissmedic.ch/en/industrie/overall.asp?
   theme = 0.00107.00003&theme_id = 528
- Instructions for Generics: Dec 2002 http://www.swissmedic.ch/files/pdf/12_2002.
   pdf
- Reference Formulations for BE/CTDs for Generics: Apr 2004 http://www.
   swissmedic.ch/files/pdf/04_2004.pdf

Thailand (FDA)
http://www.fda.moph.go.th/eng/drug/index.stm
- Instruction for the In Vivo BE Study Protocol Development: Oct 2006 http://
   wwwapp1.fda.moph.go.th/drug/zone_bioequivalence/files/be_inhuman.pdf

USA
http://www.fda.gov/cder/guidance/
http://www.fda.gov/cder/ogd/
- Guidance for Industry—Extended Release Oral Dosage Forms: Development,
   Evaluation, and Application of In Vitro/In Vivo 1997 http://www.fda.gov/cder/
   guidance/1306fnl.pdf
- Correlations Guidance for Industry SUPAC-MR: Modified Release Solid Oral
   Dosage Forms 1997—Scale-Up and Postapproval Changes: Chemistry,
   Manufacturing, and Controls; In Vitro Dissolution Testing and In Vivo
   Bioequivalence Documentation http://www.fda.gov/cder/guidance/1214fnl.pdf
- Guidance for Industry Potassium Chloride Modified-Release Tablets and
   Capsules: In Vivo Bioequivalence and In Vitro Dissolution Testing 2005 http://
   www.fda.gov/cder/guidance/5523fnl.htm
- Draft Guidance on Metformin Hydrochloride 2006 http://www.fda.gov/cder/
   guidance/bioequivalence/recommendations/
   Metformin_HCl_ERtab_21202_RC7-06.pdf
- Draft Guidance on Venlafaxine Hydrochloride 2006 http://www.fda.gov/cder/
   guidance/bioequivalence/recommendations/
   Venlafaxine_HCl_ERcap_20699_RC2-06.pdf
- http://www.fda.gov/cder/guidance/1214fnl.pdf

World Health Organization
http://www.who.int/medicines/en/
*Good Clinical Practice*
- Handbook for GCP: 2005 http://www.who.int/medicines/areas/quality_safety/
   safety_efficacy/OMS-GCP.pdf

*Generics*
- Guideline on Generics—Pharmaceutical Quality and BE

(*Continued*)

**Table 2** Selected Recent Guidelines Relevant to Modified Drug Release Registration (*Continued*)

- Annex 7, Presentation of BE Trial Information (BTIF): Aug 2005
- Supplement 1 (Dissolution testing): Jul 2005

*WHO Expert Committee on Specifications for Pharmaceutical Preparations*, Fortieth Report (WHO Technical Report Series No. 937): May 2006
- Annex 7: Multisource (generic) pharmaceutical products: guidelines on registration requirements to establish interchangeability
- Annex 8: Proposal to waive in vivo bioequivalence requirements for *WHO Model List of Essential Medicines* immediate-release, solid oral dosage forms
- Annex 9: Additional guidance for organizations performing in vivo bioequivalence studies

*Source*: Adapted from Guidance documents collated by Helmut Schütz 20 Sept 2007, http:// bebac.at/Guidelines.htm#EU.

nomenclature accords generally with the USP definition of extended release but does not specify an impact on dosing frequency. The terms *controlled release* and *extended release* are considered interchangeable in this guidance.

South Africa has also released the first part of a Dissolution Guideline in July 2007. Dissolution tests can be used to provide: a) quality assurance on the product, API test batches and on the reference products to be used in bioavailability/bioequivalence studies/pivotal clinical studies, and as a quality control tool to demonstrate consistency in product manufacture, and to infer bioequivalence. Accordingly, the guideline suggests that dissolution testing: is an essential part of product development; can support a bioequivalence waiver application; provides test batch data, including batch-to-batch and lot-to-lot consistency during manufacture, and data to establish an in vitro-in vivo correlation. Dissolution profiles are based on 15-minute or less samples using a BP or USP pharmacopoeial method for 12 units each of test and reference products, with any other method requiring approval. The USP basket, paddle and flow through methods in at least three dissolution media (e.g., pH 1, 2; 4, 5; and 6, 8 buffer) are widely referred to, with a surfactant proposed when the active drug is poorly soluble. Dissolution curves for a new and reference product are then evaluated for similarity in the percentage (%) dissolved over time using the similarity factor (f2), a logarithmic reciprocal square root transformation of the sum of squared errors. Further in vivo studies are usually not necessary if $f2 \geq 50$.

As a contrast, *Botswana* provides an example of regulatory guidelines for a less developed individual African country. Here, Drug Registration Applications (Table 2) require all specifications to be at the levels documented in the latest editions of the approved references

(BP, USP, International Pharmacopoeia, *European Pharmacopoeia* and others, as approved by the Botswana Drugs Advisory Board). In relation to pharmaceutical documentation, details need to include: specification, analytical control procedures, release criteria for both raw materials control and finished products, manufacturing procedures and in-process controls and stability studies. For established (Category B) drugs, whose safety and efficacy is well documented in standard textbooks, formulation proof of efficacy must be included and may include comparative dissolution/bio-availability data, acid neutralizing capacity and inhibition zones. More in depth safety and efficacy studies are required for Categories D and E drugs that include: new combination drugs; first line generic drug; established drug with new indication(s) and new formulation of an established drugs. Amongst the requirements are in depth investigation of safety and efficacy and includes studies confirming bioavailability, biological equivalence and/or the clinical interchangeability of pharmaceutically equivalent drugs.

## Americas

In the Americas, the United States and Canadian Regulatory Requirements for modified-release products are well developed and are described in detail elsewhere in this series. For instance Health Canada recognizes the need for rapid change in drug regulation to meet developments in drug sciences and in public expectations. It has initiated a "progressive licensing project" in which the first phase is a comparison of its regulatory documentation with those from the United States, the United Kingdom, Australia, New Zealand, Japan, and the EU. Evidence-based decision making and good planning in the definition of pre and post market studies needed are components in this strategy. Importantly, the strategy incorporates sponsor accountability within all aspects of the framework with the continued marketing of the drug dependent on compliance and on meeting regulatory benchmarks. Health Canada has been very active with its guidance documents as indicated by those published for bioavailability and bioequivalence (Table 2).

It is of particular note that bioequivalence should be demonstrated under both fasted and fed conditions for complicated (i.e., narrow therapeutic range drugs, highly toxic drugs and nonlinear drugs) drugs in immediate-release dosage form and drugs in modified-release dosage forms. The following breakfast was given as a Standard Test Meal: 2 eggs fried in butter, 2 strips of bacon, 2 slices of toast with butter, 120 gm of hash browns, and 240 mL of whole milk.

U.S. FDA guidelines are addressed separately (2) and, relevant to this chapter, include: general guidance; criteria guidance; bioanalytical guidance; biopharmaceutics classification system guidance; food-effects guidance;

general bioavailability and bioequivalence; guidance; nasal drug products (draft); oral inhalation drug products (delayed); topically applied drug products (withdrawn); dissolution testing of immediate release solid; oral dosage forms (final); extended release oral dosage forms: development, evaluation, and application of in vitro/in vivo correlations (final). It is emphasized that not all of these FDA guidances are applicable to modified-release products such as the inhalation products and topical products.

Many of the other countries in the Americas are involved in the Pan American Network for Regulatory Harmonization sponsored by the US FDA. Members at the meeting in 2006 included Bolivia, Brazil, Canada, Colombia, El Salvador, the United States, Venezuela, with observers from: Peru, Costa Rica, Aruba and Chile, and a presentation from Mexico. Table 2 shows guidelines for Argentina, Brazil, and Mexico. It is apparent that in countries such as Aruba, where there are no manufacturers or analytical laboratories, emphasis is placed on products already registered in the United States and elsewhere. In general, biopharmaceutical regulatory requirements vary among its members and, in some cases, is some way behind the United States and Canada. (http://www.paho.org/english/ad/ths/ ev/rm-4meet-agenda-eng.pdf for March, 2006).

## Europe

The EU now includes the majority of countries loosely known as "Europe." Those that are member states of the EU are covered by guidance published by the EMEA (Fig. 1). EMEA has a number of guidelines (Table 2) summarized in a later chapter. In brief, two of the key bio-availability and bioequivalence guidelines relevant to modified-release products are:

- Note for "Guidance on the Investigation of Bioavailability and Bioequivalence" CPMP/EWP/QWP/1401/98;
- Note for "Guidance on Modified Release Oral and Transdermal Dosage Forms: Section II (Pharmacokinetic and Clinical Evaluation)" CPMP/ EWP/280/96.

The later chapter also highlights regulation of devices.

It should be emphasized that not all countries in Europe are part of the EU. For instance, Switzerland remains outside the Union, as do Norway and Iceland, although these latter two countries contribute to certain EU scientific committees, and generally follow EU opinions. Certain EU Member States publish their own guidance on purely National or procedural issues, e.g., Denmark (Table 2). However, all scientific/technical guidelines relating to data requirements for the development of medicinal products are harmonized between the Member States. In addition, the EU is one of the world regions taking part in the ICH process—International

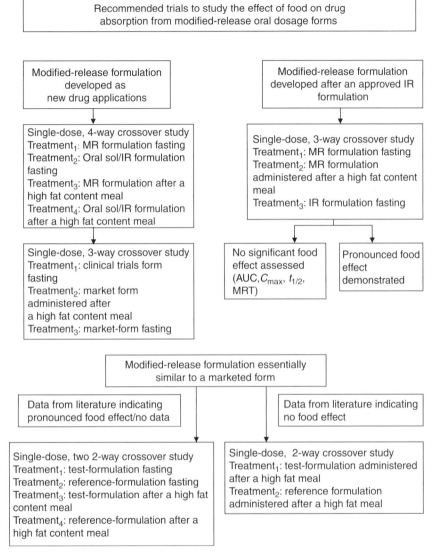

**Figure 1** EMEA guidelines for conducting food studies with modified-release products. *Abbreviation*: EMEA, European Medicines Agency. *Source*: From Ref. 7.

Conference on Harmonization (of Technical Requirements for Registration of Pharmaceuticals for Human Use)—together with the United States and Japan, and any agreements on scientific data requirements reached at this international level would be subsequently implemented in EU guidelines.

## Rest of World

In general, these counties all require chemical and pharmaceutical information, bioavailability, dissolution, and stability study data in a form that is similar to those defined by either EMEA or U.S. guidelines. Australia requests absolute bioavailability for all new entities. Table 2 provides a listing of the web pages for guidelines in Australia, India, New Zealand, Saudi Arabia, South Korea, Thailand, and Japan. Australian and Japanese guidelines are discussed in more detail in later chapters.

## DRUG SUBSTANCE

Pharmacopeias (e.g., the United States, EU, and Japanese) exist to define drug substances and a number of testing procedures in various countries. In general, most countries require detail on the description and composition of the drug product (nomenclature, properties such as melting, specific rotation, crystallinity, polymorphism, $pK_a$, partition coefficient, hygroscopicity), Manufacture, Characterization, Control of Drug Substance, Reference Standards or Materials, Container Closure System, and Stability.

## DRUG PRODUCT

The WHO seeks to apply quality standards for pharmaceutical products via a quality assessment procedure, desirably conducted in conjunction with National Drug Regulatory Authorities. This procedure evaluates whether pharmaceutical products meet WHO requirements for multisource (generic) pharmaceutical products and have been made in compliance with GMP. The procedure does depend on (*a*) National Drug Regulatory Authority information, (*b*) an understanding of manufacturer production and quality control processes, (*c*) an evaluation of manufacturer product data, possibly with a manufacturing site inspection(s), (*d*) evidence of GMP compliance, (*e*) testing of products, (*f*) adequacy of product distribution, complaint/recall handling and monitoring thereof.

Applications for regulatory approval normally require details on each of the following: (*i*) description and composition of the drug product, (*ii*) pharmaceutical development, (*iii*) manufacture, (*iv*) control of excipients, (*v*) control of drug product, (*vi*) reference standards or materials, (*vii*) container closure system, and (*viii*) stability.

## PHARMACOKINETICS AND BIOPHARMACEUTICS

The rate and extent of absorption and time to reach steady state are important. An absolute bioavailability study is valuable in order to determine the fraction of the drug that is absorbed or reaches the systemic circulation. In addition, the metabolism, elimination and distribution of a drug, including possible metabolizing enzyme induction or inhibition effects, nature of the disposition curve, e.g., bi-exponential and terminal half-life is generally expected. Interconversion of enantiomers, if they exist, dose proportionality, effect of gender and any genetic polymorphism, should be defined. This data then forms the basis for bioavailability and bioequivalence studies which need to be conducted following Good Clinical Practice, with Human Ethics Approval and using appropriately validated bioanalytical methods.

## Bioavailability and Bioequivalence—General

As expressed by the WHO (1), multisource or generic pharmaceutical products need to confirm to the same appropriate standards of quality, efficacy and safety as those required of the innovator's (comparator) product. Evidence that the multisource product is therapeutically equivalent and interchangeable with the comparator product is also required. Implementation of GMP and conformity with relevant pharmacopoeial specifications may assure interchangeability for some forms of modified-release products eg parenteral formulations of highly water-soluble compounds. In principle, the test product used should be identical to a reference (innovator—not generic) commercial product in composition, quality and in manufacturing methods, and should be from a production batch that is greater than 1/10 the final commercial product number of units. However, the reference product can be a different salt if it is an approved product. Further, it needs to be recognised that there may be a variation in synthetic route and impurity profile for generics. There have been cases where, as a consequence, the impurity profile differs from the originator so that, in certain cases, pharmacopeial limits are not always appropriate. Documentation expected include a test product certificate of analysis, batch numbers, expiry dates and a content of the active substance similar to that for the reference product ($< \pm 5\%$). In the EU, EMEA requires that the reference is from an EU country whereas the WHO specifies that the reference can be from countries such as Australia, Canada, EU Member States, Japan, the United States and Switzerland). Suitable methods to assess equivalence include (1):

- "comparative pharmacokinetic studies in humans, in which the active pharmaceutical ingredient (API) and/or its metabolite(s) are measured as a function of time in an accessible biological fluid such as blood, plasma, serum or urine to obtain pharmacokinetic measures, such as AUC and $C_{max}$ that are reflective of the systemic exposure;
- comparative clinical trials; and
- comparative in vitro tests."

EMEA (7,8) recommends that bioavailability studies enable modified drug formulation to be characterized in vivo through concentration measurements of the active substance and/or metabolite(s) (and, in some cases, acute pharmacodynamic effect) compared to a reference product by:

- the rate and extent of absorption;
- fluctuations in drug concentrations;
- variability in pharmacokinetics arising from the drug formulation and food, gastrointestinal function, diurnal rhythms and site of application (dermal);
- dose proportionality;
- factors influencing the performance of the modified drug formulation;
- the risk of unexpected release characteristics (e.g., dose dumping).

The reference product is usually the marketed immediate release product of the same active substance in the same form (e.g., salt). Studies are conducted in either healthy volunteers or in patients, with a requirement that steady state be demonstrated in multiple-dose studies.

## Bioavailability and Bioequivalence—In Vitro Testing

All regulatory systems require in vitro, e.g., dissolution; in vivo, e.g., pharmacokinetic and, in some cases, clinical data. Clinical trials assume appropriate approval through ethics committees and may have facilitated Phase 1 approval in relation to Good Manufacturing Practice requirements. Two distinct methodologies exist in relation to the in vitro dissolution testing of products: a closed system (beaker method) and an open system (flow-through method). The most common procedure defined in the United States, EU, and Japanese Pharmacopeias are the paddle and basket methods. The flow-through method is most useful in testing dosage forms in which the active ingredients are only slightly soluble. Differences in apparatus design, conditions and methodologies used, analytical methods, testing conditions and specifications exist between the three sets of guidelines. Desirably, in vitro dissolution results should be validated by in vivo data.

In vitro dissolution data enables both the determination of product quality and, in certain cases, the likely performance of a product in vivo. The latter is usually dependent on the establishment of a useful in vitro–in vivo correlation (IVIVC) whereby the in vivo input rate is related to the in vitro dissolution rate. The FDA has defined three categories of IVIVC (2,12), as follows:

1. Point-to-point relationships
2. Statistical moment correlations, e.g., mean in vivo absorption time versus mean in vitro dissolution time
3. Single point parameter relationships, e.g., $C_{max}$ versus percent dissolved at 4 hours

An appropriate IVIVC can then be used for biowaiver applications and to set meaningful dissolution specifications in terms of describing in vivo behavior.

The US has introduced a biowaiver scheme from clinical and pharmacokinetic studies for certain classes of drugs as defined by the BCS. In principle, this system is really only applicable to those oral dosage forms which have a faster release than conventional oral dose forms and not to prolonged, delayed, controlled, responsive or targeted products. This scheme recognizes that different drugs have differing absorption rate control depending on the aqueous solubility (S) and intestinal permeability (P) of the drugs:

 I.  Class I—high S, high P → gastric emptying controlled
 II. Class II—low S, high P → dissolution controlled
III. Class III—high S, low P → permeability controlled
IV. Class IV—low S, low P → case by case

Biowaivers for in vivo bioequivalence studies may be possible for many compounds in certain regulatory jurisdictions. In this context, a biowaiver defined by the BCS implies the waiving of the in vivo BE test for a better, more robust, routine and more easily implemented dissolution test. Presently, this is limited to those compounds that are solid, orally administered and immediate release (>85% release in 30 min), containing drugs with a high solubility over the pH range from 1 to 7.5 (dose/solubility ratio <250 mL) and a high permeability (fraction absorbed orally >90%) (13). It is assumed that any excipients present do not affect absorption. However, waivers for Class 3 drugs (high-solubility, low-permeability) have also been recommended (14). These authors have recently compared the provisional Biopharmaceutical Classifications of the top 200 Oral Drug Products in the United States, Britain, Spain, Japan and for the WHO essential medicine list. In doing so, they assigned a maximum dose, solubility, and log octanol-water partition coefficient for each drug and estimated a dimensionless dose number (Do) as the ratio of drug concentration in the administered volume to its saturation solubility in water (Do = maximum dose/volume of fluid/lowest aqueous solubility). A slightly higher dose number is estimated for Japan, where the volume of fluid ingested is defined as 150 mL compared to other countries, where it is defined as 250 mL (14). An alternative Biopharmaceutics Drug Disposition Classification System (BDDCS) listing based on extensively first pass metabolized drugs (>50%) having a high intestinal permeability (15) yields similar BCS and BDDCS categories for most compounds. However, there are a number of notable exceptions with, for instance, acetaminophen, caffeine, codeine, morphine, and theophylline being classified as Class 3 by BCS and Class 1 by BDDCS, using metoprolol as the reference drug for permeability classification (14). Benet et al. (26) have now reported that extensive metabolism (93.1%) better predicted BCS Class 1 than octanol water partition coefficient and have therefore recently recommended that > 90% metabolized be also used to define Class 1 marketed drugs suitable for a waiver of in vivo studies of bioequivalence.

The individual country guidelines for BCS do vary. Gupta et al. (16) have compared the regulations in relation to those for biowaivers being applied for immediate release solid oral dosage forms in the United States, EU, Japan and from the World Health Organization. Examples of differences include definitions of solubility and permeability, and addressing prior history of bioavailability problems and in method of manufacture. For instance, in Japan there can be separate qualification requirements for core versus coating layer for coated products.

## Bioavailability and Bioequivalence—Pharmacokinetics

A key aspect in any pharmacokinetic study is an appropriate study design (1). WHO (1) suggests that a two-period, two-sequence, single-dose, crossover, randomized design involving a multisource and the comparator product is the preferred design. There needs to be an adequate wash-out period between doses of each formulation to enable the elimination of the previous dose from the body, and this is usually 5 half lives so that the pre-dose level for the active is < 5% of $C_{max}$, or longer, if active metabolites exist. In general, all guidelines for modified-release products require: (*i*) a single dose, nonreplicate cross-over study in fasting conditions; (*ii*) a food effect study ruling out dose dumping; and (*iii*) multiple dose study. Food can affect modified-release preparation pharmacokinetics, efficacy and safety. In general, a two-way randomized single-dose study after fasting and with food is indicated using a marketed reference. However, the food effect for both formulations can be both different and acceptable as long as the product is deemed safe and effective under fed conditions. Any new indication requires clinical studies.

As EMEA (7,8) and WHO (1) point out, single and multiple dose studies exploring the bioequivalence of modified-release formulations seek to demonstrate that:

- the test formulation exhibits the claimed prolonged release characteristics of the reference;
- the active drug substance is not suddenly and abruptly released ("dose dumped") from the test formulation (as may occur for instance with food or an alcoholic drink);
- performance after a single dose and at steady state is equivalent for the test and the reference formulations;
- the in vivo performance is comparable for both formulations when a single dose study administered immediately after a predefined high fat meal.

WHO (1) also raises a number of issues in relation to subjects, including number (minimum 12), drop-outs, selection (usually 18 to 55 years old), monitoring and genetic phenotyping. They also emphasize the importance of study conditions, including posture, physical activity, fast for at least 10 hours with free access to water but nil in period of 1 hour before and up to hours after dosing, dosing being done with 15–250 mL water.

EMEA (7,8) requires a single dose study under fasting conditions is required for each strength when multiple strengths exist and recommends $AUC_\tau$, $C_{max}$ and $C_{min}$ be assessed using similar statistical procedures as for immediate release formulations. WHO (1) recommends at least 1–2 points before $C_{max}$, 2 points around $C_{max}$ and 3–4 points in the elimination phase and that sampling occur until about 80% of the $AUC_{0-\infty}$ is reached. WHO (1) recommends that bioavailability should be expressed in terms of rate ($C_{max}$, $t_{max}$) and extent (AUC) of absorption. For single dose studies, the key parameters are $AUC_{0-t}$, where $t$ is the last sampling point, and $C_{max}$. Other parameters of value are: $AUC_{0-\infty}$, $t_{max}$ and $t_{0.5}$ and for steady-state studies: $AUC_\tau$, $C_{max}$, $C_{min}$, and peak trough fluctuations (expressed as $100 \times (C_{max} - C_{min})/C_{max}$). Metabolites, individual enantiomer measurement, inter and intra-subject variability, dose proportionality, and risk of unexpected release behavior are also important considerations. However, there are differences between jurisdictions in, for instance, the ranges for $C_{max}$. These include: EMEA: 75–133%; South Africa: CI 75–133%; Japan: $C_{max}$ log(0.9)–log(1.11); and USA: CI 80–125%.

India has stated specific requirements for modified-release formulations likely to accumulate ($AUC_{0-t}/AUC_{0-\infty} < 0.8$). In general, these studies are similar to those required in EMEA, FDA, and WHO studies. They include single and steady state dosing with an immediate release product as a comparison, with single dose administration in both the fasting and fed state. $AUC_{0-t}$, $AUC_{0-t}$ ($=$ AUC from 0 to last quantifiable time point), $AUC_{0-\infty}$, $C_{max}$, and $k_{el}$ are required for single dose studies and $AUC_{0-(ss)}$, $C_{max}$, $C_{min}$, $C_{pd}$ ($=$ pre-dose concentration) and fluctuation for steady state. In some jurisdictions, similar in vitro dissolution profiles of products may be used to argue for bioequivalence. However, bioequivalence studies are needed when there is a narrow therapeutic index, incomplete absorption, low bioavailability, low water solubility and if therapeutic failure or toxicity is possible.

EMEA has recently published a series of answers to its 2002 bioavailability and bioequivalence guidelines (7,8). Currently the 90% confidence interval for the ratio of $C_{max}$ as a measure of relative bioavailability should lie within an acceptance range of 0.80–1.25. In exceptional, limited cases it may be increased to a small widening (0.75–1.33), providing the following applies:

1. Sufficient PK/PD data are provided to show that the proposed wider acceptance range for $C_{max}$ does not affect pharmacodynamics in a clinically significant way, or

2. If such data are not possible then compound specific clinical safety and efficacy data may be used, but
3. The proposed range is established in the planning phase—not post hoc on completion of the study.

This advice also suggests that post-hoc data exclusion may be justified under exceptional circumstances and the results of statistical analyses on data with and without the exclusions should be provided. In addition, in reiterating that "AUC and $C_{max}$ should be analysed using ANOVA after log transformation" and that nonparametric methods are recommended to analyze $t_{max}$ in the original data set, it is advised that nonparametric statistical methods and sensitivity analyses are welcome. EMEA further adds that metabolite data can only be used as an alternative to the parent compound when the latter cannot be reliably measured by state-of-the-art methods and the kinetics are linear. EMEA notes that "The standard approach to the analysis of a two-treatment, two-sequence, two-period crossover trial is an analysis of variance (ANOVA) for the log-transformed PK parameters, where the factors; formulation, period, sequence and subject nesting within sequence are used to explain overall variability in the observations. The residual coefficient of variation (CV) is a measure of the variability that is unexplained by the aforementioned factors. Amongst others, within-subject variability, formulation variability, analytical errors, and subject by formulation interaction can contribute to this residual variance. A drug product is called highly variable if its intra-individual (i.e. within-subject) variability is greater than 30%. A high CV as estimated from the ANOVA model is thus an indicator for high within-subject variability. However, a replicate design is needed to assess within-subject variability." The effect of food on bioavailability is a difficult and still a developing issue. EMEA has recommended the coadministration of the drug with food for bioequivalence studies when

1. food affects biovailability;
2. food is proposed to decrease adverse events or to improve tolerability;
3. there is a choice between fasting and fed conditions. Fasting conditions are preferred as this enables differences between a new product and its reference to be observed with more sensitivity.

## Topical Products

The vasoconstriction or blanching assay for assessment of topical corticosteroid formulations is probably the best defined for evaluation of topical products, other than by clinical trials and systemic plasma concentrations. This method was first described in 1962 by McKenzie and Stroughton (17) and defined as a regulatory guideline by FDA Guidance in 1995. The procedure relies on application of products for various periods up to 6 hours and measuring the blanching response on product removal by a chromameter over 24–28 hours. Demana et al. (18) have suggested that visual measurements are preferred to those from a chromameter. Wiedersberg et al. (19) have emphasized that the same product volume should be applied at all sites to achieve meaningful data. Keida et al. (20) has shown that an almost identical set of guidelines to the FDA created by Japan in 2003 were applicable to the Japanese population. The EMEA Guidelines, which originate from initial 1987 guidelines also refer to the FDA document. Compliance is a key determinant of topical corticosteroid efficacy that is not presently included in the regulatory requirements of various countries. Patient preference in terms of product behavior (staining, greasiness, etc) can affect outcomes (21).

## Transdermal Products

The evaluation of a testosterone liquid transdermal delivery system by plasma testosterone levels has recently been described by Chik et al. (22). The trial involved an open label, comparative, randomized placebo controlled study with 3 treatments, 3 periods and 1 week washout. Products were evaluated by examining whether the 90% confidence interval on the relative difference for the AUC (0,12 hours) and $C_{max}$ (0,12 hours) for test and reference products were within the bioequivalence limit (80, 125%) (23).

## EMERGING REGULATORY REQUIREMENTS

Regulatory requirements are in a continual process of evolution driven by the desire for harmonization across various countries. One example of this harmonization is the WHO (1) Annex 7 on pharmaceutical product registration guidelines. This document includes

- documentation of equivalence for marketing authorization;
- when equivalence studies are not necessary;
- when in vivo equivalence studies are necessary and types of studies required (in vivo studies, in vitro studies);
- bioequivalence studies in humans (general considerations, study design, subjects, study standardization, investigational product, study conduct, quantification of API, statistical analysis, acceptance ranges, reporting of results, special considerations);
- pharmacodynamic studies;
- clinical trials;
- in vitro testing (in vitro testing and the biopharmaceutics classification system, qualification for a biowaiver based on the biopharmaceutics classification system, biowaivers based on dose-proportionality of formulations, biowaivers for scale-up and post-approval changes).

It is to be noted that differences in terminology remain for bio-equivalence and equivalence (24), as follows:

- WHO "equivalence" is by PK or in vitro studies, whereas FDA "bio-equivalence" involves PK, PD, clinical and in vitro studies.
- Genotyping is considered by WHO and not the FDA
- BCS—WHO is an expansion of FDA BCS.
- WHO allows "add on" studies whereas US emphasizes "sequential BE study design."
- If the label states drug is to be given with food, WHO requires BE study done only with food, whereas FDA requires fasting plus food studies.
- Nomenclature: R = Comparator Pharmaceutical Product for WHO and R = Reference Listed Drug for FDA.

The second basis for emerging regulatory guidelines are developments arising from research. As an example, Figure 2 shows other topical corticosteroid bioequivalence methods that are still currently under evaluation. It is likely that one of these or an alternative method will emerge as a routine procedure in future drug assessments. In other areas guidelines are not well developed. For instance, USP Apparatus 4 (flow-through) device has been recommended by FIP/AAPS Guidelines for drug release testing of modified-release dosage forms. However, as Iyer et al. (25) point out, little published information is available on implants.

The third basis for emerging regulatory guidelines is the likely emergence of more sophisticated, parenteral, modified-drug delivery mechanisms will present significant challenges to the developers of the regulatory testing program. Current areas of investigation include modified-release dose forms such as nanoparticulate based slow release parenteral formulations or

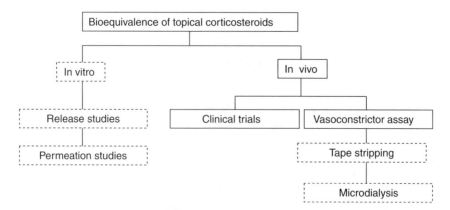

**Figure 2**  Bioequivalence methodology approved (*solid boxes*) and under evaluation (*dotted boxes*) for topical corticosteroids. *Source*: Adapted from Ref. 19.

specific target directed drug delivery mechanisms such as pegylated liposomal carriers coupled to monoclonal antibodies specific to surface proteins on a target cell population. Guidelines for such novel applications have yet to be formulated and the wide range of possible approaches make generic guidelines difficult to formulate. In considering the testing requirements for such novel products developers will need to approach the challenge from first principles specific to the application under development. As with any drug however the core issues remain quality, safety and efficacy. With these types of product however even previously well characterized active ingredients may require an extensive preclinical and pharmaceutical chemistry development program.

Modified-release parenteral formulations will alter the pharmacokinetics of the active by design, and may therefore also alter, whether intentionally or otherwise the toxicology of the active. The carrier will equally have pharmacokinetic and toxicological characteristics of its own and where the intent is to target specific cells or tissues the efficacy and specificity of the targeting will need to be demonstrated. One concern raised for nanoparticulate carriers is that of persistence of nonbiodegradable carriers in tissues leading, through free radical generation as one example, to malignancy long after the drug product has been utilized. Although such concerns are readily amenable to thoughtful pharmaceutical development, ensuring for example that carriers are degradable to normal body constituents or readily excretable moieties over a relatively short period, this nonetheless needs to be demonstrated in the preclinical data package. Clearly the stability and reliability of he product not just in its packaging but also after administration to a patient, need to be demonstrated over its life span. In many cases the component parts of such products may need to be combined just prior to administration further complicating quality issues. Developers of such products need to be in close consultation with regulatory agencies early in the development process to ensure that testing programs meet their requirements.

## CONCLUSION

While the landscape for regulation of modified products shows considerable variation, there is a convergence of guidelines with harmonization under the WHO banner. In addition, scientific principles are now being more widely applied leading to a lessening of the need to conduct in vivo human studies on every occasion but, at the same time, providing more consistent quality assurance of products for modified-release products.

## REFERENCES

1. WHO (World Health Organization) Technical Report Series, No. 937, 2006 Annex 7 Multisource (generic) pharmaceutical products: guidelines on registration requirements to establish interchangeability.

2.  Marroum PJ. Regulatory Issues Relating to Modified Release Drug Formulations, 2007, this book.
3.  Wade G, Keitel S, Korakianiti1 E. Regulatory Aspects of Delivery Systems in the EU. 2007, this book.
4.  Nagai N, Toyoshima T. Japanese Regulatory Issues on Modified-Release Drug Products, 2007, this book.
5.  Ghani S, Lee, D. Canadian Regulatory Requirements of Drug Approval, 2007, this book.
6.  Bartholomaeus A, Rolls C. Roberts MS. Australian Regulatory Requirements of Drug Approval, 2007, this book.
7.  EMEA European Medicines Agency, for the Evaluation of Medicines for Medicinal Products. Committee for Proprietary Medicinal Products: Modified-release Oral and Transdermal Dosage forms. London, 2: July 1999. Doc. Ref. CPMP/EWP/280/96.
8.  EMEA European Medicines Agency: Evaluation of Medicines for Human Use CHMP Efficacy Working Party Therapeutic Subgroup on Pharmacokinetics (EWP-PK). Questions and Answers on the Bioavailability and Bioequivalence Guideline. London, 27 July 2006. Doc Ref: EMEA/CHMP/EWP/40326/2006.
9.  EMEA European Medicines Agency: Committee for Medicinal Products for Human Use (CHMP). Questions and answers on guideline title: clinical investigation of corticosteroids intended for use on the skin. Doc. Ref. CHMP/EWP/21441/2006 London, 16 November 2006 http://www.emea.europa.eu/pdfs/human/ewp/2144106en.pdf
10. WHO Web site: Drug regulation 2007 http://www.who.int/medicines/areas/quality_safety/regulation_legislation/en/
11. WHO Drug Information. Improving the quality and usefulness of drug regulatory authority websites. 2001; 15(3 and 4): 163–8.
12. Lindenberg M, Kopp S, Dressman JB. Classification of orally administered drugs on the World Health Organization Model List of Essential Medicines according to the biopharmaceutics classification system. Eur J Pharm Biopharm 2004; 58(2):265–78.
13. Uppoor VR. Regulatory perspectives on in vitro (dissolution)/in vivo (bioavailability) correlations. J Control Release. 2001 May 14; 72(1–3):127–32.
14. Takagi T, Ramachandran C, Bermejo M, Yamashita S, Yu LX, Amidon GL. A provisional biopharmaceutical classification of the top 200 oral drug products in the United States, Great Britain, Spain, and Japan. Mol Pharm 2006; 3 (6):631–43.
15. Wu CY, Benet LZ. Predicting drug disposition via application of BCS: transport/absorption/elimination interplay and development of a biopharmaceutics drug disposition classification system. Pharm Res 2005; 22(1):11–23.
16. Gupta E, Barends DM, Yamashita E, et al. Review of global regulations concerning biowaivers for immediate release solid oral dosage forms. Eur J Pharm Sci 2006 Nov; 29(3–4):315–24. Epub 2006.
17. McKenzie AW, Stoughton RB. A method for comparing percutaneous absorption of steroids. Arch Dermatol 1962; 86:608–10.

18. Demana PH, Smith EW, Walker RB, Haigh JM, Kanfer I. Evaluation of the proposed FDA pilot dose-response methodology for topical corticosteroid bioequivalence testing. Pharm Res 1997; 14(3):303–8.

19. Wiedersberg S, Leopold CS, Guy RH. Bioavailability and bioequivalence of topical glucocorticoids. Eur J Pharm Biopharm 2007 Aug 8; [Epub ahead of print].

20. Keida T, Hayashi N, Kawashima M. Application of the Food and Drug Administration (FDA) bioequivalent guidance of topical dermatological corticosteroid in yellow-skinned Japanese population: validation study using a chromameter. J Dermatol 2006; 33(10):684–91.

21. Hodari KT, Nanton JR, Carroll CL, Feldman SR, Balkrishnan R. Adherence in dermatology: a review of the last 20 years. J Dermatolog Treat 2006; 17(3): 136–42.

22. Chik Z, Johnston A, Tucker AT, Chew SL, Michaels L, Alam CA. Pharmacokinetics of a new testosterone transdermal delivery system, TDS-testosterone in healthy males. Br J Clin Pharmacol 2006; 61(3):275–9.

23. Pabst G, Jaeger H. Review of methods and criteria for the evaluation of bio-equivalence studies. Eur J Clin Pharmacol 1990; 38(1):5–10.

24. Williams RL. Bioequivalence Harmonization and International BioWaivers at SFBC Anapharm Understanding Bioequivalence of Generic Drugs: A World-Wide Review, 2005, http://www.anapharm.com/sfbc/upload/sfbc/Generateur/WilliamsRogers.pdf

25. Iyer SS, Barr WH, Karnes HT. Profiling in vitro drug release from subcutaneous implants: a review of current status and potential implications on drug product development. Biopharm Drug Dispos 2006; 27(4):157–70.

26. Benet LZ, Amidon GL, Barends DM, et al. The use of BDDCS in classifying the permeability of marketed drugs. Pharm Res 2008; [E pub ahead of print].

# 34

# Regulatory Issues in the United States Relating to Modified-Release Drug Formulations

Patrick J. Marroum

*Division of Pharmaceutical Evaluation I, Office of Clinical Pharmacology, Center for Drug Evaluation and Research, Food and Drug Administration, Silver Spring, Maryland, U.S.A.*

## INTRODUCTION

In recent years the use of modified-release drug formulations has increased considerably. This is partly due to advances in formulation technologies enabling one to design formulations that provide a better control of the release of the drug to the site of action. Controlled-release formulations provide several advantages over conventional immediate release formulations of the same drug such as a reduced dosing frequency, a decreased incidence and or intensity of side effects, a greater selectivity of pharmacologic activity and a reduction in drug plasma fluctuation resulting in a more constant or prolonged therapeutic effect.

However, modified-release formulations provide unique challenges from a formulation and manufacturing point of view requiring specific studies to characterize the controlled-release nature of the formulation. In this chapter the regulatory considerations that come into play in approving and maintaining such formulations on the market will be discussed with an emphasis on the laws, regulations and guidances that pertain to this type of drug delivery formulations.

The views expressed in this chapter are those of the author. No official support or endorsement by the Food and Drug Administration is intended or should be inferred.

The requirements discussed in this chapter cover all types of controlled-release dosage forms. The primary focus will be on oral controlled-release drug products, which are the most common type of controlled-release dosage form. Requirements for other types of controlled-release drug products, such as transdermal patches or implants, are similar to those described in this chapter.

## DEFINITIONS

Before beginning a discussion of the regulatory requirements of controlled-release products it is useful to understand several commonly used definitions for these types of products:

- *Controlled-release dosage forms*: A class of pharmaceuticals or other biologically active products from which a drug is released from the delivery system in a planned, predictable and slower than normal manner (1).
- *Modified-release dosage form*: Refers, in general, to a dosage form for which the drug release characteristics of time course and or location are chosen to accomplish therapeutic or convenience objectives not offered by conventional dosage forms (1).
- *Extended-release dosage form*: This is a specific type of modified-release dosage form which allows at least a twofold reduction in dosage frequency as compared to that drug presented as an immediate (conventional) release dosage form (1).
- *Delayed-release dosage form*: This is a specific type of modified-release dosage form, which releases a drug at a time other than promptly after administration. An example is enteric-coated tablets (1).
- *Proportional similarity*:
    *Definition 1*: All active and inactive ingredients are in exactly the same proportion between different strengths (e.g., a tablet of 50 mg strength has all the inactive ingredients exactly half that of a tablet of 100 mg strength and twice that of a tablet of 25 mg strength) (2).
    *Definition 2*: The total weight of the dosage form remains nearly the same for all strengths (within 5% of the total weight of the strength on which a biostudy was performed), the same inactive ingredients are used for all strengths, and the change in any strength is obtained by altering the amount of the active ingredient and one or more of the inactive ingredients. For example, with respect to an approved 5 mg tablet, the total weight of new 1 and 2.5 mg tablets remain nearly the same, and the changes in the amount of active ingredient are offset by a change in one or more inactive ingredients. This definition is generally applicable to high potency drug substances where the amount of active drug substance in the dosage form is relatively low (2).

- *Dose dumping*: Dose dumping is defined as the disruption of the modified-release characteristics leading to significantly higher availability of the drug in the gastrointestinal (GI) tract resulting in altered bioavailability.

## CONTROLLED-RELEASE NEW DRUG APPLICATIONS

A fundamental question in evaluating a controlled-release product is whether formal clinical studies of the dosage form's safety and efficacy are needed or whether only a pharmacokinetic evaluation will provide adequate evidence for approval. A rational answer to this question must be based on evaluation of the pharmacokinetic properties and plasma concentration/ effect relationship of the drug. Where there is a well-defined predictive relationship between the plasma concentrations of the drug and the clinical response (regarding both safety and efficacy), it may be possible to rely on plasma concentration data alone as a basis for the approval of the controlled-release product. In the following situations, it is expected that clinical safety and efficacy data be submitted for the approval of the controlled-release New Drug Application (NDA):

- When the controlled-release product involves a drug which is an unapproved new molecular entity, since there is no approved reference product to which a bioequivalence claim could be made
- When the rate of input has an effect on the drug's efficacy and toxicity profile
- When a claim of therapeutic advantage is intended for the controlled-release product
- When there are safety concerns with regards to irreversible toxicity
- Where there are uncertainties concerning the relationship between plasma concentration and therapeutic and adverse effects or in the absence of a well-defined relationship between plasma concentrations and either therapeutic or adverse clinical response
- Where there is evidence of functional (i.e., pharmacodynamic) tolerance
- Where peak to trough differences of the immediate release form are very large

In all the above instances where there is already an immediate release formulation of the drug, a 505(b)(2) NDA could be submitted for approval to the FDA. The regulations for a 505(b)(2) NDA are covered under 21CFR 314.54. These regulations state that any person seeking approval of a drug product that represents a modification of a listed drug, e.g., a new indication or a new dosage form, and for which investigations other than bioavailability or bioequivalence studies are essential to the approval of the changes, may submit a 505(b)(2) application. However, such an application may not be submitted under this section of the regulations for a drug product whose only difference from the reference listed drug is that the extent of absorption or rate of absorption is less than that of the reference listed drug or if the rate of absorption is unintentionally less than that of the reference listed drug (3).

## CODE OF FEDERAL REGULATIONS: BIOAVAILABILITY STUDY REQUIREMENTS FOR CONTROLLED-RELEASE PRODUCTS

The bioavailability requirements for controlled-release products are covered in the U.S. Code of Federal Regulations under 21 CFR 320.25(f) (4).

The aims of these requirements are to determine that the following conditions are met:

- The drug product meets the controlled-release claims made for it.
- The bioavailability profile established for the drug product rules out the occurrence of clinically significant dose dumping. This is usually achieved by the conduct of a food effect study where by the drug is administered with and without a high fat breakfast.
- The drug product's steady-state performance is equivalent to a currently marketed noncontrolled-release or controlled-release drug product that contains the same active drug ingredient or therapeutic moiety and that is subject to an approved full new drug application.

The drug product's formulation provides consistent pharmacokinetic performance between individual dosage units.

The reference material for such a bioavailability study shall be chosen to permit an appropriate scientific evaluation of the controlled-release claims made for the drug product. The reference material is normally one of the following:

- A solution or suspension of the active drug ingredient or therapeutic moiety.
- A currently marketed immediate release drug product containing the same active drug ingredient or therapeutic moiety and administered according to the dosage recommendations in the labeling of immediate release drug product.
- A currently marketed controlled-release drug product subject to an approved full new drug application containing the same active drug ingredient or therapeutic moiety and administered according to the dosage recommendations in the labeling proposed for the controlled-release drug product.

Guidelines for the evaluation of controlled-release pharmaceutical dosage forms provide assistance to those designing, conducting, and evaluating studies. However, a drug may possess inherent properties that require considerations specific to that drug and its dosage form which may override the generalities of these Guidelines. Guidances related to the evaluation of controlled-release drug products as well as many other types of Guidances are available on the Internet, at the Center for Drug Evaluation and Research website (http://www.fda.gov/cder/).

## GENERAL APPROACHES FOR EVALUATING CONTROLLED-RELEASE PRODUCTS

### Demonstration of Safety and Efficacy Primarily Based on Clinical Trials

In general, for drugs where the exposure–response relationship is not established or is unknown, applications for changing the formulation from immediate release to modified release will require the demonstration of the safety and efficacy of the product in the target patient population. Typically the approval of such applications will be based on the results of the pivotal clinical trials (at least two trials that are deemed pivotal to the assessment of the drug product from a clinical point of view).

In these cases, the pharmacokinetic and biopharmaceutics studies conducted are for descriptive purposes (5) and in certain cases will help in the initial dose selection. The types of pharmacokinetic studies generally include the following:

- Single-dose relative bioavailability
- Multiple-dose relative bioavailability
- Food effect study
- Single-dose BE studies (clinical vs. market formulations, different dosage strengths, etc.)
- Dosage strength proportionality
- Dose proportionality study
- In vivo–in vitro correlation (IVIVC)
- PK-PD evaluation

When a new molecular entity is developed as an MR formulation additional studies to characterize its clinical pharmacology and ADME characteristics are recommended.

#### Example of an NDA with Clinical Data

This NDA for this once-a-day formulation of diltiazem is a typical example of an application with clinical data. The clinical portion of the NDA consisted of three clinical trials. The first trial was a randomized double-blind placebo run in parallel group pilot study with 36 patients with mild to moderate hypertension (24 on diltiazem 360 mg and 12 placebo) to investigate the time effect relationship of this diltiazem formulation. The second trial was considered to be one of the 2 pivotal trials and was a dose response trial in patients with mild to moderate hypertension. This was a multicenter randomized double blind placebo controlled fixed dose response trial: 90, 180, 360, and 540 mg once a day diltiazem and placebo. 229 patients participated in this study which consisted of a 4-week run in phase followed by a 4-week active treatment period. The third trial was a multicenter dose titration trial for the treatment of mild to moderate hypertension. This pivotal trial was a multicenter randomized double blind placebo controlled parallel study comparing optimally titrated doses ranging from 120 to 360 mg of diltiazem to placebo in a total of 117 patients (6).

The biopharmaceutics and clinical pharmacology portion of the NDA consisted of four studies:

■ A single-dose relative bioavailability study comparing the controlled-release formulation to the approved immediate release formulation
■ A pivotal steady state relative bioavailability and dose proportionality study
■ A food effect and absorption profile study

The sponsor also conducted a pilot relative bioavailability study to select the formulation with optimal release characteristics and also used the data obtained from this study to develop a multiple level C IVIVC (7).

It is to be noted that the approval was mainly based on the results of the safety and efficacy trials where the biopharmaceutics studies were undertaken to characterize the release properties of the formulation and ensure that no dose dumping is occurring.

## Demonstration of Safety and Efficacy Based on PK, PK/PD Trials

"The Guidance for Industry—Providing Clinical Evidence of Effectiveness for Human Drug and Biologic Products" indicates that in certain cases, the clinical efficacy of a modified-release dosage form or different dosage forms can be extrapolated from existing studies, without the need for additional well-controlled clinical trials. The Guidance states that this may be possible because other types of data allow the application of known effectiveness to the new dosage form.

> Sometimes clinical efficacy of modified-release dosage formulations can be extrapolated from existing studies, without the need for additional well-controlled clinical trials because other types of data allow the application of known effectiveness to the new dosage form. Even in the cases where blood levels are quite different, if there is a well-understood relationship between blood concentration and response, including an understanding of the time course of that relationship, it may be possible to conclude that the new dosage form is effective on the basis of pharmacokinetic data without an additional clinical efficacy trial (8).

The types of studies and requirement will depend on whether the nature of the exposure-response relationship and whether the therapeutic window is defined, as outlined below.

### No Prior Knowledge of the Exposure-Response Relationship or Therapeutic Window; Approval Solely Based on Plasma Concentrations

Such an approach although being used in developing an MR product, is not encouraged. In such a case strict bioequivalence between the IR and MR product is required in terms of $C_{max}$, $C_{min}$, and AUC at steady state.

The impact of differences in the shapes of the plasma concentration-time profile for the IR and MR products should be assessed depending on the knowledge of the drug, the therapeutic class and the proposed indication for the drug.

In certain instances, a MR product may be developed to actually mimic the performance of an IR product and its dosing regimen (e.g., Repetabs). The MR product is designed to simulate actual multiple single dose administrations, which would correspond to individual dosage administrations of the IR product. Under such circumstances, with or without PK/PD information, it is conceivable that approval of the MR product could be based strictly on bioequivalence determinations for the pharmacokinetic parameters. When deviations in the steady-state pharmacokinetic profiles are seen between the MR and IR product regimens, more dependence on PK/PD information or clinical studies would be required for approval rather than
on simple bioequivalence of the pharmacokinetic parameters of AUC, $C_{max}$, and $C_{min}$.

### No Quantitative Exposure-Response Relationship but Well-Defined Therapeutic Window in Terms of Safety and Efficacy

In the case where the rate of input is known not to influence the safety and efficacy profile, the following criteria have to be met for the approval of such a product:

- The 90% confidence interval for the log-transformed ratio of the $AUC_{ss}$ of the controlled-release formulation relative to the immediate release approved formulation should be between 80 and 125.
- The $C_{max,ss}$ should be equal to or below the upper limit of the defined therapeutic window.
- The $C_{min,ss}$ should be equal or above the lower limit of the defined therapeutic window.
- In the case where the rate of input is known to influence the safety and efficacy profile or is unknown the approval criteria are the same as

above. In addition, studies investigating the impact of the rate of input
on the pharmacodynamics of the drug in terms of safety and efficacy
should be investigated.

### Well-Defined Quantitative Exposure-Response Relationship Using Different Input Rates of IR or the MR Product

Under such circumstances, where adequate efficacy and safety PK/PD
relationships exist, further safety and efficacy studies may not be required.
The exposure–response relationship should be established with the intended
clinical end point. The safety profile of the drug should be well understood.
In such situations, steady state comparative BA/BE study(s) would be
required to demonstrate that the MR product performs in a manner that
ensures safety and efficacy under the labeled dosing conditions. In addition,
the standard PK/BA studies would also be required for descriptive and
labeling purposes

Under circumstances where clinical responses or surrogates of such
responses related to efficacy or safety have been preliminarily related to
pharmacokinetic parameters or dose, further safety or efficacy studies may
be required to confirm the preliminary PK/PD relationships. It is anticipated that such additional safety or efficacy studies would not be of the
same scale where no preliminary PK/PD relationships had been shown. The
standard PK/BA studies would also be required for descriptive and labeling
purposes in such situations.

If the exposure-response relationship is established with a validated
surrogate end point, the surrogate end point used should be accepted as a
validated marker for clinical efficacy. In addition, the safety profile of the
drug should be well understood.

### Example of the Approval of New CR Formulation Based on PK/PD Study

Immediate release Coreg (carvedilol) is approved for the treatment of
hypertension as well as the treatment of congestive heart failure and left
ventricular dysfunction following myocardial infarction. The MR formulation of Coreg would inherit the same indications as the immediate
release on the basis of sustained effects on blood pressure (demonstrated in
one ABPM study) and a demonstration of beta blockade throughout the
inter-dosing interval.

For that effect the sponsor conducted one ABPM study to demonstrate the effects on systolic and diastolic blood pressure throughout the
inter-dosing interval. In addition the sponsor conducted a PK/PD study
showing that the effects of the MR formulation on exercise heart rate in
hypertensive patients were within the 80–125 % confidence limits of the IR

for both area under the curve and maximal effect. The study also demonstrated that the relationship between exposure and effect on heart rate stays the same irrespective of the formulation used and that the rate of input of carvedilol does not alter this relationship.

From a biopharmaceutics point of view, the sponsor conducted the necessary study to demonstrate the controlled release aspect of the formulation, a food effect study to rule out dose dumping, a pharmacokinetic study in heart failure subjects showing that the pharmacokinetic characteristics in the target population are the same as in healthy adults. Moreover, the sponsor conducted an in-vivo alcohol drug interaction to rule out that the modified-release characteristics are not dramatically altered in the presence of alcohol. Such a study was warranted based on in vitro data showing that the release characteristics of this formulation might be affected by the amount of alcohol present. An attempt to establish an IVIVC was undertaken but was unsuccessful.

## GENERAL CONSIDERATIONS IN EVALUATING PK/PD RELATIONSHIPS FOR CONTROLLED-RELEASE DRUG PRODUCTS

In assessing PK/PD relationships for controlled-release products, it is important to not only establish concentration effect relationships, but it is also important to determine the significance of differences in the shape of the steady state concentration versus time profile for a MR product regimen as compared to the approved IR product regimen. In this regard, any differential effects based on the rate of absorption and/or the fluctuation within a profile as related to safety and/or efficacy should be determined. Issues of tolerance to therapeutic effects and toxic effects related to drug exposure, concentration, absorption rate, and fluctuation should also be examined as part of the PK/PD assessment.

In certain cases minimizing fluctuation in a steady state profile for a MR product may be desirable to reduce toxicity, while maintaining efficacy as compared to the IR product regimen (i.e., theophylline products). In other cases, minimizing fluctuation in a steady state profile for a MR product may reduce efficacy (i.e., nitroglycerin-fosters tolerance) as compared to the IR product regimen's profile where higher fluctuation is observed. It is therefore important and necessary to know or study the profile shape versus PD relationships. Commonly made assumptions regarding therapeutic superiority or equivalency through fluctuation minimization in an MR product regimen versus an IR product regimen must be verified.

## IMPORTANT FORMULATION CONSIDERATIONS

The performance of the modified-release formulation is a crucial aspect in contributing to the therapeutic advantage that a controlled-release formulation is providing. Two important aspects both from a regulatory and clinical point of view in evaluating MR formulations are: (*i*) the possibility of dose dumping and (*ii*) the assurance that the formulation is providing consistent performance from one unit to the other.

## Dose Dumping Due to Food or Alcohol Ingestion

It is important to evaluate the potential for dose dumping for any new modified-release formulation. Depending on the therapeutic index and the clinical indication of a drug product, dose dumping can pose a significant risk to patients either due to safety or diminished efficacy or both.

The most common type of dose dumping occurs usually in the presence of food. However, the potential of dose dumping after ingestion of alcohol is present. The most recent example of dose dumping of hydromorphone (Palladone) with its associated potential risk lead to the new requirement that every new modified-release formulations be tested for potential alcohol dose dumping. Some modified release oral dosage forms contain drugs and excipients that exhibit higher solubility in alcoholic solutions compared to aqueous solutions. Such products may exhibit a more rapid dissolution, release rate and an increased rate of systemic absorption in the presence of ethanol. Therefore it is recommended that in vitro dissolution testing in the presence of physiologically relevant alcohol concentrations be always conducted. Based on the results of the in vitro dissolution testing and the associated potential risks, an in vivo study of the effect of alcohol on the modified-release formulations might be warranted.

## Consistency in the Performance of the Formulation

A prime consideration when evaluating and approving a new modified-release formulation is how consistently it releases the drug from one unit to the other. Considerable variation in the release characteristics of the dosage form can lead to a reduced therapeutic benefit and greater potential for adverse events. Erratic release patterns can be a major issue in considering the approval of the new formulation. The consistency of the formulation is usually evaluated by determining the variability associated with the dissolution profiles along with the assessment of both inter and intra subject variability in the plasma concentration time profiles. The most definitive way of verifying the consistency of the formulation is to test the new formulation in vivo using a replicate design study that allows the determination of intra-subject variability in the pharmacokinetic parameters of interest (usually $C_{max}$ and AUC). An intrasubject variability much greater than what was observed with either the immediate release version of the same drug or other modified-release formulations is usually an indication of the erratic release characteristics. Alternatively, a less optimal approach than can be used to assess the ruggedness of the new formulation is the comparison of the inter-subject variability across the various approved formulations. An unusually high inter-subject variability is an indication that the formulation is introducing additional variability to the plasma levels. Such inconsistent formulations would have a bigger hurdle for approvability compared to a well-behaved formulation.

## GENERIC EQUIVALENT OF AN APPROVED CONTROLLED-RELEASE PRODUCT

The Drug Price Competition and Patent Term Restoration Act amendments, of 1984, to the Food, Drug and Cosmetic Act, gave the Food and Drug Administration statutory authority to accept, and approve for marketing, abbreviated new drug application (ANDAs) for generic substitutes of pioneer products, including those approved after 1962. To gain approval according to the law, ANDAs for a generic controlled-release drug product must, among other things, be both pharmaceutically equivalent and bioequivalent to the innovator controlled-release product, which is termed the reference listed drug product as identified in FDA's Approved Drug Products with Therapeutic Equivalence Ratings (The Orange Book). Pharmaceutical Equivalence

As defined in the Orange Book, to be pharmaceutically equivalent, the generic and pioneer formulations must (*i*) contain the same active ingredient; (*ii*) contain the same strength of the active ingredient in the same dosage form; (*iii*) be intended for the same route of administration; and (*iv*) be labeled for the same conditions of use. FDA does not require that the generic and reference listed controlled-release products contain the same excipients, or that the mechanism by which the release of the active drug substance from the formulation be the same (9). For substitution purposes the two products have to be pharmaceutical equivalents.

### Bioequivalence Requirements

The same bioequivalence requirements apply to, the establishment of the equivalence of the formulation used in efficacy trials if it is different from the formulation intended for marketing, and generic controlled-release product approval. For modified-release products submitted as ANDA, the following studies are recommended (2):

1.  A single dose replicate fasting study comparing the highest strength of the test and reference listed drug product
2.  A food effect nonreplicate study comparing the highest strength of the test and reference product . A typical meal consists of the following: 2 eggs fried in butter, 2 strips of bacon, 2 slices of toast with butter, 4 ounces of hash brown potatoes, 8 ounces of whole milk (10). Alternatively, other

meals with 1000 calorie content, with 50% of the calories derived from fat, could be used. The dosage form should be administered immediately following the completion of the breakfast or meal.

Since single dose studies are considered more sensitive in addressing the primary question of bioequivalence (11) (release of the drug at the same rate to the same extent), multiple dose are no more recommended even in instances where nonlinear kinetics are present (12). This is departing from the long standing policy that was outlined in the 1993 guidance issued by the Office of Generic Drugs to also require controlled-release generic products to also be bioequivalent under steady state conditions (13).

For controlled-release formulations marketed in multiple strengths, a single dose bioequivalence study under fasting conditions is required only on the highest strength, provided that the compositions of the lower strengths are proportional to that of the highest strength, and all strengths are manufactured under the same conditions. Single dose bioequivalence studies may be waived for the lower strengths on the basis of acceptable dissolution profiles. For controlled-release products that are not compositionally proportional, a single dose bioequivalence study is required for each strength. This requirement can also be waived in the presence of an in vivo in vitro correlation whose predictability has been established. For the waiver to be granted on the basis of an acceptable IVIVC, the following conditions have to be met:

■ Have the same release mechanism
■ Have similar in vitro dissolution profiles
■ Are manufactured using the same type of equipment, the same process and at the same site as other strengths that have bioavailability data

In addition one of the following situations should exist:

■ Bioequivalence has been established for all strengths of the reference listed product.
■ Dose proportionality has been established for the reference listed product, and all reference product strengths are compositionally proportional, have the same release mechanism and the in vitro dissolution profiles for all strengths are similar.
■ Bioequivalence is established between the generic product and the reference listed product at the highest and lowest strengths, and for the reference listed product, all strengths are compositionally proportional or qualitatively the same, have the same release mechanism and the in vitro dissolution profiles are similar.

The criteria for granting such waivers is that the difference in predicted means of $C_{max}$ and AUC is no more than 10 % based on dissolution profiles of the highest strength and the lower strength product (14).

## SCALE UP AND POST-APPROVAL CHANGES FOR MODIFIED-RELEASE FORMULATIONS

In September 1997, the FDA issued a guidance on scale and post approval changes for modified-release formulations. The purpose of the guidance was to provide recommendations for sponsors of NDAs and ANDAs on the type of information needed for components and composition changes, scale up and scale down changes, site of manufacture changes and process and equipment manufacturing changes (15). The guidance also improved the consistency of the review process by making the requirements uniform across the reviewing divisions within the FDA.

For each type of change the Guidance defines three levels. A level I change is defined as a change that is unlikely to have any detectable impact on formulation quality and performance and is usually reported in the annual report.

A level II change could have a significant impact on formulation quality and performance and is usually reported in a change being affected supplement.

A level III change is likely to have a significant impact on quality and performance and is usually included in a prior approval supplement.

Tables 1–12 summarize the level for each type of change along with the regulatory requirements for each level of change for both extended and delayed release formulations.

Where the "Guidance for Industry SUPAC-MR: Modified Release Solid Oral Dosage Forms; Scale-Up and Postapproval changes: Chemistry, Manufacturing, and Controls, In Vitro Dissolution Testing, and In Vivo Bioequivalence Documentation" (14) recommends a biostudy, biowaivers for the same changes made on lower strengths are possible without an IVIVC if (*i*) all strengths of the tablets are compositionally proportional or qualitatively the same, (*ii*) in vitro dissolution profiles of all strengths are similar, (*iii*) all strengths have the same release mechanism, (*iv*) bioequivalence has been demonstrated on the highest strength (comparing changed and unchanged drug product and the dissolution profiles of the changed and unchanged product are similar in three media (0.1N HCl, phosphate buffer pH 4.5 and 6.8). For beaded capsule formulations the comparability of the dissolution profiles should only be established in the approved dissolution method using the approved dissolution medium.

## IN VITRO DISSOLUTION FOR MODIFIED-RELEASE FORMULATIONS

### In Vitro–In Vivo Correlations

Since the release of the drug is the rate-limiting step of the appearance of the drug in the systemic circulation for controlled-release formulations, it is therefore possible to establish a relationship between the in vitro dissolution

(*Text continues on p. 410*)

**Table 1** Summary of the Requirements for the Levels of Changes in Release Controlling Components and Composition for Extended-Release Dosage Forms

| Level | Classification | Therapeutic range | Test documentation | Filing documentation |
|---|---|---|---|---|
| I | = 5% w/w change based on total release controlling excipient (e.g., controlled release polymer, plasticizer) content No other changes | All drugs | Stability Application/compendial requirements No biostudy | Annual report |
| II | Chance in technical grade and/or specifications = 10% w/w change based on total release controlling excipient (e.g., controlled release polymer, plasticizer) content No other changes | Non-narrow | Notification and updated batch record Stability Application/compendial requirements plus multi-point dissolution profiles in three other media (e.g., water, 0.1N HCL, and USP buffer media at pH 4.5 and 6.8) until = 80% of drug released or an asymptote is reached[a] Apply some statistical test(F2 test) for comparing dissolution profiles[b] No biostudy | Prior approval supplement |
| | | Narrow | Updated batch record Stability Application/compendial (profile) requirements Biostudy or IVIVC[a] | Prior approval supplement |
| III | >10% w/w change based on total release controlling excipient (e.g., controlled release polymer, plasticizer content | All drugs | Updated batch record Stability Application/compendial (profile) requirements Biostudy or IVIVC[a] | Prior approval supplement |

[a]In the presence of an established IVIVC only application/compendial dissolution testing should be performed.
[b]In the absence of an established IVIVC.
*Abbreviation*: IVIVC, in vitro–in vivo correlation.

**Table 2** Summary of the Requirements for the Levels of Changes in Nonrelease Controlling Components and Composition for Extended-Release Dosage Forms

| Level | Classification | Therapeutic range | Test documentation | Filing documentation |
|---|---|---|---|---|
| I | Complete or partial deletion of color/flavor<br>Change in inks, imprints<br>Upto SUPAC-IR level 1 excipient ranges<br>No other changes | All drugs | Stability<br>Application/compendial requirements<br>No biostudy | Annual report |
| II | Change in technical grade and/or specifications<br>Higher than SUPAC-IR level 1 but less than level 2 excipient ranges<br>No other changes | All drugs | Notification and updated batch record<br>Stability<br>Application/compendial requirements plus multi-point dissolution profiles in three other media (e.g., water, 0.1N HCL, and USP buffer media at pH 4.5 and 6.8) until $=80\%$ of drug released or an asymptote is reached[a]<br>Apply some statistical test (F2 test) for comparing dissolution profiles[b]; no biostudy | Prior approval supplement |
| III | Higher than SUPAC-IR level 2 excipient ranges | All drugs | Updated batch record<br>Stability<br>Application/compendial (profile) requirements<br>Biostudy or IVIVC[a] | Prior approval supplement |

[a]In the presence of an established IVIVC only application/compendial dissolution testing should be performed.
[b]In the absence of an established IVIVC.
*Abbreviation*: IVIVC, in vitro–in vivo correlation.

**Table 3** Summary of the Requirements for the Levels of Changes in Equipment for Extended-Release Dosage Forms

| Level | Classification | Change | Test documentation | Filing documentation |
|---|---|---|---|---|
| I | Equipment changes No other changes (all drugs) | Alternate equipment of same design and principle Automated equipment | Updated batch record Stability Application/compendial requirements No biostudy | Annual report |
| II | Equipment changes No other changes (all drugs) | Change to equipment of a different design and operating principle | Updated batch record Stability Application/compendial requirements plus multi-point dissolution profiles in three other media (e.g., water, 0.1N HCL, and USP buffer media at pH 4.5 and 6.8) until = 80% of drug released or an asymptote is reached[a] Apply some statistical test (F2 test) for comparing dissolution profiles[b] No biostudy | Prior approval supplement |

[a]In the presence of an established IVIVC only application/compendial dissolution testing should be performed.
[b]In the absence of an established IVIVC.
*Abbreviation*: IVIVC, in vitro–in vivo correlation.

**Table 4** Summary of the Requirements for the Levels of Changes in Manufacturing Site for Extended-Release Dosage Forms

| Level | Classification | Therapeutic range | Test documentation | Filing documentation |
|---|---|---|---|---|
| I | Single facility Common personnel No other changes | All drugs | Application/compendial requirements No biostudy | Annual report |
| II | Same contiguous campus Common personnel No other changes | All drugs | Identification and description of site change, and updated batch record Notification of site change Stability Application/compendial requirements plus multi-point dissolution profiles in three other media (e.g., water, 0.1N HCL, and USP buffer media at pH 4.5 and 6.8) until = 80% of drug released or an asymptote is reached[a] Apply some statistical test (F2 test) for comparing dissolution profiles[b] No biostudy | Changes being effected supplement |
| III | Different campus Different personnel | All drugs | Notification of site change Updated batch record Stability Application/compendial (profile) requirements Biostudy or IVIVC[a] | Prior approval supplement |

[a]In the presence of an established IVIVC only application/compendial dissolution testing should be performed.
[b]In the absence of an established IVIVC.
*Abbreviation:* IVIVC, in vitro–in vivo correlation.

**Table 5** Summary of the Requirements for the Levels of Changes in Manufacturing Process for Extended-Release Dosage Forms

| Level | Classification | Change | Test documentation | Filing documentation |
|---|---|---|---|---|
| I | Processing changes affecting the non-release controlling excipients and/or the release controlling excipients No other changes | Adjustment of equipment operating conditions (e.g., mixing times, operating speeds, etc.) Within approved application ranges | Updated batch record Application/compendial requirements No biostudy | Annual report |
| II | Processing changes affecting the non-release controlling excipients and/or the release controlling excipients No other changes | Adjustment of equipment operating conditions (e.g., mixing times, operating speeds, etc.) Beyond approved application ranges | Updated batch record Stability Application/compendial requirements plus multi-point dissolution profiles in three other media (e.g., water, 0.1N HCL, and USP buffer media at pH 4.5 and 6.8) until $= 80\%$, of drug released or an asymptote is reached[a] Apply some statistical test (F2 test) for comparing dissolution profiles[b] No biostudy | Changes being effected supplement |
| III | Processing changes affecting the non-release controlling excipients and/or the release controlling excipients | Change in the type of process used (e.g., from wet granulation direct compression) | Updated batch record Stability Application/compendial (profile) requirtments Biostudy or IVIVC[a] | Prior approval supplement |

[a]In the presence of an established IVIVC only application/compendial dissolution testing should be performed.
[b]In the absence of an established IVIVC.
*Abbreviation*: IVIVC, in vitro–in vivo correlation.

**Table 6** Summary of the Requirements for the Levels of Changes in Scale Up/Scale Down for Extended-Release Dosage Forms

| Level | Classification | Change | Test documentation | Filing documentation |
|---|---|---|---|---|
| I | Scale-up of bio-batch(s) or pivotal clinical batch(s) No other changes | −10 × (all drugs) | Updated batch record Stability Application/compendial requirements No biostudy | Annual report |
| II | Scale-up of bio-batch(s) or pivotal clinical batch(s) No other changes | > 10 × (all drugs) | Updated batch record Stability Application/compendial requirements plus multi-point dissolution profiles in three other media (e.g., water, 0.1 N HCL and usp buffer media at pH 4.5 and 6.8) until = 80% of drug released or an asymptote is reached[a] Apply some statistical test (F2 test) for comparing dissolution profiles[b] No biostudy | Changes being effected supplement |

[a]In the presence of an established IVIVC only application/compendial dissolution testing should be performed.
[b]In the absence of an established IVIVC.
*Abbreviation:* IVIVC, in vitro–in vivo correlation.

**Table 7** Summary of the Requirements for the Levels of Changes in Scale Up/Scale Down for Delayed-Release Dosage Forms

| Level | Classification | Change | Test documentation | Filing documentation |
|---|---|---|---|---|
| I | Scale-up of bio-batch(es) or pivotal clinical batch(es) No other changes | −10× (all drugs) | Updated batch record Stability Application/compendial requirements No biostudy | Annual report |
| II | Scale-u p of bio-batch(es) or pivotal clinical batch (es) No other changes | >10× (all drugs) | Updated batch record Stability Application/compendial requirements plus multi-point dissolution profiles in additional buffer stage testing (e.g., USP buffer media at pH 4.5–7.5) under standard and increased agitation conditions until =80% of drug released or an asymptote is reached[a] Apply some statistical test (F2 test) for comparing dissolution profiles[b] No biostudy | Changes being effected supplement |

[a]In the presence of an established IVIVC only application/compendial dissolution testing should be performed.
[b]In the absence of an established IVIVC.
*Abbreviation*: IVIVC, in vitro–in vivo correlation.

**Table 8** Summary of the Requirements for the Levels of Changes in Manufacturing Site for Delayed-Release Dosage Forms

| Level | Classification | Therapeutic range | Test documentation | Filing documentation |
|---|---|---|---|---|
| I | Single facility Common personnel No other changes | All drugs | Application/compendial requirements No biostudy | Annual report |
| II | Same contiguous campus Common personnel No other changes | All drugs | Identification and description of site change and updated batch record Notification of site change Stability Application/compendial requirements plus multi-point dissolution profiles in additioonal buffer stage testing (e.g., USP buffer media at pH 4.5–7.5) under standard and increased agitation conditions until $= 80\%$ of drug released or an asymptote is reached[a] Apply some statistical test (F2 test) for comparing dissolution profiles[b] No biostudy | Changes being effected supplement |
| III | Different campus Different personnel | All drugs | Notification of site change Updated batch record Stability Application/compendial (profile) requirements Biostudy or IVIVC[a] | Prior approval supplement |

[a]In the presence of an established IVIVC only application/compendial dissolution testing should be performed.
[b]In the absence of an established IVIVC.
*Abbreviation*: IVIVC, in vitro–in vivo correlation.

**Table 9**  Summary of the Requirements for the Levels of Changes in Nonrelease Controlling Components and Composition for Delayed-Release Dosage Forms

| Level | Classification | Therapeutic range | Test documentation | Filing documentation |
|---|---|---|---|---|
| I | Complete or partial deletion of color/flavor<br>Change in inks, imprints<br>Upto SUPAC-IR level 1 excipient ranges<br>No other changes | All drugs | Stability<br>Application/compendial requirements<br>No biostudy | Annual report |
| II | Change in technical grade and/ or specifications<br>Higher than SUPAC-IR level 1 but less than level 2 excipient ranges<br>No other changes | All drugs | Notification and updated batch record<br>Stability<br>Application/compendial requirements plus multi-point dissolution profiles in additional buffer stage testing (e.g., USP buffer media at pH 4.5–7.5) under standard and increased agitation conditions until = 80% of drug released or an asymptote is reached[a]<br>Apply some statistical test (F2 test) for comparing dissolution profiles[b]<br>No biostudy | Prior approval supplement |
| III | Higher than SUPAC-IR Level 2 excipient ranges | All drugs | Updated batch record<br>Stability<br>Application/compendial (profile) requirements<br>Biostudy or IVIVC[a] | Prior approval supplement |

[a]In the presence of an established IVIVC only application/compendial dissolution testing should be performed.
[b]In the absence of an established IVIVC.
*Abbreviation*: IVIVC, in vitro–in vivo correlation.

**Table 10** Summary of the Requirements for the Levels of Changes in Equipment for Delayed-Release Dosage Forms

| Level | Classification | Change | Test documentation | Filing documentation |
|---|---|---|---|---|
| I | Equipment changes No other changes (all drugs) | Alternate equipment of same design and principle Automated equipment | Updated batch record Stability Application/compendial requirements No biostudy | Annual report |
| II | Equipment changes No other changes (all drugs) | Change to equipment of a different design and operating principle | Updated batch record Stability Application/compendial requirements plus multi-point dissolution profiles in additional buffer stage testing (e.g., USP buffer media at pH 4.5–7.5) under $=80\%$ of drug released or an asymptote is reached[a] Apply some statistical test (F2 test) for comparing dissolution profiles[b] No biostudy | Prior approval supplement |

[a]In the presence of an established IVIVC only application/compendial dissolution testing should be performed.
[b]In the absence of an established IVIVC.
*Abbreviation*: IVIVC, in vitro–in vivo correlation.

**Table 11** Summary of the Requirements for the Levels of Changes in Manufacturing Process for Extended-Release Dosage Forms

| Level | Classification | Change | Test documentation | Filing documentation |
|---|---|---|---|---|
| I | Processing changes affecting the nonrelease controlling excipients and/or the release controlling excipients No other changes | Adjustment of equipment operating conditions (e.g., mixing times, operating speeds, etc.) Within approved application ranges | Updated batch record Application/compendial requirements No biostudy | Annual report |
| II | Processing changes affecting the nonrelease controlling excipients and/or the release controlling excipients No other changes | Adjustment of equipment operating conditions (e.g., mixing times, operating speeds, etc.) Beyond approved application ranges | Updated batch record Stability Application/compendial requirements plus multi-point dissolution profiles in additional buffer media (e.g., water, 0.1 N HCL, and USP buffer media at pH 4.5–7.5) until = 80%, of drug released or an asymptote is reached[a] Apply some statistical test (F2 test) for comparing dissolution profiles[b] No biostudy | Changes being effected supplement |
| III | Processing changes affecting the nonrelease controlling excipients and/or the release controlling excipients | Change in the type of process used (e.g., from wet granulation direct compression) | Updated batch record Stability Application/compendial (profile) requirements Biostudy or IVIVC[a] | Prior approval supplement |

[a]In the presence of an established IVIVC only application/compendial dissolution testing should be performed.
[b]In the absence of an established IVIVC.
*Abbreviation:* IVIVC, in vitro–in vivo correlation.

**Table 12** Summary of the Requirements for the Levels of Changes in Release Controlling Components and Composition for Extended-Release Dosage Forms

| Level | Classification | Therapeutic range | Test documentation | Filing documentation |
|---|---|---|---|---|
| I | = 5% w/w change based on total release controlling excipient (e.g., controlled release polymer, plasticizer) content no other changes | All drugs | Stability<br>Application/compendial requirements<br>No biostudy | Annual report |
| II | Change in technical grade and/or specifications<br>= 10% w/w change based on total release controlling excipient (e.g., controlled release polymer, plasticizer) content | Non-narrow | Notification and updated batch record<br>Stability<br>Application/compendial requirements plus multi-point dissolution profiles in additional buffer stage testing (e.g., USP buffer media at pH 4.5–7.5) under standard and increased agitation conditions until = 80% of drug released or an asymptote is reached[a]<br>Apply some statistical test (F2 test) for comparing dissolution profiles[b]<br>No biostudy | Prior approval supplement |
| | No other changes | Narrow | Updated batch record<br>Stability<br>Application/compendial (profile) requirements<br>Biostudy or IVIVC[a] | Prior approval supplement |
| III | >10% w/w change based on total release controlling excipient (e.g., controlled release polymer, plasticizer) content | All drugs | Updated batch record<br>Stability<br>Application/compendial (profile) requirements<br>Biostudy or IVIVC[a] | Prior approval supplement |

[a]In the presence of an established IVIVC only application/compendial dissolution testing should be performed.
[b]In the absence of an established IVIVC.
*Abbreviation*: IVIVC, in vitro–in vivo correlation.

of the drug and its in vivo performance. A USP PF Stimuli Article published in 1988 (16) established three levels of correlations:

*Level A Correlation*: is defined as a point-to-point relationship between the in vitro dissolution profile and the in vivo input rate (usually expressed as the fraction of drug absorbed vs. time). This type of correlation is considered to be the most useful from a regulatory point of view.

*Level B Correlation*: uses the principles of statistical moment analysis. In such a correlation, e.g., the mean in vitro dissolution time is correlated with the mean residence time or the mean absorption time in vivo. Such a correlation suffers from the fact that a number of different in vivo profiles can produce the same mean absorption time in vivo. Thus, level B correlations are considered of little value from a regulatory point of view.

*Level C Correlation*: establishes a relationship between the amount of drug dissolved at a certain time with a certain pharmacokinetic parameter. A multiple level C correlation on the other hand relates one or more pharmacokinetic parameter such as AUC or $C_{max}$ to the amount of drug dissolved at several time points of the dissolution profile.

In September of 1997, the FDA issued a guidance on this topic to provide recommendations for the development Evaluation and applications of IVIVCs.

## Development of IVIVC

Human data should be utilized for regulatory consideration of an IVIVC. Bioavailability studies for IVIVC development should be performed with enough subjects to characterize adequately the performance of the drug product under study. Although crossover studies are preferred, parallel studies or cross-study analyses may be acceptable. The reference product in developing an IVIVC may be an intravenous solution, an aqueous oral solution, or an immediate release product. IVIVCs are usually developed in the fasted state. When a drug is not tolerated in the fasted state, studies may be conducted in the fed state. Any in vitro dissolution method may be used to obtain the dissolution characteristics of the oral controlled-release dosage form but the same system should be used for all formulations tested (17). The preferred dissolution apparatus is USP apparatus I (basket) or II (paddle), used at compendially recognized rotation speeds (e.g., 100 rpm for the basket and 50–75 rpm for the paddle). In other cases, the dissolution properties of some oral controlled-release formulations may be determined with USP apparatus III (reciprocating cylinder) or IV (flow through cell). An aqueous medium, either water or a buffered solution preferably not exceeding pH 6.8, is recommended as the initial medium for development of an IVIVC. For poorly soluble drugs, addition of surfactant (e.g., 1 % sodium lauryl sulfate) may be appropriate (18–20).

IVIVCs are established in two stages. First, the relationship between dissolution characteristics and bioavailability characteristics needs to be determined. Second, the reliability of this relationship must be tested. The first stage may be thought of as developing an IVIVC, whereas the second stage may involve evaluation of predictability. The most commonly seen process for developing a Level A IVIVC is to (*i*) develop formulations with different release rates, such as slow, medium, fast, or a single release rate if dissolution is condition independent; (*ii*) obtain in vitro dissolution profiles and in vivo plasma concentration profiles for these formulations; (*iii*) estimate the in vivo absorption or dissolution time course using an appropriate deconvolution technique for each formulation and subject (e.g., Wagner-Nelson, numerical deconvolution) (21). These three steps establish the IVIVC model. Alternative approaches to developing level A IVIVCs are possible. The IVIVC relationship should be demonstrated consistently with two or more formulations with different release rates to result in corresponding differences in absorption profiles. Exceptions to this approach (i.e., use of only one formulation) may be considered for formulations for which in vitro dissolution is independent of the dissolution test conditions (e.g., medium, agitation, pH) (22).

The in vitro dissolution methodology should adequately discriminate among formulations. Dissolution testing can be carried out during the formulation screening stage using several methods. Once a discriminating system is developed, dissolution conditions should be the same for all formulations tested in the bioavailability study for development of the correlation and should be fixed before further steps towards correlation evaluation are undertaken. During the early stages of correlation development, dissolution conditions may be altered to attempt to develop a 1-to-1 correlation between the in vitro dissolution profile and the in vivo dissolution profile.

Time scaling may be used as long as the time scaling factor is the same for all formulations (23).

### Evaluation of an IVIVC

An IVIVC that has been developed should be evaluated to demonstrate that predictability of the in vivo performance of a drug product from its in vitro dissolution characteristics is maintained over a range of in vitro dissolution release rates and manufacturing changes. Since the objective of developing an IVIVC is to establish a predictive mathematical model describing the relationship between an in vitro property and a relevant in vivo response, a logical evaluation approach focuses on the estimation of predictive performance or, conversely, prediction error. Depending on the intended application of an IVIVC and the therapeutic index of the drug, evaluation of prediction error internally and/or externally may be appropriate. Evaluation of internal predictability is based on the initial data used to develop the IVIVC model. Evaluation of external predictability is based on additional test data sets.

Figure 1 shows the procedure by which one predicts the plasma concentration time profile of a modified-release formulation from its in vitro dissolution (24).

The dissolution profiles are fitted to a mathematical function. The cumulative dissolution profiles are converted to dissolution rates by taking the first derivative of this function. The dissolution rate is then converted into an absorption rate by using the IVIVC relationship. The predicted plasma concentrations are then obtained by convolving the absorption rates with the disposition function of the drug.

For internal predictability, the IVIVC is deemed acceptable if the average prediction errors for all the formulations used to develop the correlation for $C_{max}$ and AUC is less than 10% with none exceeding 15%. If the criteria for internal predictability are not met, then one would proceed to the evaluation of external predictability. If the prediction errors are less than 10% the IVIVC is deemed acceptable, if the prediction errors are more than 15% on average, the IVIVC is deemed inconclusive and further evaluation would be needed. This can be accomplished by attempting to predict additional data sets. If the prediction errors are on average above 20%, the IVIVC is considered to be of poor predictive ability and is considered unacceptable from a regulatory point of view (14).

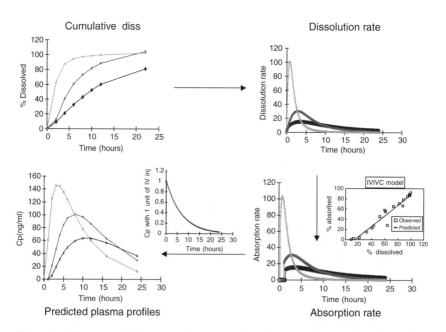

**Figure 1** The convolution procedure to predict plasma concentrations from dissolution profiles.

Applications of IVIVCs

Once a predictive IVIVCs has been developed, in vitro dissolution can not only serve as (*i*) an important tool for providing process control and quality assurance, (*ii*) determining stable release characteristics over time and facilitating the determination of minor formulation changes on the release characteristics of the drug product but can also serve as a surrogate for the in vivo performance of the product. This will in turn reduce the regulatory burden on the industry by reducing the number of studies required for the approval and maintenance on the market of a controlled-release product.

With an IVIVC, waivers for more significant changes are possible. A biowaiver will likely be granted for an oral controlled-release drug product using an IVIVC for (*i*) Level 3 process changes as defined in SUPAC-MR; (*ii*) complete removal of or replacement of nonrelease controlling excipients as defined in SUPAC-MR; (*iii*) Level 3 changes in the release controlling excipients as defined in SUPAC-MR; and (*iv*) a level 3 site change.

The criteria for granting an in vivo bioavailability/bioequivalence waiver are that the predicted mean $C_{max}$ and AUC for the test and reference formulation should not differ by no more than 20% as illustrated in Figure 2 (25).

If an IVIVC is developed with the highest strength, waivers for changes made on the highest strength and any lower strengths may be granted, if these strengths are compositionally proportional or qualitatively the same, the in vitro dissolution profiles of all the strengths are similar, and all strengths have the same release mechanism.

This biowaiver is applicable to strengths lower than the highest strength, within the dosing range that has been established to be safe and effective, provided that the new strengths are compositionally proportional or qualitatively the same, have the same release mechanism, have similar in vitro dissolution profiles, and are manufactured using the same type of

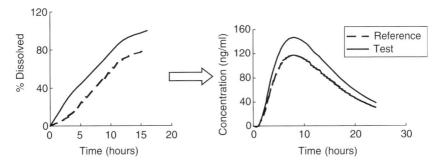

**Figure 2** Criteria for granting biowaivers based on a level A IVIVC.

equipment, and the same process at the same site as other strengths that have bioavailability data available.

Certain changes generally always necessitate in vivo bioavailability testing and in some cases might necessitate clinical trials, even in the presence of an IVIVC. These include the approval of a new formulation of an approved oral controlled-release drug product when the new formulation has a different release mechanism, approval of a dosage strength higher or lower than the doses that have been shown to be safe and effective in clinical trials, approval of another sponsor's oral controlled-release product even with the same release controlling mechanism, and approval of a formulation change involving a nonrelease controlling excipient in the drug product that may significantly affect drug absorption.

## Setting Dissolution Specifications

### No IVIVC Present

The dissolution test is an important tool from a quality control point of view. In the past, the dissolution specifications were set based on the performance of the clinical/bio lots. Therefore if the release characteristics of the formulation were variable and not well controlled, then one would end up with dissolution specifications that are somewhat wider than a formulation with good release characteristics. The end result of this practice was the possibility of the introduction on the market of potentially highly variable formulations with different in vivo performance. This might result in widely fluctuating plasma concentration profiles leading to a variable therapeutic effect and increased incidence of adverse effects and therapeutic failures. The FDA guidance attempted to change this less than optimal practice. The FDA guidance stipulates that the maximum allowable width of a dissolution specifications be no more than 20 %, ± 10 % deviation from the dissolution profile of the desired target formulation (Fig. 3).

The guidance recommends that the dissolution specifications include at least 3 time points, one covering the initial part of the profile, the second one the middle part and the last one should be where 80 % dissolution has occurred or where the plateau has been reached if one is unable to obtain complete dissolution. Specifications should be set to pass USP stage II of testing (based on average data). However, if dissolution specifications wider than 20 % are desired, then one would have to conduct a bioequivalency study to show that lots at the upper and lower limit of the specifications are bioequivalent (13).

### Level A IVIVC Present

In the presence of an IVIVC, the criteria are shifted from the in vitro side to the in vivo side. In this case, the IVIVC is used to predict the plasma

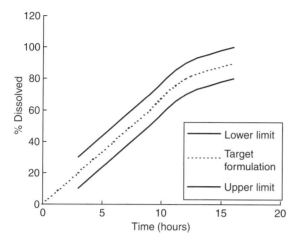

**Figure 3** Dissolution specifications in the absence of IVIVC.

concentration time profile that corresponds to lots that are on the upper and lower limit of the dissolution specifications.

Acceptable dissolution specification limits are limits that do not result in plasma concentration time profiles that differ by more than 20 % in the area under the plasma concentration time (AUC) and peak plasma concentrations ($C_{max}$) (usually ± 10 % of the target clinical/bio formulation). Therefore, it is possible to obtain dissolution specification limits that are wider than 20 % if the predicted limits do not result in plasma concentration time profiles that are different in their mean predicted $C_{max}$ or AUC by more than 20%. However, the guidance does not penalize sponsors if the 20% width in the limits results in more than a 20% difference in the predicted pharmacokinetic parameters. Tighter limits than the case where no IVIVC is present will only be required for drugs with narrow therapeutic index to avoid potentially serious toxicities (26).

With a multiple C correlation, the relationship between the amount of drug dissolved at each time point and the relevant PK parameter such as $C_{max}$ and AUC should be used to set the dissolution specification limits in such a way that the upper and lower limit do not result in the release of batches than differ by more than 20% in their plasma concentration time profiles.

### Release Rate Specifications

The FDA guidance also allows for a novel approach in setting dissolution specifications for formulations exhibiting a zero order release characteristic.

An example of such a formulation is the osmotic delivery system commonly referred to as GITS (gastrointestinal therapeutic systems). If these formulations are designed to deliver the drug at a constant rate that can be described by a linear relationship over a certain period of time, then one can set a release rate specification to describe the performance of the formulation.

This release rate specification can be in addition to or instead of the cumulative dissolution specifications that one usually sets for a modified-release product.

Having a release rate specification will provide for a better control of the in vivo performance of the drug because it is the release characteristics of the formulation that will determine the rate of appearance in the systemic circulation. This can be described more appropriately by the release rate compared to the cumulative amounts of drug dissolved at a certain interval of time.

As an illustration of this point, let's consider the dissolution profiles of two lots of the same formulation (Fig. 4) with similar release rates but are on the upper and lower limits of the cumulative dissolution specifications. Assuming a level A correlation for this product, the predicted plasma concentration time profile corresponding to these two lots are similar, differing only in the time to achieve peak plasma concentration.

On the other hand if one examines the case presented in Figure 5 whereby the two lots are very close in their cumulative dissolution profiles (both at the upper limit of the dissolution specifications) but markedly different in their release rates, one can clearly see that the predicted plasma profiles corresponding to these lots are very different and considered not to be bioequivalent.

## CONCLUSION

The current increase in the number of controlled-release formulations available on the market is the results of the recent advances in drug delivery

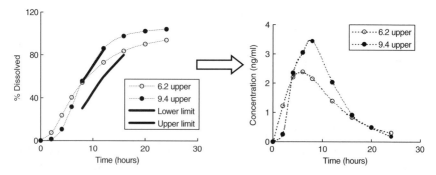

**Figure 4**   Influence of the release-rate specifications on plasma levels: inequivalent plasma profiles.

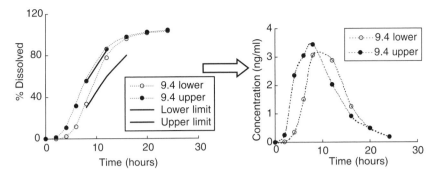

**Figure 5** Influence of the release-rate specifications on plasma levels: equivalent plasma profiles.

technologies and well as the availability of sensitive analytical assays. The establishment and understanding of the relationship between the plasma concentrations and/or input rate and the pharmacodynamic properties of the drug (whether desired or adverse) plays an important role in facilitating the development of such formulations. The use of PK/PD model for certain drug products could alleviate the regulatory burden since it would decrease the number of studies needed for both the understanding of the pharmacokinetic and pharmacodynamic properties of the drug product and its approval. Moreover, the establishment of an IVIVC will enable one to predict the plasma concentration time profile from its in vitro dissolution characteristics therefore enabling the dissolution test to act as a surrogate for the bioavailability of the drug product. This will in turn decrease the number of bioavailability/bioequivalence studies that are needed for the approval and maintenance of the controlled-release product on the market. In addition the establishment of a predictive IVIVC will enable one to obtain wider dissolution specifications without compromising on the quality of the in vivo performance of the formulation.

## REFERENCES

1. Marroum PJ. Bioavailability/Bioequivalence for Oral Controlled Release Products, Controlled Release Drug Delivery Systems: Scientific and Regulatory Issues, Fifth International Symposium on Drug Development, East Brunswick, NJ, May 1997; 15–7.
2. Guidance on BA and BE Studies for Orally Administered Drug Products—General Considerations. Center for Drug Evaluation and Research, Food and Drug Administration, August 2000.
3. Code of Federal Regulations 21 314.54.
4. Code of Federal Regulations 21 320.25.

5.  Skelly JP. Division Guidelines for the Evaluation of Controlled Release Drug Products. Center for Drug Evaluation and Research, Food and Drug Administration, April 1984.
6.  Duarte C, Cardizem CD. Medical review, Division of Cardio-Renal Drug Products. Center for Drug Evaluation and Research, Food and Drug Administration, February 1991.
7.  Marroum PJ. Clinical Pharmacology and Biopharmaceutics review. Center for Drug Evaluation and Research, Food and Drug Administration, June 1991.
8.  Guidance for Providing Clinical Evidence of Effectiveness for Human Drug and Biological Products. Center for Drug Evaluation and Research, Food and Drug Administration, May 1998.
9.  Approved Drug Products with Therapeutic Equivalence Evaluations, 20th ed. Center for Drug Evaluation and Research, Food and Drug Administration, 2000: vii–xxi.
10.  Guidance on the Food-Effect Bioavailability and Bioequivalence Studies. Center for Drug Evaluation and Research, Food and Drug Administration, October 1997.
11.  El-Tahtawy A, Jackson A, Ludden T. Evaluation of bioequivalence of highly variable drugs using Monte Carlo simulations. I. Estimation of rate of absorption for single and multiple dose trails using Cmax. Pharm Res 1994; 11 (9):1330–6.
12.  Guidance on Bioavailability and Bioequivalence Studies for Orally Administered Drug Products—General Considerations. Center for Drug Evaluation and Research, Food and Drug Administration, October 2000.
13.  Guidance for Oral Extended (Controlled) Release Dosage Forms: In Vivo Bioequivalence and In Vitro Dissolution Testing. Office of Generic Drugs, Center for Drug Evaluation and Research, Food and Drug Administration, 1993.
14.  Malinowski H, Marroum PJ, Uppoor R, et al. Dissolution Technologies. Extended Release Oral Dosage Forms: Development, Evaluation and Application of In Vitro/In Vivo Correlations 1997; 4(4):23–32.
15.  Guidance for Modified Release Solid Oral Dosage Forms, Scale Up and Post Approval Changes: Chemistry and Controls: In Vitro Dissolution Testing and In Vivo Bioequivalence Documentation, Center for Drug Evaluation and Research, Food and Drug Administration, July 1997.
16.  In vitro and in vivo evaluation of dosage forms. US Pharmacopoeia 1088, 1995; 23:1924–9.
17.  Malinowski H. ER Guidance. In Amidon G, Robinson JR, Williams RL, eds. Scientific Foundations for Regulating Drug Product Quality. Alexandria VA: AAPS Press, 1997; 259–73.
18.  Siewert M. Perspective of in vitro dissolution tests in establishing in vivo/on vitro correlations. Eur J Drug Metab Pharmacokinet 1993; 18(1):7–18.
19.  Skelly JP, Shiu GF. In vitro/in vivo correlations in biopharmaceutics: scientific and regulatory implications. Eur J Drug Metab Pharmacokinet 1993; 18(1): 121–9.
20.  Blume HH, McGilvery I, Midha KK. Bio-International 94 Conference on Bioavailablity, Bioequivalence and Pharmacokinetic studies and Pre-Conference Satellite on In Vivo/In Vitro Correlation. Eur J Pharm Sci 1995; 3:113–24.

21. Wagner J. Absorption analysis and bioavailability. In: Wagner J, ed. Pharmacokinetics for the Pharmaceutical Scientist. Lancaster: Technomic Publishing Company 1993; 159–205.
22. Marroum P. Development of In Vivo In Vitro Correlations, SUPAC-MR/IVIVC guidance FDA Training Program Manual, Center for Drug Evaluation and Research, Food and Drug Administration, July 1997; 62–76.
23. Brockmeier D, Voegele D, Hattingberg HM. Drug Res 1983; 33(1):598–601.
24. Uppoor R. Evaluation of Predictability of In Vitro In Vivo Correlations, SUPAC-MR/IVIVC guidance FDA Training Program Manual, Center for Drug Evaluation and Research, Food and Drug Administration, July 1997; 97–110.
25. Marroum PJ. Regulatory examples: dissolution specifications and bio-equivalence product standards. In: Amidon G, Robinson JR, Williams RL, eds. Scientific Foundations for Regulating Drug Product Quality. Alexandria VA: AAPS Press, 1997; 305–19.
26. Marroum P. Role of in vitro in vivo correlations in setting dissolution specifications. Am Pharm Rev 1999; 2(4):39–42.

# 35

# Japanese Regulatory Issues on Modified-Release Drug Products

## Naomi Nagai and Satoshi Toyoshima

*Pharmaceuticals and Medical Devices Evaluation Center,
Pharmaceuticals and Medical Devices Agency, Tokyo, Japan*

## INTRODUCTION

The recent progress of drug delivery technologies has been contributing to the increase in the number and variety of modified-release drug products approved in Japan. Those products have many clinical benefits for pharmacotherapy, such as reducing dosing frequency, maintaining therapeutic effect, decreasing side effect/toxicity, and increasing pharmacological selectivity/specificity. For a successful drug design and clinical development of this type of drug products, adequate planning and step-by-step evaluation is very important.

This chapter summarizes several regulatory issues relating to modified-release drug products to be approved under the Pharmaceutical Affairs Law of Japan. Although the points described in this chapter are mainly focused on oral extended release drug products, the basic concepts and procedures can be applied to other types of modified-release drug products.

## CLASSIFICATION OF PHARMACEUTICAL PRODUCTS

The classification of prescription drugs and data category for submission for approval applications are shown in Table 1. The data required for approval application depends upon the situations of each drug product as follows: whether the drug product contains a new active pharmaceutical ingredient (API), whether the drug product has a new route of administration, whether

**Table 1**  Classification of Prescription Drugs and Category of Data Submitted with Approval Applications

| Category of data | Classification of drugs[a] | | | | | | | | |
|---|---|---|---|---|---|---|---|---|---|
| | (1) | (2) | (3) | (4) | (5) | (6) | (7) | (8) | (9) |
| A. Data on origin, details of discovery, use in foreign countries, etc. | | | | | | | | | |
| 1. Data on origin and details of discovery | ○ | ○ | ○ | ○ | ○ | ○ | ○ | ○ | × |
| 2. Data on use in foreign countries | ○ | ○ | ○ | ○ | ○ | ○ | ○ | ○ | × |
| 3. Data on characteristics and comparison with other drugs | ○ | ○ | ○ | ○ | ○ | ○ | ○ | ○ | × |
| B. Data on physical and chemical properties, specifications testing methods, etc. | | | | | | | | | |
| 1. Data on determination of structure, physical and chemical properties, etc. | ○ | × | × | × | × | × | × | × | × |
| 2. Data on manufacturing process | ○ | ○ | ○ | × | ○ | × | ○ | ○ | △ |
| 3. Data on specifications and testing methods | ○ | ○ | ○ | × | ○ | × | ○ | ○ | ○ |
| C. Data on stability | | | | | | | | | |
| 1. Data on long-term storage test | ○ | ○ | ○ | × | ○ | × | △ | ○ | × |
| 2. Data on severe test | ○ | ○ | ○ | × | ○ | × | △ | ○ | × |
| 3. Data on acceleration test | ○ | ○ | ○ | × | ○ | × | ○ | ○ | ○ |
| D. Data on pharmacological action | | | | | | | | | |
| 1. Data on effectiveness | ○ | ○ | ○ | ○ | × | ○ | × | △ | × |
| 2. Data on general/safety pharmacology | ○ | △ | △ | × | × | × | × | △ | × |
| 3. Data on other pharmacology | △ | △ | △ | × | × | × | × | × | ○ |
| E. Data on absorption, distribution, metabolism, and excretion | | | | | | | | | |
| 1. Data on absorption | ○ | ○ | ○ | △ | ○ | ○ | × | × | × |
| 2. Data on distribution | ○ | ○ | ○ | △ | ○ | ○ | × | × | × |
| 3. Data on metabolism | ○ | ○ | ○ | △ | ○ | ○ | × | × | × |

| | (1) | (2) | (3) | (4) | (5) | (6) | (7) | (8) | (9) |
|---|---|---|---|---|---|---|---|---|---|
| 4. Data on excretion | ○ | × | △ | ○ | ○ | △ | ○ | × | × |
| 5. Data on bioequivalence | × | × | × | × | × | × | × | ○ | × |
| 6. Data on other pharmacokinetics | △ | △ | △ | △ | △ | × | △ | × | × |
| **F. Data on toxicity** | | | | | | | | | |
|   1. Data on single dose toxicity | ○ | ○ | ○ | × | × | × | × | ○ | × |
|   2. Data on repeated dose toxicity | ○ | ○ | ○ | × | × | × | × | △ | × |
|   3. Data on mutagenicity | ○ | × | × | × | × | × | × | × | × |
|   4. Data on carcinogenicity | △ | × | △ | × | × | × | × | × | × |
|   5. Data on reproductive and developmental toxicity | ○ | ○ | △ | × | × | × | × | △ | × |
|   6. Data on local irritation | △ | △ | △ | △ | △ | × | △ | △ | × |
|   7. Data on other toxicities | △ | △ | △ | × | × | × | × | × | × |
| G. Data on results of clinical trials | ○ | ○ | ○ | ○ | ○ | ○ | ○ | ○ | ○ |

[a]Classification of drugs: Yakushokushin in No.0331009. March 2005.

(1) Drugs with new API
(2) New combination prescription drugs
(3) Drugs with new routes of administration
(4) Drugs with new indications
(5) Drugs with new dosage forms
(6) Drugs with new doses
(7) Drugs with additional dosage forms
(8) Combination prescription drugs with similar formulations
(9) Miscellaneous drugs

*Abbreviations:* ○, data shall be submitted; ×, data may be omitted; △, data submission shall be determined depending upon the conditions of drugs.

the drug product has a new indication, whether the drug product has a new dosage form, and whether the drug product has a new dosage and administration.

Modified-release drug products with an unapproved new API are categorized into the classification (1). For drugs of the classification (1), almost a full package of data shown in Table 1 is generally required. Modified-release drug products that contain an approved API are categorized into either classification (3), (5), or (9). Modified-release products with a new route of administration, for an example, levonorgestrel intrauterine system instead of solid oral dosage forms are categorized as the classification (3). When a new dosage form with the same route of administration gives an influence on efficacy and/or safety, such as extended-release products that have been changed from immediate release ones, the new drug application is categorized into the classification (5). For these three classification (1), (3), and (5), the efficacy and safety data of the modified-release drug product based on the formal clinical trials should be submitted. Although the classification (7) is also related to an additional application of dosage form, the drug product classified into (7) is usually approved with in vivo bioequivalence (BE) study as the human data, and has the same dosage and administration as those of approved products. Since modified-release property influences clinical outcome and is usually accompanied by change of dosage and administration, the classification (7) does not correspond as an approval application for modified-release drug products. The classification (9) is for generic drugs, with the same API, dosage form, quality, dosage and administration as those of the corresponding approved products.

## RELATED GUIDELINE AND TERMINOLOGY

The Japanese guide, "Guidelines for the Design and Evaluation of Oral Prolonged Release Dosage Forms" is the fundamental guideline. It covers all general issues and factors to be studied for the development and approval application of extended-release drug products (1). "Guideline for Bioequivalence Studies of Generic Products," "Guideline for Bioequivalence Studies for Different Strengths of Oral Solid Dosage Forms," "Guideline for Bioequivalence Studies for Formulation Changes of Oral Solid Dosage Forms," and "Draft Guideline for Bioequivalence Studies for Manufacturing Changes of Oral Solid Dosage Forms" provide the qualification procedures and acceptance criteria of in vivo BE studies and in vitro dissolution tests (2–6). The Japanese regulatory document "Clinical Pharmacokinetic Studies of Pharmaceuticals" describes the scope and basic principles of clinical pharmacokinetic (PK) studies necessary for submitting new drug applications and re-examining approved drugs, which is useful for evaluating the PK property and pharmacokinetic/pharmacodynamic (PK/PD) relationship of the drug products (7,8). The Japanese clinical trial guidelines have been published to provide rational guidance for conducting clinical trials and evaluating efficacy/safety data for the following therapeutic drugs: arrhythmia, angina pectoris, analgesics, cerebral circulation/metabolism, lipidemia, anxiety, anesthetics, cardiac failure, hypertensive, cancer, dementia, infection, impairment of cerebral blood vessels, osteoporosis, and over active bladder. The International Conference on Harmonization (ICH) of Technical Requirement for Registration of Pharmaceuticals for Human Use guideline Q6A, "Guideline for Specifications: Test Procedures and Acceptance Criteria for New Drug Substances and New Drug Products" and JP Pharmacopeia should be considered to establish test procedures and acceptance criteria of the final product (9,10). The Ministry of Health, Labour and Welfare (MHLW) pays an attention to global harmonization, therefore, accepts foreign clinical data if it meets Japanese regulations (11). Those guidelines and regulatory documents are available through the Web sites of MHLW, National Institute of Health Sciences (NIHS) and Pharmaceuticals and Medical Devices Agency (http://www.mhlw.go.jp, http://www.nihs.go.jp, http://www.pmda.go.jp)

The following terminologies in this chapter are defined in the documents (2,7,9):

*Modified-Release (MR):* Release characteristics of time course and/or location are chosen to accomplish therapeutic or convenience objectives not offered by conventional dosage forms such as a solution or an immediate release dosage form. Modified-release solid oral dosage forms include both delayed and extended release drug products.

*Delayed-Release (DR):* Release of a drug (or drugs) at a time other than immediately following oral administration. One example dosage form is enteric-coated drug products.

*Extended-Release (ER):* Release allows the drug available over an extended period after administration.

*Immediate-Release (IR):* Release allows the drug to dissolve in the gastrointestinal (GI) contents, with no intention of delaying or prolonging the dissolution or absorption of the drug.

*Final Product (or Final Formulation):* Pharmaceutical preparation that has the same formulation as the product on the market and is manufactured in the same way and on/at least one-tenth of the scale of the actual lot of production.

*Innovator Products:* Products being approved as new drugs by clinical trials or relating drug products.

*Generic Products*: Products whose API strengths, dosage forms and regimen are the same as those of innovator products.

## GENERAL CONSIDERATIONS RELATING TO APPROVAL
## APPLICATIONS FOR MODIFIED-RELEASE DRUG PRODUCTS

### New Drug Products

"Guidelines for the Design and Evaluation of Oral Prolonged Release Drug Forms" outlines general principles for designing and developing oral ER drug products, mainly as new dosage forms: classification (5). However, many of the issues are also applicable to other MR drug products.

In order to achieve rational development of ER drug products, the following three points should particularly be considered: (*i*) the property of API has clear rationale for developing ER dosage form, (*ii*) the ER drug product is designed based on sufficient studies for both API and product formulation, (*iii*) the standards for in vitro dissolution test is appropriately established. This guideline is composed of two sections, one of which addresses the factors to be studied in dosage form design and the other addresses those to be evaluated for the final product.

The following properties of API, (*i*) absorption site, (*ii*) first pass effect, (*iii*) elimination half life, and (*iv*) adverse reactions are especially thought to be critical factors in ER formulation, because (*i*) if the absorption site is limited, decrease in absorption and large variability in

**Table 2**   Factors to be Studied in Dosage Form Design

| |
|---|
| **(A) Active Pharmaceutical Ingredient** |
| *Pharmacodynamics* |
|    Average minimum effective concentration, optimal therapeutic concentration, toxic concentration, intra- and intersubject variabilities |
| *Biopharmaceutics* |
|    Major absorption sites and specificity in the site of absorption, absorption rate, elimination half-life, existence of nonlinear absorption due to first pass effects, etc., existence of nonlinear elimination due to saturation of metabolism, etc., inactivation or metabolism in the body including GI tract |
| *Chemistry/Physicochemistry* |
|    Chemical and physicochemical properties (especially, pH dependent solubility) |
| **(B) Physiological Condition** |
| *GI tract transit characteristics* |
|    Formulation (size, form, gravity, adhesion), physiological factors (length, size and motility of GI tract, composition and volume of GI content), food, diseases, posture, stress |
| *GI tract physiology* |
|    Volume, composition, pH, surface tension and viscosity of GI content, GI motility |

*Abbreviation*: GI, gastrointestinal.

bioavailability (BA) may occur, (*ii*) BA of the drug with extensive first pass effect may be impaired, if the release rate is retarded, (*iii*) the drug with long elimination half life is generally undesirable for ER dosage form, (*iv*) undesirable adverse reactions may be developed by ER formulation. Therefore, the properties of API should be sufficiently studied. Table 2A shows factors to be studied for API in dosage form design.

The ER drug products are generally more susceptible to physiological conditions in the GI tract than IR drug products. The possible effects of those factors listed in Table 2B should be considered in the dosage form design.

Finally, the appropriate final product should be selected from all the prototype dosage forms, based on the fully tested for both release characteristics and PK profile. The most excellent final product can maintain appropriate concentrations with minimal influence of food and physiological factors of the GI tract, and minimal inter- and intra-individual variabilities.

**Table 3**   Factors to be Studied in the Final Product

---

**(A) Evaluation of the Final Product**

*Release characteristics*

In vitro release characteristics under many conditions: multiple levels of pH, agitation rate, wettability, ionic strength and composition of the test medium, different kind of apparatus and methods

Specification for dissolution testing

Stability test for long-term storage test specimens

*Pharmacokinetics*

Comparative PK study with IR drug product

Single-dose PK study

Parameters to be compared: area under the concentration time curve (AUC), duration of minimum ($C_{max}$), or optimal effective concentration

Others: Time to reach maximum concentration ($T_{max}$), absorption rate constant, elimination rate constant, clearance, mean residence time, etc.

Repeated-dose PK study

Parameters to be compared: Peak and trough concentration at steady state, ratio of peak/trough concentration, duration of minimum or optimal effective concentration

Effect of dosing condition/physiological factors: food effect, diurnal change

Clinical efficacy/safety profile

**(B) Establishment of Dosing Regimen**

*Factors to be considered*

Overdose, dose dumping, disease state, combination therapy

*Dosing guideline (dosage and administration)*

Dosing conditions, frequency of dosing per day, dose levels (initial dose, maintenance dose, dose adjustment, maximum tolerable dose)

---

Table 3 shows the factors be studied in the final product. In order to sufficiently grasp factors that may affect in vivo release rate, it is necessary to examine results of in vitro test conducted under as many conditions as possible. The specifications for dissolution test which can appropriately evaluate in vivo concentration–time profile should be established for quality assurance of the ER drug product. The PK of the ER drug product should be evaluated in healthy subjects based on the plasma (or serum/blood) data in comparison with PK of either approved IR drug product or a solution of API. Food effect is particularly an important factor, therefore, PK under the both conditions of fasting and after a meal should be compared. When a remarkable food effect is observed, that should be reflected in the dosage and administration. Clinical benefits of ER drug product should be clarified based on efficacy/safety data of clinical trials using an appropriate referential product such as either already approved IR drug product or ER drug product (if a better ER profile is claimed) in the target population.

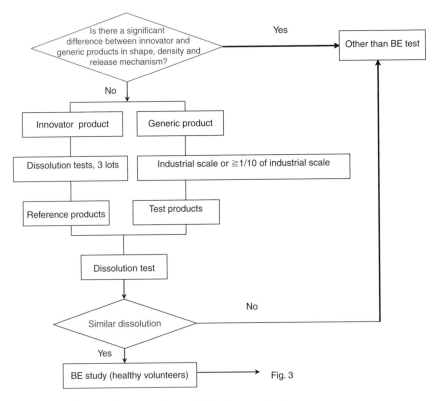

**Figure 1**   Bioequvalence study: oral ER drug products.

The appropriate guidance for dosage and administration should be established based on clinical trial results. Especially, overdose and dose dumpling, physiological changes in hepatic, renal, gastrointestinal and cardiac function, combination therapy are more carefully considered for establishing dosage and administration of ER drug products. The dosing conditions, frequency of dosing per day and dose levels (initial dose, maintenance dose, dose adjustment, maximum tolerable dose) should be established based on both PK data and clinical data. The management and rescue methods for toxic signs or adverse events should be demonstrated in the dosing guideline.

## Generic Drug Products

The generic drug products must have both pharmaceutical equivalence and BE as compared with the corresponding innovator drug products. For the first approval of an oral generic drug product, in vivo BE between generic

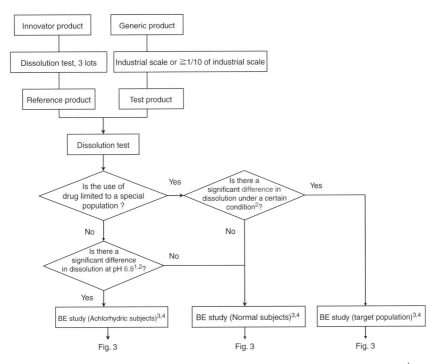

**Figure 2** Bioequivalence study: oral IR drug products and DR drug products.[1] pH 3.0–6.8 for basic drugs.[2] Go to "No" when drug products are DR drug products.[3] Patients should be enrolled, if healthy subjects are inappropriate.[4] Subjects with high clearance should be enrolled, if there is genetic polymorphism. *Abbreviations*: ER, extended-release; IR, immediate-release.

and innovator drug products are always required in Japan (2,12). The decision trees and acceptance criteria of BE studies, and the procedure of dissolution tests for DR and ER drug products are shown in Figures 1–6, and Tables 4 and 5. In considering dissolution profile for BE evaluation, similar dissolution is essential for both IR and DR drug products. While, as for ER drug products, similar dissolution profile is needed for conducting BE study in human, and equivalent dissolution is essential for BE evaluation. If the BE studies are not appropriate and feasible, PD or clinical studies are needed.

## Changes in Formulation, Strength, or Manufacturing Process

As for the formulation development and line extensions of a new drug product (additional strengths, changes in composition, components and manufacturing process) and post-approval changes both for innovator and generic products, their BE to the reference products should be demonstrated. When the change is expected to influence drug quality such as PK properties of the drug, in vivo BE study is required. When the change is slight and is not expected to affect drug quality, the basic requirement is dissolution test, therefore, the biowaiver option may be eligible. A series of

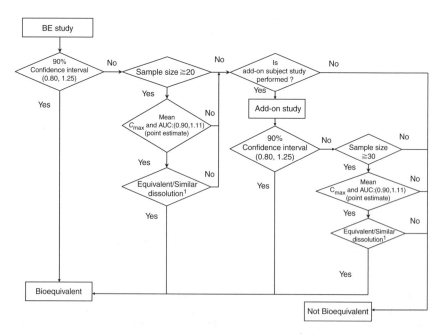

**Figure 3** Acceptance criteria for bioequivalence study. [1]Figure 4 for oral IR drug products and DR drug products. [2]Figure 5 and 6 for oral ER drug products.

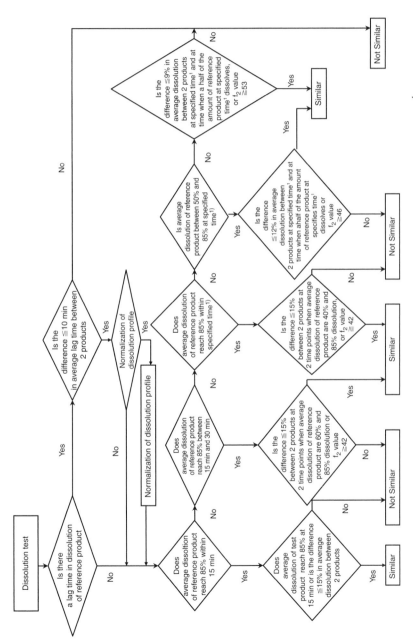

**Figure 4** Acceptance criteria for similarity in dissolution: oral IR drug products and DR drug products. [1] The testing time is specified in "Guideline for BE Studies of Generic Products."

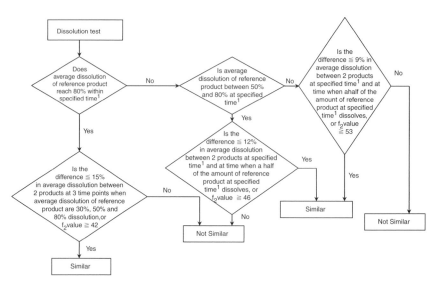

**Figure 5** Acceptance criteria for similarity in dissolution: oral ER drug products.

guidelines for BE studies defined several types of changes categorized as levels A–E or levels 1 –3[3]~[6]. The requirements are based on the magnitude of the change, the therapeutic index of the API, and the dissolution of the drug product and the solubility of the API. Tables 6 and 7 summarize the levels and BE requirements.

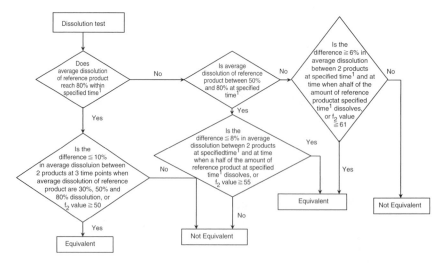

**Figure 6** Acceptance criteria for equivalence in dissolution: oral ER drug products.

**Table 4** Dissolution Test Conditions for DR Drug Products

1. No. of units: 12 units or more for each testing condition
2. Testing time: 2 hr in pH 1.2, and 6 hr in other test solutions. The test can be ended at the time when the average dissolution of reference product reaches 85% release.
3. Testing conditions:
   Apparatus: JP paddle apparatus
   Volume of test solution: Usually 900 mL
   Temperature: $37 \pm 0.5°C$
   Test solutions: The first and second fluids for the dissolution test (JP15) as pH 1.2 and 6.8 test solutions. Diluted McIlvaine buffers (0.05M disodium hydrogen-phosphate/0.025M citric acid) for other pH solutions. Other suitable test fluids can be used when the average dissolution of reference product does not reach 85% at 6 hr in the McIlvaine buffers
   Agitation: 50 rpm/pH 1.2; 50 rpm/pH 6.0; 50 rpm/pH 6.8; 100 rpm/pH 6.0
      DR drug products containing low solubility drugs should be tested by adding polysorbate 80 to the test solution 50 rpm/pH 6.0; 50 rpm/pH 6.8; and 100 rpm/pH 6.0.

## CONCLUSION

Since physical and chemical properties, pharmacology, PK, toxicity, and clinical practice are different among drugs, it is needed to plan and conduct appropriate development for each MR drug product, with the optimum balance between scientific qualification and time/cost performance. The progress and innovation of pharmaceutical technologies, scientific background and regulatory guidelines contribute to rational development

**Table 5** Dissolution Test Conditions for ER Drug Products

1. No. of units: 12 units or more for each testing condition
2. Testing time: 2 hr in pH 1.2, and 24 hr in other test solutions. The test can be ended at the time when the average dissolution of reference product reaches 85% release.
3. Testing conditions:
   Apparatus: JP paddle apparatus and either rotating basket or disintegration testing apparatus can be selected, the reason of which should be stated
   Agitation: JP paddle: 50 rpm/pH 1.2; 50 rpm/pH 3.0–5.0[a]; 50 rpm/pH 6.8–7.5[a]; 50 rpm/
      water; 50 rpm/pH 6.8–7.5 with polysorbate 80 (1.0w/v%) 100 rpm/pH 6.8–7.5; 200 rpm/pH 6.8–7.5
   Rotating basket: 100 rpm/pH 6.8–7.5; 200 rpm/pH 6.8–7.5
   Disintegration: 30 cpm/pH 6.8–7.5 with and without disk
      Volume, temperature and test solutions: same as those for DR drug products

[a]The testing solution providing the slowest dissolution in the pH range which give average 85% dissolution or more within 24 hr should be selected. If the average dissolution from the reference product does not reach 85% at 24 hr in any test solutions, the test solution providing the fastest dissolution should be used.

**Table 6** Levels of Formulation Changes and Qualification of BE

| Level[a] | Dosage form[b] | Therapeutic range | Solubility[c] | Dissolution | Qualification of BE |
|---|---|---|---|---|---|
| A | — | — | — | — | A single dissolution test[d] |
| B | — | — | — | — | Multiple dissolution tests[e] |
| C | IR, DR | Not narrow | Not low | — | Multiple dissolution tests |
|  |  |  | Low | — | In vivo BE study according to "Guideline for BE Studies of Generic Products" |
|  |  | Narrow | Not low | ≥85%/30 min | Multiple dissolution test |
|  |  |  | Not low | <85%/30 min | In vivo BE study according to "Guideline for BE Studies of Generic Products" |
|  | ER | Not narrow | — | — | Multiple dissolution test |
|  |  | Narrow | — | — | In vivo BE study according to "Guideline for BE Studies of Generic Products" |
| D | IR | Not narrow | Not low | ≥85%/30 min | Multiple dissolution test |
|  |  |  | Not low | <85%/30 min | In vivo BE study according to "Guideline for BE Studies of Generic Products" |
|  |  |  | Low | — | In vivo BE study according to "Guideline for BE Studies of Generic Products" |
|  | DR, ER | Narrow | — | — | In vivo BE study according to "Guideline for BE Studies of Generic Products" |
| E | IR, DR, ER | — | — | — | In vivo BE study according to "Guideline for BE Studies of Generic Products" |

[a] Level A–E are categorized as follows [3,4]: A: ratio of components identical, or addition/deletion of trace excipients; B: total change in excipients 5%, C: total change in excipients 10%, D: total change in excipients 15%; E: change exceeding the range of D.

[b] IR, immediate release; DR, delayed release; ER, extended release.

[c] Low solubility: Dissolution from the reference product does not reach 85% at 2 hr at pH 1.2 and 6 hr at other pHs by paddle method at 50 rpm without surfactants.

*[d] Dissolution test performed under specification conditions.

[e] Dissolution test performed under multiple conditions.

**Table 7** Levels of Manufacturing Changes and Qualification of BE

| Level[a] | Change | Content | Qualification of BE | Stability |
|---|---|---|---|---|
| Level 1 (Minor) | Lot size | Change in manufacturing scale which unlikely affect drug quality | 1. To meet the requirement, if rational dissolution specification is established according to ICH Q6A Guideline<br>2. Other: multiple dissolution tests | Long term (1 lot) |
| | Site | Same equipment, SOP, environmental condition and controls, education and training | | |
| | Equipment | Same design and operation principle | | |
| | Manufacturing process | Process changes within application and validation ranges | | |
| Level 2 (Moderate) | Physicochemical property | Change in physicochemical properties (crystal form or particle size, etc.) | 1. Equivalent dissolution profile under the specification test condition, if rational dissolution specification is established according to ICH Q6A Guideline<br>2. Other: multiple dissolution tests | Long term (1 lot)<br>Accelerated (3 months, 1 lot) |
| | Lot size | Change in manufacturing scale which may affect drug quality | | |
| | Site | Site change (same equipment, SOP, environmental condition, and controls, but different education and training) | | |
| | Equipment | Different design and operating principle | | |
| | Process | Process change outside of application and validation ranges | | |
| Level 3 (Major) | Process and site | Change exceeding the above change which will give a significant impact on drug quality | In vivo BE study according to "Guideline for BE Studies of Generic Products" | Long term (3 lots)<br>Accelerated (3 months, 3 lots) |

[a]Level A–E are categorized as follows [5,6]:
Level 1: The changes which unlikely give impacts on the quality of pharmaceutical dosage forms.
Level 2: The changes which may give impacts on the quality of pharmaceutical dosage forms.
Level 3: The changes which will give significant impacts on the quality of pharmaceutical dosage forms.

for MR drug products. It is also expected continuously international harmonization of regulations for globally simultaneous development of MR drug products.

## ACKNOWLEDGMENTS

We thank Dr. N. Aoyagi, Pharmaceuticals and Medical Devices Agency for the useful comments.

## NOTICE

The views expressed do not necessarily represent those of the Ministry of Health, Labour and Welfare and Pharmaceuticals and Medical Devices Agency.

## REFERENCES

1. Guidelines for the design and evaluation of oral prolonged release dosage form. Yakushin 1–5, March 1988. http://www.nihs.go.jp/drug/be-guide(e)/CR-new.pdf.
2. Guideline for bioequivalence studies of generic products and Q&A. Iyakushin No487, December 1997 and Jimurenraku, October 1998. Both were amended in November 2006 and May 2007. http://www.nihs.go.jp/drug/be-guide(e)/Generic/be97E.pdf.
3. Guideline for bioequivalence studies for different strengths of oral solid dosage forms and Q&A. Iyakushin No 64, February, 2000 and Jimurenraku, May, 2000. Those were amended in November 2006 and May 2007. http://www.nihs.go.jp/drug/be-guide(e)/strength/strength.PDF.
4. Guideline for bioequivalence studies for formulation changes of oral solid dosage forms and Q&A. Iyakushin No. 67, February, 2000 and Jimurenraku, May 2000. Those were amended in November 2006 and May 2007. http://www.nihs.go.jp/drug/be-guide(e)/form/form-change.PDF.
5. Aoyagi N, Morikawa K, Sonobe H, et al. Guideline (draft) for bioequivalence studies for manufacturing changes of oral solid dosage forms: conventional and enteric coated products. Iyakuhin Kenkyu, 2004; 35(6):295–317. http://www.nihs.go.jp/drug/Drug Div-Jhtml. (in Japanese).
6. Guideline (draft) for bioequivalence studies for manufacturing changes of oral solid dosage forms: controlled release products. http://www.nihs.go.jp/drug/DrugDiv-J (in Japanese).
7. Clinical Pharmacokinetic Studies of Pharmaceuticals. Iyakushin No 796, June, 2001.
8. Nagai N. Japanese guidance on clinical pharmacokinetic studies and review of the new drug applications. Xenobio Metabol Disp 2001; 16:187–92.
9. Specifications: test procedures and acceptance criteria for new drug substances and new drug products. Iyakushin No 568, May 2001 (ICHQ6A).
10. JP Pharmacopeia 15 2006.
11. Ethnic factors in the acceptability of foreign clinical data (ICH E5) and Q and A, 1998, 2003.
12. Aoyagi N. Japanese guidance on bioavailability and bioequivalence. Eur J Drug Metab Pharmacokinet 2000; 25(1):28–31.

# 36

# Regulatory Aspects of Delivery Systems in the European Union

## George Wade and Evdokia Korakianiti

*European Medicines Agency (EMEA), London, U.K.*

## Susanne Keitel

*European Directorate for the Quality of Medicines (EDQM),
Strasbourg, France*

## INTRODUCTION

This chapter addresses regulatory issues that have an impact on the pharmaceutical development of delivery systems for medicines to be used in humans. It deals with current European Union (EU) regulations and guidelines relating to the physicochemical/technical aspects of a delivery system which have to be optimized and controlled in vitro in order to achieve a desirable and consistent clinical response in patients. Furthermore, since EU law allows a number of possible routes to market, with some routes being optional and others mandatory, it appears that the EU regulatory picture may be more diverse than that in the United States, and therefore it is appropriate to at least mention the regulatory options.

The standard dosage forms and routes of administration of many medicinal products have remained largely unchanged for many years. The standard capsule, tablet and injection are well known and depend for the

The views expressed in this article are the personal views of the authors and may not be used or quoted as being made on behalf of, or reflecting the position of, any national competent authority, the European Medicines Agency (EMEA) or one of its committees or working parties.

activity on systemic delivery, in the main. On the other hand, the application of technology allows pharmaceutical scientists to do better—they can talk in terms of "focused" delivery, drug targeting etc. In other words, the use of an appropriate delivery system allows for optimization of the efficacy and/or safety of a particular product, ensuring the active substance reaches those places where it is indeed active—at the right time, in the required amounts—and, as far as possible, is kept away from places where it may have only undesirable activity, such as side effects. These are the main challenges facing industry in the development of new delivery systems, and the results will determine the claims that a given company makes concerning the advantages of their product.

On the regulatory side, the same principles that apply to the development are also utilized in the evaluation of such systems by the EU competent authorities. It largely depends upon what is claimed for the system in question, and in some cases the rather optimistic claims from the company's side are not realized when the application for a marketing authorisation is evaluated. If companies make excessive claims for specificity in one form or another, this will certainly be challenged by the authorities, and the claimed benefits will be evaluated in real terms (this usually means in *clinical* terms).

There is no guarantee of approval, and the inherent risk of failure may be very expensive in the event of a negative outcome. For many years, the regulatory authorities in Europe have been well aware of these negative outcomes and, not surprisingly, the authorities speak in terms of incomplete development leading to a premature dossier, or complete development but unfortunately carried out along the wrong lines. There are also those cases where a complete and sound development program is undermined in the end by results that unfortunately do not support reasonable expectations of efficacy or safety. Whilst not much can be done in this last case, it may be possible to reduce the occurrence of the first two, and the FDA and EU approaches are slightly different in this regard.

## ROUTES TO THE EU MARKET

A description of the detailed particulars of the EU regulatory system is outside the scope of this chapter, but as a start, it may be useful to highlight some basic principles so that developers of novel delivery technology can at least form an idea of where their product may ultimately end up.

A medicinal product cannot be marketed in the EU until it receives a marketing authorisation. Suffice it to say that there are three basic routes (procedures) to authorisation—at the national, de-centralised, and centralised (i.e., EU-wide) levels. The centralised route was set up in 1995 to deal primarily with new technology, new clinical indications etc., although many innovative products are authorised nationally with subsequent mutual recognition. American colleagues often ask why there are so many different procedures; the answer is that they are different to take into account the different types of product and the different marketing strategies foreseen by applicants. Within limits, companies can choose to market either in a localized, small number of EU Member States or in a pan-EU market. The latter requires more coordination and management, and may be beyond the resources of a small company. However, several small companies do indeed manage pan-EU authorisations for their products, and the number is expected to increase—in part through the dedicated support provided to small-and medium-sized enterprises (SMEs) provided by the EMEA. In some cases, regardless of the size or intentions of the applicant, EU legislation requires a mandatory submission through the centralised procedure, coordinated by the EMEA.

## Mandatory Centralised Route

The Annex to Regulation (EC) No 726/2004 (1) defines those products that must be submitted through the EMEA for a centralised authorisation (officially called a "community marketing authorisation"). Since 20 November 2005, companies who are developing products containing a new active substance whose ultimate clinical indication is for the treatment of the following diseases must file centrally:

- AIDS (including patients who are HIV+)
- Cancer
- Neurodegenerative disorders
- Diabetes

The mandatory scope will be extended to include auto-immune diseases and other immune dysfunctions, so that dossiers relating to these submitted on or after May 20, 2008 must also be submitted centrally.

The spirit of the older legislation [Council Regulation (EEC) No. 2309/93] has been retained in that the centralised route is also mandatory for medicinal products developed by a number of biotechnological processes, primarily recombinant DNA technology, but also including controlled gene expression and hybridoma and monoclonal antibody methods.

Medicinal products that are designated as orphan medicinal products according to Regulation (EC) No. 141/2000 must also be filed centrally.

## Optional Centralised Route

Companies seeking a pan-EU marketing authorisation for products that are not included in the above lists are not necessarily excluded and may still consider the option of a central filing. Articles 3(2)(a) and 3(2)(b) of Regulation (EC) No. 726/2004 open the door to:

- products containing a new active substance, i.e., one that was not authorised in the EU prior to 20 November 2005;
- products that are shown to constitute a significant therapeutic, scientific or technical innovation.

In these cases, prospective applicants have to prove their claims for "eligibility" by providing a reasoned justification to the EMEA, which will be judged by the EMEAs Committee for Medicinal Products for Human Use (CHMP), or by its veterinary equivalent in the case of products for veterinary use.

### Article 3(2)(b)—Significant Therapeutic, Scientific, or Technical Innovation

In the context of this chapter on delivery systems, especially *novel* delivery systems, option 3(2)(b) is very relevant. As with the old legislation, novelty or innovation can now provide a basis for a central, pan-EU authorisation, if this is what the applicant company wants. The difficulty lies in the definition of what exactly is a scientific or technical innovation, and what is regarded as significant. There may also be circumstances where an application could be regarded as indeed innovative but not significantly so—thus closing the centralised door.

The authors would propose the following points to consider in this context:

**Basic (short) definition:** Significant scientific or technical innovation refers to the application of new scientific principles or new technologies to the development of medicinal products, leading to a novel product having some clinically relevant or useful properties directly arising from this application, and having a benefit/risk balance at least identical to that of established treatments in the same therapeutic area.

**"Scientific or technical":** For the purposes of this document, no *practical* distinction is made between scientific innovation and technical innovation; they are taken together as the same entity in practice. Technology may be regarded as the practical application of "pure" scientific principles in the real world, and they are thus intimately linked. Conversely, the application of new technologies allows further refinement of underlying scientific principles.

**"Significant":** Concerning the old legislation, the CHMPs interpretation was that the application of new technology (specifically in the form of a new delivery system) should lead to some form of "significant" change, which needed to be justified in terms of clinical benefit in order to gain access to the centralised procedure. In principle, this has carried into the new legislation. The application of new scientific principles in the form of innovative technologies may be enough to gain access to the centralised procedure, provided they are clinically relevant. Developments that are merely points of detail, and that may be regarded as cosmetic or aesthetic, would not be classified as significant in this context.

**"Innovation":** Innovations have a fixed lifetime: what is regarded as an innovation today will eventually become old-fashioned in time. In the particular context of innovative medicinal products, the technology could in theory remain innovative for a number of years, even after authorisation of a product utilizing the same technology but applied to a different active substance. For chemical substances, the CHMP has traditionally taken the view that even established technology may be accepted as new or innovative if used for the first time for the active substance in question, regardless of whether there are any previous authorisations, including national ones. It is proposed that such a definition be carried over into the new legislation. Such arguments are probably not necessary in the case of biological/biotechnology products.

From a procedural point of view (as in the case of "new delivery systems" under the old legislation), eligibility for the centralised procedure on the grounds of significant scientific/technical innovation is normally judged by CHMP on a case-by-case basis, involving the Committee's scientific working parties as necessary.

## DECENTRALISED PROCEDURE AND MUTUAL RECOGNITION

For those products, which do not fall under the mandatory scope of the centralised procedure but are eligible for this route of submission, the applicant has the choice between different options. In this situation, as soon as it is the intention to market a product in more than one member state of the European Union, the applicant can choose between the centralised and the decentralised procedure. The decentralised procedure, newly introduced with the revision of the EU pharmaceutical legislation in November 2005, offers the advantage of short processing timelines (a decision on the marketing authorisation is made after 210 days, plus a potential time for a clock stop allowing the applicant to answer any questions the competent authorities may have raised during their assessment) with the free choice of the number of Member States to be involved in the respective procedure.

If a product has already been authorised in one Member State and the marketing authorisation holder wishes to change their marketing strategy to include additional Member States, the mutual recognition procedure has to be followed. Based on an assessment report issued by the competent authority of the Member State which had already authorised the product, all additional Member States selected by the applicant are supposed to recognize this first national authorisation, unless they identify a "potential serious risk to public health" which in consequence would lead to clarification and/or arbitration by the relevant regulatory and scientific committees, e.g., the Coordination Group for Mutual Recognition and Decentralised Procedures (CMD) and the CHMP.

## National Procedures

For the sake of completeness, the national marketing authorisation procedure needs to be listed as well. Only those products are eligible for this route of submission that do not fall under the mandatory scope of the centralised procedure and where it is the intention of the applicant to only market the product in one Member State. In the context of novel delivery systems, this is a rather unlikely route to be taken. More common is for the company to apply for the national authorisation to be accepted or "mutually recognised" by a selected group of Member States.

It is important to stress that, regardless of the procedure applicable or selected for the submission of a dossier, the same requirements have to be fulfilled as regards the description of an adequate quality of a medicinal product. EU quality guidelines are equally valid for the centralised, decentralised and national procedures.

## MEDICAL DEVICES

There is a convergence of technology in the area of those drug delivery systems that are an integral part of a medicinal product (drug-device combinations), and delivery systems that are medical devices in their own right. In some cases the boundary between them is very narrow indeed. Yet another group of products consists of medical devices whose function is improved in some way by the addition of a medicinal substance—an "ancillary substance" in terms of the EU medical devices legislation. Coronary stents coated with a taxane or an immune-modulating anti-rejection substance are well-known cases in point. These may be called device-drug combinations.

A major issue in the EU for companies and regulators alike is classification. In the United States, the recently created Office of Drug Device Combinations will help in answering the question "medicinal product or medical device?", although nothing so specific exists in the EU at present. It is important because the regulatory approval systems for medicinal products and devices are quite different, with a general belief on the part of industry that the device route would be easier, and less onerous in terms of data requirements. With this belief, industry would probably be more content with a classification in terms of medical device, but, unfortunately, at the time of writing there is no single regulatory ombudsman with the power to settle such potential classification disputes in the EU (see later section on classification).

## Medical Devices as Delivery Systems

To take the simplest example, delivery can also mean administration, and delivery systems taken in a wider context may include systems that have more in common with medical devices as administration systems. Drug delivery (administration) by means of a simple, separate device is a relatively easy case to define, and would include the parenteral administration of pharmacologically active drugs in solution by means of syringes, in-dwelling catheters, adapters, giving sets, etc. There is nothing novel about this, and it is not exactly targeted delivery, but without the device elements the solution would be useless. From a regulatory point of view the two elements are quite clear and distinct. The parenteral solution is a medicinal product and the syringe or giving set is a medical device, and each is evaluated according to separate "core" EU legislation:

| | |
|---|---|
| Medicinal products: | Directive 2001/83/EC (as amended by Directives 2002/98/EC, 2004/24/EC and 2004/27/EC), hereafter referred to as the pharmaceuticals directive (PD); |
| Medical devices: | Council Directive 93/42/EEC (currently under revision), hereafter referred to as the medical devices directive (MDD). |

### Example 1

If a separate (empty) syringe is included in the presentation of a medicinal product for "administration" (with reference to the MDD, Article 1(3), first paragraph), then the empty syringe must comply with the requirements of the MDD and must be CE-marked (1). However, the presentation as a whole remains a medicinal product following the pharmaceuticals legislation and does not need to be CE-marked on the outer package. (To understand what is meant by the term "presentation" in the EU, it is useful to think of it in terms of those items you see when you open the box, including the box itself.)

### Example 2

However, if the device delivery or administration element is intimately connected to the medicinal product element in some way, such that they cannot readily be disentangled and still retain any useful function, then this is regarded as "single integral use" of the product (cf. MDD Article 1(3), second paragraph), and the requirements of the MDD do not apply. In line with this, a case of single integral use would be a pre-filled syringe. Contrary to Example 1, the syringe in this case would not need to be CE-marked. The following examples in Figure 1 and Figure 2 expand on these ideas in the case of a transdermal iontophoretic system.

Single integral use debates usually center around the degree of separation of the device element and the "active" element in the presentation of the product. There are sophisticated cases where an apparent medical device aspect is less easy to disentangle from the functionality of the product entity as a whole. This immediately raises the question of classification of the entity to be developed and marketed—medicinal product or medical device?—and opens up the possibility of classification disputes.

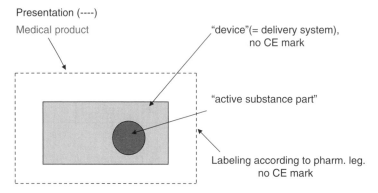

**Figure 1**  Iontophoresis system, with integrated drug reservoir.

Speaking of drug delivery, we should also keep in mind that drug "targeting" may be achieved in other ways, without recourse to a specific delivery system for the active substance. It may be feasible to systemically disseminate a drug and to focus its activity at a specific locus by means of an external influence, e.g., magnetic field, laser light radiation, ultrasound, etc. These external activating influences would be classified as medical devices. The point is that a growing number of medicinal products rely for their proper function on the involvement of a medical device in one way or another.

Classification

The definition of a medicinal product and a medical device in the relevant legislation does not automatically lead to a clear "demarcation" between the

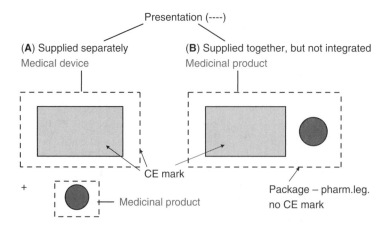

**Figure 2**  Iontophoresis system, with nonintegrated drug reservoir (notation as in Fig. 1).

two. The current definition of a (human) medicinal product exists in Article 1(2) of Directive 2001/83/EC, as amended:

1.  Any substance or combination of substances presented as having properties for treating or preventing disease in human beings; or
2.  Any substance or combination of substances which may be used in or administered to human beings either with a view to restoring, correcting or modifying physiological functions by exerting a pharmacological, immunological or metabolic action, or to making a medical diagnosis.

It has been said that these definitions could equally well apply in some cases to medical devices. Essentially, this definition has a mechanistic basis—it is important to begin with the question, what is the mechanism of action of the entity in question? If it acts by means of a pharmacological, immunological or metabolic action, then this is a good basis for a provisional conclusion in favor of medicinal product. However, we know there are medicinal products where this is not the case—where the utility of the product rests on physical rather than pharmacological activity. The intravenous ultrasound diagnostic agents used in echocardiography display diagnostically useful information only when they interact with externally applied ultrasound; receptor-based pharmacological interaction is not required and may even be a disadvantage in this particular case. This is the "physical vs pharmacological" debate over mechanism, and in fact these products are cited as exceptions in the EU guideline on these demarcation issues, MEDDEV 2.1/3 rev, section A4.2 (2).MEDDEV gives examples to assist in classification but this is probably in need of updating. National interpretations of MEDDEV may also be consulted, e.g., the UK guidance document published on the website of the Medicines and Healthcare products Regulatory Agency (3).

Generally, it is too simplistic to say that physical action = medical device, and pharmacological action = medicinal product.

The application of nanotechnology in the field of drug delivery poses interesting regulatory questions of classification. It is interesting to speculate on the regulatory possibilities in a published example in the public domain: a case described by Bergey et al. (4) consists of nano-size iron oxide particles coated in silica and attached by a ligand to a targeting molecule. The targeting molecule binds to a tumor cell surface and the whole is internalized. It is then activated by the application of an externally applied oscillating magnetic field, which disturbs the iron nanoparticles, leading to inter alia some disruption of the tumor. Figure 3 summarizes the mechanisms at work in this complicated system.

Mechanism is crucial to classification, and it is tempting to speak of the "primary" or main mechanism of action as a deciding factor, but unfortunately this is not in the medicinal products legislation at present.

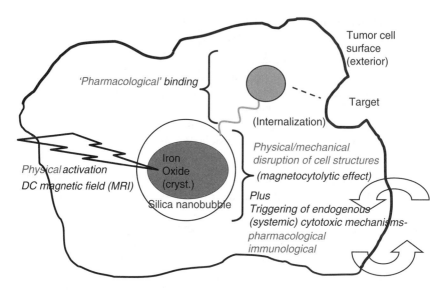

**Figure 3**   Mechanisms: physical and pharmacological.

Taking the above case further, a more difficult hypothetical situation would arise if simple coated iron nanoparticles were injected intratumorally (i.e., without the targeting molecule) then activated magnetically. The authors of this chapter think it is difficult to see any clear pharmacological activity in this situation, although, on the other hand, the effects of cytokine release on cell damage may invoke an immunological mechanism and may possibly provide a basis for classification as a medicinal product.

## Device-Drug Combinations

In these cases, it is accepted a priori that the clinical usefulness is due to the medical device (e.g., a mechanical activity, but not necessarily). Medicinal substances may be included for added value but the activity of the medicinal substance is only a secondary or "ancillary" activity: the medical device could have acceptable clinical usefulness and safety without it. Coronary stents and coated coronary stents, e.g., with sirolimus, are a case in point. In these cases the MDD applies; i.e., to say they are authorised as medical devices, but the so-called ancillary substance must be evaluated by a competent authority for medicinal products (through what is called a "Notified Body consultation procedure").

For ancillary substances that are blood derivatives, a separate legislation applies and mandatory consultation with the EMEA is required; an opinion will be given by the CHMP. For other substances, the MDD Annex I (Essential Requirements), II.7.4, has historically not been so specific in requiring a mandatory EMEA consultation, and applicants/Notified Bodies have so far had a choice about which medicines authority they appoint to do the evaluation of the substance. However, at the time of writing, this part of the MDD is currently under revision, and there may be new provisions to extend the mandatory centralised consultation for certain ancillary substances apart from blood derivatives, e.g., a substance that has been previously evaluated by the CHMP as a new active substance in a medicinal product that was subsequently granted a Community marketing authorisation. Readers are advised to check the latest revision of Annex I to the MDD in order to find out to which competent authority they should submit their dossiers.

In summary, we can only repeat the message at the beginning: there is a need for an EU body to take charge of classification issues. Presently, the EMEA has no official mandate in this regard, but it does have the Innovation Task Force (ITF), which apart from looking at new technologies, can also give, in liaison with the CHMP and European Commission where appropriate, advice on whether a product could be eligible for EMEA procedures. The ITF, the CHMP and its working parties will look into the mechanism of action of the entity in question, as proposed by the applicant, and will issue a report on whether it contains elements that could be considered to fall within the scope of the definition of a medicinal product according to Articles 1 and 2 of Directive 2001/83/EC, as amended (5).

## NEW (EMERGING) TECHNOLOGIES

Concerning the very wide spectrum of emerging technology, it is perhaps unreasonable for companies to expect the regulators to foresee and be prepared for the details of every new system with a ready-made guideline to facilitate the development and guarantee authorisation of their individual product. Sometimes the authorities come late into the picture, since the precise details of the technology may be protected during development for obvious reasons. In addition, the premature development of guidelines might constrain innovative scientific approaches by setting pre-defined boundaries while there is still inadequate experience. It is believed that regulations should follow science and not define it. Few EU guidelines exist at present in this area, and therefore initially at least, the authorities will have to approach these problems using basic principles applied to targeted medicines in general. In addition, the EMEA has the Innovation Task Force, as mentioned above, to coordinate a response from the CHMP in the domain of new technology.

### Nanotechnology in Drug Delivery

Concerning the nanoworld, a number of nanoscale medicinal products are already authorised, including liposomes, nanometer-sized colloidal dispersions of iron salts for magnetic resonance imaging, and nanosize liposomal systems, neither of which are particularly new. Obviously, the regulatory evaluation of such systems involved an emphasis on the measurement and control of disperse phase size distribution; this is especially important since it can affect the disposition and, in the case of the iron salts, can determine the diagnostic indication. We have yet to see a marketing authorisation for a product whose nanoscale properties lead directly to surprising and unforeseen biological effects and novel indications; the published antimicrobial effects of apparently simple paraffin emulsions is an example, but there are still no dossiers.

Many of the short-term nanotechnology applications in medicine are geared towards drug delivery. An area where the application of nanotechnology seems advantageous is the use of micellar and biodegradable polymeric nanoparticles as potential carriers for DNA, gene, protein and peptide delivery. The development of nonviral vectors (the delivery tools) is attractive due to the potential for improved safety, reduced ability to provoke an immune response, ease of manufacturing and scale-up, and the ability to accommodate larger molecules compared to viral vectors. However, synthetic systems such as polymer-, lipid-, and peptide-based gene carriers are typically much less efficient in delivering genes compared to viral vectors. These nanodelivery systems seem to be in an early development phase at present.

The major trend and novelty seems to be the development of multifunctional platforms that combine both detection and drug delivery properties and can be controlled by external signals or local environment stimuli. Nanoparticles usually form the core of these platforms. Their shape may vary from cylindrical, as in the case of carbon nanotubes, to spherical, as in the case of magnetic nanoparticles. The nanoparticles may also consist of several layers and can be multifunctional. Such an example is a nanoparticle consisting of magnetic and luminescent layers that would allow both particle detection with imaging techniques and particle manipulation using an external magnetic field. The active substance may be encapsulated in the nanoparticles "cores" or absorbed on their surface. To ensure biocompatibility, nanoparticles are usually covered by layers of biocompatible coating. Silica has often been used for this purpose, among other coatings. The problem of the specific drug targeting is addressed by adding onto the external surface of the nanoparticles reactive molecules that are linked to targeting agents, e.g., monoclonal antibodies, proteins or sugars, aimed at targeting specific receptors.

Such complicated systems will present new regulatory challenges, not least of which could be a medicinal-product/medical-device dispute. At the moment, there is in the EU no guidance specific to nanomedicinal products. This would not be feasible at this point of time since nanotechnology is a very broad term that embraces many different scientific and engineering principles;

it is not a single technology, but a cross-disciplinary collaboration on a variety of applications. Once clearly defined areas emerge, and experience with such products is gained, then the need to develop new guidance or adjust the existing guidance will be considered. However, as mentioned above, the evaluation of nano-scale medicinal products has already been carried out over a number of years, using established and robust procedures to ensure quality, safety and efficacy, by means of experts in the national authorities acting with external specialists in the normal way. Therefore, the evaluation and pre-vention of potential hazards related to the use of any given medicinal product containing nanoparticles is already foreseen under the existing pharmaceut-ical legislation and evaluation systems. As for any other medicinal product, the EU competent authorities will evaluate any application to place a nano-medicinal product on the market utilising established principles of benefit/risk analysis, rather than solely on the basis of the technology per se. However, having said this, we can foresee the need for some additional foci of attention in the evaluation of these systems.

A number of issues still need to be addressed, mainly relating to the safety of nanoparticles with regard to human health and the environment. Due to their very small size, nanoparticles may pass through physiological barriers such as the blood-brain barrier. There is insufficient knowledge and data concerning the fate (and especially the persistence) of nanoparticles in humans and in the environment, and concerning all aspects of toxicology and environmental toxicology related to nanoparticles, to allow satisfactory risk assessments for humans and ecosystems to be performed. The existing methodologies seem to be able to address most, but not all, the potential hazards, and might need to be adapted and new methods might need to be devised.

Nanoparticles' characterization and measurement is another critical issue. A different approach is needed compared to small molecules. Besides parameters that are usually investigated, like the size, size distribution, molecular weight, purity, chemical composition, stability and solubility, there are some other parameters that might need to be considered in addi-tion, like the surface characteristics and functionality, or the possible aggregation in biologically relevant media. In addition, there might be a need to use different or additional characterization methods compared to the standard practice [e.g., microscopy (AFM, SEM, TEM), electrophoresis, zeta-potential measurements, fluorimetry]. It is likely that the main focus of attention will be on risk, taking into account issues such as translocation and persistence.

In view of the growing interest in the field of nanotechnology, the European Commission has developed a number of initiatives to stimulate research and facilitate commercialization of new technologies (6). Among these initiatives is a consultation on nanotoxicology and nanoecotoxicology, a round table promoted by the European Group of Ethics in Science and New Technologies, and the development of a Strategic Research Agenda of the European Technology Platform. In parallel, the European Commission has requested the independent experts of the Scientific Committee on Emerging and Newly Identified Health Risks (SCENIHR) to evaluate "the appropriateness of existing methodologies to assess the potential risks associated with engineered and adventitious products of nanotechnologies."

It remains to be seen how this will develop.

## Gene Transfer

Gene transfer (sometimes loosely called "gene therapy") represents a special case of targeted delivery, aimed at delivering large nucleotides not only into the cell, but into the nucleus, which presents an additional technological challenge. Many delivery systems are described in the scientific literature, including large synthetic cationic macromolecules. Others are complex biological systems such as viral vectors, with possible additional problems related to safety.

The rather disappointing results obtained in the early clinical trials in gene transfer indicates the enormous quality, efficacy and safety issues to be overcome. Current EU guidance exists (7), and since research has continued and may be expected to increase, it is likely that the current guidance will develop as a consequence.

## SCIENTIFIC ADVICE

Furthermore, companies often take the opportunity to meet with national agencies independently, to get an informal impression of the likely scientific difficulties that may lie ahead during development of their product, often prior to seeking confirmation from the SAWP on the acceptability of their proposed plans from a pan-European perspective.

Advice from the SAWP is not binding, and may be reviewed based on the evolution of the state of the art, or on specific amendments in the company's development program. It can include all aspects of development: pharmaceutical, nonclinical and clinical.

Current timelines allow for a 40-day procedure or a 70-day procedure. In both cases, initial reports from the assessors (coordinators) are prepared at day 20, and, if necessary, the longer procedure allows for an additional report at day 50, and also the possibility of a revised final report at day 63. Fees for scientific advice are published on the EMEA website (8).

From the patterns emerging from individual scientific advice requests, it is a natural step to develop "class" guidelines on specific topics to assist the development of new systems, or at least to reduce the risk of unpleasant surprises occurring during the evaluation for a marketing authorisation.

The usual pattern is: individual case requests → clusters → guidelines.

In the case of orphan medicinal products, scientific advice takes a different terminology: "protocol assistance." The term can be misleading, implying that the procedure is limited to clinical trials. This is not the case, as it can also include requests for quality and nonclinical advice.

It has to be noted that in addition to the centralised scientific advice offered by EMEA/CHMP, all national competent authorities of the EU Member States offer their own scientific advice. However, in any case where the applicant intends to file their submission via the centralised procedure, use of the CHMP scientific advice procedure is highly recommended. In any case, scientific advice or protocol assistance from the CHMP is available only for medicinal products.

## CURRENT GUIDELINES

It is not the intention of this section to simply revisit and recite current EU guidelines in this context. Guidelines relevant to delivery systems are of course mentioned and the main messages are summarized in this section. A complete listing of ICH and CHMP quality guidelines may be found on the EMEA website (9).

EU guidelines developed by the CHMP exist for some of the standard delivery systems—modified release oral systems, transdermal systems and pulmonary delivery systems. CHMP guidelines are harmonized; i.e., to say they reflect a harmonized EU point of view that transcends any single, national view. It is also worth mentioning that guidelines are not legal requirements; they are, as the title suggests, suggestions and proposals for EU norms or standard cases, and applicants may diverge from such guidelines where this can be justified in a special case. However, EU pharmaceutical legislation requires the quality part of a marketing authorisation dossier to be state-of-the-art at all times. Thus, guidelines which define state-of-the-art requirements play a crucial role in the EU regulatory system.

Trade and professional organizations are always at liberty to present their views to the Commission, the national EU authorities, the EMEA and specialist CHMP working parties concerning their problems or need for new or revised guidelines.

### General Requirements

As the marketing authorisation application for all medicinal products in the European Union is legally required to follow the structure of the Common Technical Document (CTD), regardless of whether they are innovative drug delivery systems or generics, the guideline of the ICH on the CTD should be considered as a starting point (ICH M4). Although it is the clear intention of this document to describe format rather than requirements on the content of a submission, the illustrative examples provided in this guideline may be very helpful, e.g., in case of the use of novel excipients. More detailed information on the documentation requirements for excipients is outlined in the recently revised guideline on excipients in the dossier for application for marketing authorisation of a medicinal product. In addition, special care needs to be taken as regards restrictions to the use of certain excipients or additional labeling requirements as outlined in the Commission guideline "Excipients in the labe and package leaflet of medicinal products for human use," a document contained in the Notice to Applicants, Volume 3B.

## Pharmaceutical Development

The recently published ICH guideline on pharmaceutical development (ICH Q8) describes the baseline requirements to pharmaceutical development of any medicinal product in very broad terms. In addition, it introduces the notion of a design space based on an enhanced and multidimensional understanding of formulation and process parameters, including their interaction. An established and approved design space allows the applicant/marketing authorisation holder to freely move within the described boundaries without necessitating the submission of variations. However, at present, there are only few examples of the practical application of this new concept available. In addition, they are mainly based on "conventional" dosage forms, e.g., immediate release tablets. While offering a lot of advantages and flexibility post-approval, it has to be noted that the establishment of such a design space for a complex dosage form will require substantial investments in the product's development. Thus, EU regulatory authorities leave it entirely up to the applicant/MAH to decide whether they wish to make this investment or whether they decide to meet baseline requirements only.

In contrast to the United States and Japan, the EU has a long-standing tradition of requiring information on pharmaceutical development of a medicinal product in the submission. Before the introduction of the CTD, the description of the pharmaceutical development of a product and thus a summary of its history constituted one of the first parts of the dossier, which provided assessors with the background knowledge for the assessment of the adequate quality of the active ingredient and excipients. The CHMP guideline "Note for guidance on development pharmaceutics" describes general requirements to pharmaceutical development which nowadays could be classified as baseline requirements according to the International Conference on Harmonization (ICH) document, e.g., compatibility studies, physico-chemical characterization and parameters. However, in addition it provides more detailed information on the requirements for specific dosage forms, i.e., liquid and semi-solid, solid dosage forms and a variety of others, e.g., transdermal patches, pressured metered dose preparations (pMDIs) or dry powders (DPIs) for inhalation. For all sterile products, the decision tree for the selection of sterilization methods as outlined in the annex to this document, may be noteworthy. Although the methods of choice for sterilization are clearly those where the product is terminally sterilized in its final container, alternative methods may be of special relevance for drug delivery systems. In this context, the two guidance documents on the limitations to the use of ethylene oxide and on the use of ionising radiation in the manufacture of medicinal products should be taken into consideration.

## Packaging Material

The selection of the container/closure system needs to be addressed in the framework of pharmaceutical development, information on the composition, construction and routine quality control should be included in the relevant parts of the CTD. In the European Union, in addition to the legally binding requirements described in the respective monographs of the *European Pharmacopoeia*, the requirements as outlined in the guideline on plastic immediate packaging materials should be considered. Especially in the case of products intended for inhalation, parenteral, or ophthalmic application, there is a clear need for results of studies investigating the potential of interaction between filling and the immediate plastic packaging material. The document provides guidance on the general information requested as well as on specific extraction and interaction studies.

## Manufacture of the Medicinal Product

All three ICH regions require manufacture of medicinal products to be conducted under the application of the rules of good manufacturing practices (GMPs). The requirements may differ between the regions, however, when it comes to the need to include or have on site information on the validation of the manufacturing process at the time of submission or prior to granting a marketing authorisation. In the European Union, there are several guidance documents available which describe the different scenarios, depending on the specifics of the medicinal product.

The guideline on the manufacture of the finished dosage forms describes in rather general terms the requirements as regards the description of the manufacturing process itself in the dossier. In the context of drug delivery systems it has to be noted that the more complex a dosage form and thus the manufacturing process gets, the more details are required to be submitted to the regulatory authorities. At the same time, the guideline make a clear statement that unnecessary details should be avoided in order to prevent overburdening both applicant/MAH and regulatory authorities with variation applications on minor details. Thus, the decision on the degree of detail on the actual manufacturing process to be included in the dossier remains a tightrope walk which very much depends on the specifics of the product and the complexity of its manufacturing process.

As regards the need to include process validation information in the submission, the EU clearly differentiates between "standard" and "nonstandard" manufacturing processes. An explanation of what may be considered a nonstandard manufacturing process is outlined in annex II "Nonstandard processes" to the note for guidance on process validation. Examples of nonstandard manufacturing processes are the manufacture of specialized pharmaceutical dosage forms (e.g., MDIs and DPIs, prolonged release preparations and other specialized dosage forms such as parenteral depot preparations based on biodegradable polymers as well as liposomal or micellar preparations), new technologies incorporated into a conventional process, specialized processes which involve new technologies or an established process know or likely to be complex, thus requiring special care, as well as nonstandard methods of sterilization. For all these nonstandard processes, there is a clear requirement in the the EU to submit data of successful process validation at the intended production scale in the dossier. For the future, it will be important to observe further development in the area of ICH Q 8. With the development of new concepts such as design space, there may be a potential to change from the typical "three batch"-validation to continuous process verification with a clear impact on the amount of data to be included in the dossier.

For all other products and manufacturing processes, the EU requires submission of a so-called validation scheme with the dossier. The validation scheme should form the bridge between the information on pharmaceutical development and product history in the dossier, to be evaluated by the licensing authority, and the more GMP-related information on the actual details and validation of the manufacturing process, to be reviewed by the inspectors of the supervisory GMP authority. Thus, it is required that the applicant submits their intended validation protocol with the dossier. However, it has to be noted that the EU GMP clearly requires manufacture of all medicinal products to be validated prior to the release of the first batch to the market.

### Dosage Form–Specific Guidance

As outlined in the introduction to this section, the CHMP has published two additional guidance documents on specific dosage forms, namely the quality of modified release products and of inhalation and nasal products. Both put special emphasis on safeguarding the desired performance of the medicinal product. The first document is separated into respective sections on oral and transdermal dosage forms and is complemented by a second part, a guidance document on the pharmacokinetic and clinical evaluation of these types of products. It includes information on the requirements on prolonged and delayed release dosage forms, with a focus on specific requirements on pharmaceutical developments, specification setting and control tests (in-process as well as at time of batch release). An annex covers details of how to develop the different levels of in vivo/in vitro correlation and their respective predictability and use.

The guideline on the pharmaceutical quality of inhalation and nasal products is an example of an interesting collaborative exercise. It represents the outcome of a joint Health Canada/EU drafting group. Thus, it does not only reflect EU requirements but is equally applicable for products to be submitted to the Canadian health authorities. The document is complementary to a guideline on the clinical evaluation of orally inhaled products. It covers all aspects relevant to the pharmaceutical development and submission of products intended to administer active substances to the lungs, e.g., pMDIs, DPIs, products for nebulization. Given the nature of all inhalation and nasal products which contain an active substance in an undissolved form, special emphasis is put on the particle size determination and specification of the active substance.

## EU INITIATIVES FOR SMALL- AND MEDIUM-SIZED ENTERPRISES

### Small- and Medium-Sized Enterprises

Innovative ideas for the development of new delivery systems are often conceived in academia or in small start-up and spin-out companies. Unfortunately, though, great ideas are quite often wasted or never translated into practical applications, particularly in the case of small companies that are mainly research-based and have neither the funds nor the infrastructure to develop a medicinal product in accordance with the current regulatory requirements. The lack of in-depth knowledge of the pharmaceutical regulatory framework might also lead to a poor development, thus hindering the future commercialization of the product. A common strategy that several small companies follow is to protect their intellectual rights by acquiring a patent and then hopefully to form a partnership or sell their ideas to a larger company with an established regulatory affairs function to take over the regulatory burden which they perceive to be large (it is). But even in doing so, it is essential to be aware of and have a good understanding of the regulations. For example, if the product under development is a multifactional nanoparticle platform that exhibits its action through a combination of physical, pharmacological, metabolic or immunological mechanisms, then it is vital for the company to understand from the early stages of the development whether it will fall under the remit of the pharmaceutical or the medical device legislation.

With the aim of supporting innovation and the development of new medicinal products by SMEs, the European Commission has adopted Commission Regulation (EC) No. 2049/2005, which implements new provisions favorable for SMEs.

According to Commission Recommendation 2003/361/EC, the category of micro, SMEs is made up of enterprises that employ fewer than 250 persons and have an annual turnover not exceeding EUR 50 million, and/or have an annual balance sheet total not exceeding EUR 43 million.

In order to help SMEs navigate through the regulatory maze, the EMEA has established an "SME Office" with the remit of offering assistance to SMEs (10). The SME Office responds to practical or procedural enquiries, monitors applications, and organizes workshops and training sessions for SMEs on regulatory aspects. The office is also responsible for coordinating the granting of a number of incentives foreseen by the Regulation. These include:

- administrative and procedural assistance from the SME Office of the EMEA;
- fee reductions for scientific advice, inspections and (for veterinary medicines) establishment of maximum residue limits;
- fee exemptions for certain administrative services of the EMEA;
- deferral of the fee payable for an application for marketing authorisation or related inspection;
- conditional fee exemption where scientific advice is followed and a marketing authorisation application is not successful;
- assistance with translations of the product-information documents submitted in the application for marketing authorisation.

## ANNEX: RELEVANT EU GUIDELINES

### Quality

Modified Release

The "parent' guidelines:
CPMP/QWP/604/96 Note For Guidance on Quality of Modified Release Products:A.Oral Dosage Forms; B. and Transdermal Dosage Forms; Section I (Quality).
To be read in conjunction with CPMP/EWP/280/96 Section II (Pharmacokinetics and Clinical aspects)

Inhaled Products

CPMP/QWP/2845/00 Note for Guidance on Requirements for Pharmaceutical Documentation for Pressurized Metered Dose Inhalation Products (adopted March 02).
CHMP/QWP/49313/05 Guideline on the Pharmaceutical Quality of Inhalation and Nasal Products (CHMP adopted March 2006).
EMEA/CHMP/CVMP/QWP/103155/06 Overview of comments received on draft Guideline on the Pharmaceutical Quality of Inhalation and Nasal Products.
CPMP/QWP/158/96 Note for guidance on Dry Powder Inhalers.

## Safety Toxicology

EMEA/273974/05 Note for Guidance on the Quality, Preclinical and Clinical aspects of Gene Transfer Medicinal Products—Annex on Non-Clinical testing for Inadvertent Germline transmission of Gene Transfer Vectors (Released for consultation November 2005).

## Clinical

CPMP/EWP/280/96 Note For Guidance on Modified Release Oral and Transdermal Dosage Forms: Section II (Pharmacokinetic and Clinical Evaluation)

CPMP/EWP/282/02 Position Paper on the Regulatory Requirements for the Authorization of low-dose Modified Release as a Formulations in the Secondary Prevention of Cardiovascular Events (Final).

CPMP/180/95 Guideline for PMS Studies for Metered Dose Inhalers with New Propellants.

CPMP/EWP/QWP/1401/98 Note For Guidance on the Investigation of Bioavailability and Bioequivalence (Adopted July 2001).

CHMP/EWP/40326/06 Questions & Answers on the Bioavailability and Bioequivalence Guideline. And also the addendum to this guidance:

CHMP/EWP/147231/06 Concept Paper for an addendum to the Note for Guidance on the investigation of bioavailability and bioequivalence: Evaluation of bioequivalence of highly variable drugs and drug products (Released for consultation April 2006).

CPMP/EWP/239/95 Note for Guidance on the Clinical Requirements for Locally Applied, Locally Acting Products containing Known Constituents (CPMP adopted November 95).

CHMP/EWP/18463/06 Concept Paper on the Development of new Products for the Treatment of Ulcerative Colitis (Released for consultation January 2006).

CHMP/EWP/18446/06 Concept Paper on the Revision of the CHMP Points to Concider on Clinical Investigation of Medicinal Products for the Management of Crohn's disease (Released for consultation January 2006).

## MEDICAL DEVICES: ANCILLARY SUBSTANCES

CHMP/EWP/56477/06 Concept Paper on the Development of a CHMP Guideline on the evaluation of nonclinical and clinical data on the medicinal substances contained in drug-eluting (medicinal substance eluting) coronary stents within the framework of a consultation procedure for combination products (Released for consultation February 2006).

## GENE TRANSFER

CPMP/BWP/3088/99 Note for Guidance on the quality, preclinical and clinical aspects of gene transfer medicinal products.
CPMP/BWP/2458/03 Guideline on Development and Manufacture of Lentiviral Vectors (CHMP adopted May 2005).

## REFERENCES

1. "CE" is the European conformity marking for products, which indicates that the product complies with the essential requirements of the relevant European health, safety and environmental-protection legislation. See: http://ec.europa. eu/enterprise/medical_devices/index_en.htm
2. See http://ec.europa.eu/enterprise/medical_devices/meddev/2_1_3____07-2001. pdf
3. MHRA website: http://www.mhra.gov.uk
4. Biomedical Microdevices, 4:4, 293–9 (2002).
5. For further information, search for Innovation Task Force on the EMEA website: www.emea.europa.eu
6. See European Commission's nanotechnology homepage: http://cordis.europa. eu/nanotechnology
7. See the Note for Guidance on the quality, preclinical and clinical aspects of gene transfer medicinal products http://www.emea.europa.eu/pdfs/human/ bwp/308899en.pdf and the current guideline on lentiviral vectors (CPMP/ BWP/2458/03)
8. See: http://www.emea.europa.eu/htms/general/admin/fees/fees1.htm
9. See: http://www.emea.europa.eu/htms/human/humanguidelines/quality.htm
10. SME Office section of the EMEA website: http://www.emea.europa.eu/SME/ SMEoverview.htm

# 37

# Canadian Regulatory Requirements for Drug Approval

Sultan Ghani and David Lee

*Drugs and Health Products, Health Canada, Ottawa, Ontario, Canada*

## BACKGROUND

### Social Aspect of Government Regulation

The history of the evolution of pharmaceutical regulations is, in fact, the history of the social and economic development of North America. During the 19th century when relative political stability was attained, economic life started to grow. The growth of farming communities, establishment of industries, increase in trading activity, necessitated the gradual development of laws and regulations to organize and regulate the national standards and requirements.

The multinational character and background of the new settlers, produced a hotchpotch of culture, habits, and traditions, which, together with the factors of greed and self-interest, endangered the quality of products, and jeopardized an acceptable standard of service. The task of assimilating all the people and thus all the professions, to adhere to a certain minimum nationally acceptable standard further necessitated the existence of a central authority to devise and implement regulations.

The United States, because of the larger population and greater economic activity, was in a better shape to develop a central authority which would oversee the ethical side of manufactured products, i.e., to satisfy the minimum standards set for the manufactured products. Existence and effective control of such an authority was all the more necessary in order to be able to compete well with the more industrialized and well-established countries of Europe.

To be able to appreciate how important a role the sound economic condition of a country plays in the development of industrial health, and how imperceptibly government agencies are summoned to work on establishing necessary standards to ensure safety and protection of the consumers, we have to have some brief insight into the economic history of Canada and the United States of the past 200 years.

Canada having been a colony of Britain, had its economic and trade policies always modified and influenced by the primary interest of Britain: "The character of importers in relation to exports was, in part, determined by the mercantile policy which directly governed the industry of the colony. This policy, calculated to benefit primarily the mother country, could not fail to arouse opposition in a growing colony" (1, p. 71).

A quick glimpse of 19th century Canada shows tanning, whisky distilling and brewing industries, paper factories, and glass manufacturing activities going on in Canada. In fact, the overall industrial activity was very minor. "The scarcity of technical skill and capital, and the smallness of demand for high class goods, in part accounted for the fact that Canadian manufacturers in each department of industry were of low grade" (1, p. 162). "We have not hitherto brought any kind of manufacture except Ashes, to the degree of perfection, which enables us to compete with other nations in foreign markets" (2).

Diffused economic activity, scarce skilled human resources, and lack of educational consciousness contributed towards the slow pace of establishing educational institutions. Thus we notice practically no meritable high degree institution of learning in the field of medicine and pharmaceutics, and practically no research activity in 18th and 19th century Canada.

The backwardness of the American people in the pre-independence period can be discerned by the fact that ".... in case of illness the village doctor was not summoned unless the numerous home remedies and nostrums failed to bring relief, for every family had its Jerusalem oak, pennyroyal, wormwood, sweet basil, rhubarbs, salts, and calomel, not to mention patent medicines. Every springtime each member of the household was dosed with various concoctions so that the blood might be purified and 'the system toned up'" (3). The first medical school on the American continent was established in Philadelphia in 1765.

Pharmacy, as a profession, was still in its infancy in 1800. Generally, the doctors were their own apothecaries. Sometimes, people would work as apprentices to a physician, where they would qualify themselves to engage in the unregulated and unlicensed business of pharmacy.

"The few important drug discoveries that occurred before the twentieth century included nitrous oxide, ether, and chloroform as anaesthetics; amyl nitrate and nitroglycerine for anginal pain; chloral hydrate and barbiturates for sedation; and antipyrene, acetanilid, acetophenitidin and aspirin for the control of pain and fever" (4).

A very direct and positive result of the political and socio-economic stability achieved in the latter part of the nineteenth century was the growth in the number of educational and research institutions which could now be adequately funded by the growth financial resources. A new consciousness and an invigorated awareness started to surface to initiate research in all fields of human knowledge, including medicine, to guarantee the perpetuation of economic growth, and attain high standards of living. This included also a provision of quality medical care and protection against harmful, and ineffective pharmaceutical products. Substandard drugs, and improperly trained doctors failed to address the health care needs of the growing population. The need to protect the consumers from such an undesirable situation became too demanding on the governments. It was this pressing factor which stimulated governments of Canada and the United States to start regulating the medical profession and the pharmacies, which now could be better administered and supervised in view of greater financial resources and the availability of better-trained scientists. Regulations to control the quality of pharmaceutical products did exist in one form or another almost at all times; however, the newer researches in the scientific, medical and pharmaceutical fields, and the availability of the more sophisticated automated manufacturing and analytical equipment put the onus on manufacturers, pressured by the stricter and more stringent demands by the regulatory bodies, to produce better and better quality of their product. In essence, this could not have been possible if the economic growth had not been proportionate to support the highly expensive requirements by the government regulations, which themselves evolved as part of economic growth, widespread educational facilities, and a general consciousness concerning improvements in quality products and quality living.

The above discourse thus shows the role of political, social, educational and other factors in the formulation and implementation of industrial regulations.

## Historical Precedence

The development of Federal statutes on medicine, so-called First Canadian Drugs Act, was mainly modeled on English laws. In order to develop a clear understanding of the administration and development of federal statutes on medicine, it is necessary to have an appreciation of English laws and the conditions prevailing in Canada at the time of the passage of the first Food & Drugs Act.

The influence of the pattern of early English statutes appears to be quite prevalent in many aspects of Canadian Food & Drugs Act, as well as on Acts of many other countries belonging to the Commonwealth.

It is interesting to note that the situation which prompted development of the first English statute was the urgent need to deal with the problem of beverage, food and medicines adulteration which was prevalent in the middle of the nineteenth century. The efforts of John Postage in the early

1850s, as cited in Beeston's papers, and published in *Food & Drug News Canada,* April 1952, may be considered as the first documented reference towards the eradication of harmful adulteration.

A resultant enquiry on adulteration confirmed the prevalence of adulteration within consumer products to the extent that "not only is the public health in danger, and pecuniary fraud committed on the whole community, but the public morality is tinted, and high commercial character of the country seriously lowered, both at home or in the eye of the foreign country."

A Bill for preventing the adulteration of articles of food and drink was eventually passed in Britain in 1860, after initial impediments. This was entitled "An Act For Preventing the Adulteration of Articles of Food and Drinks."

A section of the Law stated as follows:

> Every person who shall sell an article of food or drink with, to the knowledge of such person, any Ingredient or Material injurious to the Health of Persons eating or drinking such article, has been mixed, and every person who shall sell as pure or unadulterated, or not pure, shall for every such offence ... forfeit and pay a penalty ...

From the above British legislation, it is conspicuous to note that firstly this legislation deals only with the actual sales of foods and not the manufacturer; and secondly that this legislation does not include drugs as part of its subject matter.

Later, in the year 1872, some of the shortcomings of the 1860 legislation were modified and the Act was amended to include drugs. Eventually the Acts of 1860 and 1872 were replaced by the Food & Drugs Act (Great Britain) of 1875. This is the law that was put into force in many Commonwealth countries. The most important section of this Act is Section 6, which is reported as follows:

> No person shall sell to the prejudice of the purchaser any article of food or any drug which is not of the nature, substance, and quality of the article demanded by such purchaser, under a penalty not exceeding twenty Pounds; provided that an offence shall not be deemed to be committed under this section in the following cases; i.e., to say,
>
> (1) where any matter or ingredient no injurious to health has added to the food or drug because the same is required for the production and preparation thereof as an article of commerce, in a state fit for carriage or consumption, and not prudently to increase the bulk weight, or measure of the food or drug, or conceal inferior quality thereof;
>
> (2) where the drug or food is a proprietary medicine, or is the subject of a patent in force, and supplied in a state required by the specifications of a patent;

(3) where the food or drug is compounded as in this Act mentioned;
(4) where the food or drug is unavoidably mixed with some extraneous matter in the process of collection or preparation.

Although the Act provided a legal tool to control the prevalent problem of adulteration, it failed to address the two important issues—defining the term "adulteration," and specifying legal standards of quality or identity for foods or drugs.

A history of development of legislations related to medicine in North America provides an opportunity to evaluate not only the existing regulations in terms of the past, but also gives an understanding of the present circumstances which are influencing the drug laws on this Continent.

Laws are developed to regulate or monitor the activity of people. The drug laws, like all the other laws, are not different in this respect, although they exert much greater influence on the public starting from the point of its manufacture to distribution and eventually to sales. They have social and economical implications, and they influence both national and international trade, particularly where free economic enterprise exists and where there is competition within business.

As with any other Drug Act, Canada's Food & Drugs Act is designed to give effective protection to consumers from ineffective and unsafe medicine. This is achieved by prohibiting the sale of drugs that might cause harm to consumers, and providing protection from fraud in sales and controlling manufacturing and distribution.

In order to have a clear perception of the Administration and Development of federal statutes of medicine in Canada, it is important to have an understanding of Canadian Constitution as it relates to the subject of Food & Drug Laws. An attempt will be made, in a preliminary way, to review the constitutional status of the Food & Drug Laws in Canada, and the subsequent legal problems that have arisen consequent to it.

The government of Canada is divided into Federal and Provincial governments under the old BNA Act and this is perpetuated in the Canadian Constitution of 1984, which provides for the legislative powers to be exercised in Canada by both the Federal and Provincial governments.

Because the subject of food and drugs was not covered by the BNA Act, there arose the difficulty of deciding which of the two levels of government had the legislative authority to deal with situations arising out of problems in this respect. Because of the exclusion of Judiciary as the interpretative authority in situations of legislative conflict between the provinces and the federal government, all matters of conflict had to be referred to the Privy Council; however, since 1950, the Supreme Court of Canada has been the final resort in all civil and criminal matters, and the Federal Government has been chosen as the body to administer the Federal Food and Drugs Act, and create, promulgate and, if necessary, enforce the regulations arising from the Act. The Food & Drugs Act, in Canada, is administered under Criminal Law.

The Act and Regulations provide working documents of specifications which are used by the regulatory agencies, and which must be familiar to the manufacturers and distributors of drugs. The evolution of The Canadian Food & Drugs Act and Regulations, when looked at in perspective, will be found to be interesting and challenging, but sometimes subject to subjective interpretation. An attempt will be made to present an overview of the legislative upheavals and the various developmental stages the Act underwent to reach its present form.

## FOOD & DRUGS ACT AND REGULATIONS

The Food & Drugs Act requires that all drugs, biologics, natural health products, cosmetics and medical devices, meet the requirements of the Act and Regulations whether they are manufactured or imported into Canada. Like any other act and regulations, the objective of the Food & Drugs Act and Regulations is to ensure safety and to prevent fraud with respect to food, drugs, cosmetics and medical devices by monitoring their sale.

Some of the key components included in the first section of the Act are drugs, devices, food, and cosmetics. This section also contains the general prohibition of advertising, packaging, labeling and sale of drugs, food, cosmetics, and devices. Basically, the Act is divided into two parts and schedules. The Parts deal with the prohibition and the Schedule deals with the specific subjects, e.g., Schedule A is a list of diseases and abnormal physical states.

### Parts

Part I deals with the general provision of prohibition of sale, advertising, packaging and labelling of drugs, foods, cosmetics and medical devices in Canada.

Part II deals with administration, compliance and enforcement.

### Schedules

Schedule A includes a list of diseases or disorders that require a physician or
    a healthcare professional for treatment.
Schedule B includes a list of publication of standards, e.g., USP, BP, etc.
Schedule C deals with radiopharmaceuticals
Schedule D deals with biologics and blood products
Schedule E deals with artificial sweeteners
Schedule F deals with prescription drugs
Schedule G, repealed in 1997
Schedule H, repealed in 1997

## Regulations—Part II

The Regulations are further divided into parts and divisions. Each part deals with a specific subject matter, e.g.,

Part A deals with the general administration of Regulations
Part B deals with the food
Part C deals with the drugs
Part D deals with the vitamins, minerals, etc.
Part E deals with artificial sweeterners
Part G deals with controlled drugs
Part J deals with restricted drugs

> There are separate regulations that deal with cosmetics, distribution of semen, medical devices, and natural health products.
> As mentioned previously, there are three parts and each part has various divisions.
> Under Part A, the Regulations deal with general administration of drugs, food, cosmetics and medical devices.
> Under Part B, the Regulations deal with food and is not part of this presentation.
> Part C is the part that deals with Regulations related to drugs and consists of ten divisions:

Division 1 General
Division 2 Good Manufacturing Practices
Division 3 Schedule C Drugs—Radiopharmaceuticals
Division 4 Schedule D Drugs—Biologicals
Division 5 Clinical Trials involving humans
Division 6 Canada Standard drugs
Division 7 Repealed
Division 8 New Drugs
Division 9 Nonprescription Drugs
Division 10 Repealed

> Division 1

There are various sections in this division which deal in general with various aspects of Regulations from the definition of drugs to drug recall reporting. Some of the key sections are briefly discussed here.

C.01.014   This section deals with drug identification number (DIN). A DIN is an eight-digit number that identifies a drug product that is sold in Canada. When a drug is approved for sale in Canada, this number is issued.
C.01.016 and C.01.017   These sections basically deal with the reporting requirements of adverse drug reactions.
C.01.051   This section deals with product recall reporting requirements.

### Division 1a

This is a fairly new division that deals with the requirements of Establishment Licences (EL). EL are issued to establishments that fabricate, package, label, distribute and test drugs. The condition of issuing EL is based on the compliance of Good Manufacturing Practices (GMP) in accordance with Division 2 of the Food and Drugs Regulations. The licenses are issued for a period of one year and are reviewed annually. These licenses are basically issued to Canadian establishments; however, establishments outside Canada, involved in the fabrication, packaging, processing, labeling and testing, are subject to GMP compliance and it is the responsibility of the Canadian license holder to register and include the name of these establishments in their licenses.

### Division 2

This division describes the requirements of Good Manufacturing Practices.

### Division 3

This division deals with the requirements of licensing of Schedule C drugs (radiopharmaceuticals).

### Division 4

This division deals with the requirements and licensing of Schedule D drugs (biologics). The division includes various sections outlining requirements such as storage, lot release, specific regulations for vaccines, toxins, antisera, etc. Also included are products from human sources, as well as blood products and insulin.

### Division 5

This division includes the requirements of drugs used in clinical trials. This includes the data requirements when filing a clinical trial application. There is a 30-day default period. In other words, a sponsor can commence the study after 30 days' filing if a No Objection Letter is received from the Department. This division further provides direction on how clinical trial supplies be labeled. Good Clinical Practices (GCP) and inspection of the trial site are also followed. For GCP, ICH harmonized guidelines are closely followed.

### Division 6

This division provides Canadian standards for drugs such as conjugated estrogen and thyroid

### Division 8

This is the most important piece of regulatory requirements dealing with new drugs submissions as well as abbreviated new drugs submissions. This division describes the requirements of drug submissions from both innovator and generic companies.

Division 9

This division deals with regulatory requirements of nonprescription drugs.

**Part D:** This part deals with vitamins, minerals and amino acids. These products are now regulated under the new legislature of natural health products.

**Part E:** This part deals with batch release.

**Parts F, H, and I:** These parts have been repealed.

**Parts G and J:** These parts deal with controlled drugs and are now part of the regulations under the Controlled Drugs and Substances Act.

The Federal Government is responsible for setting and administering national principles or standards for the healthcare system. It is responsible for health-related functions such as health protection, disease prevention and health promotion. It regulates the safety, efficacy and quality of drugs. Other Federal legislations, besides the Food & Drugs Act and Regulations, are Patent Medicine Linkage Regulations, Financial Administration Act, Access to Information and Privacy Act, Controlled Drugs and Substances Act, and various policies and guidelines.

## ORGANIZATIONAL ROLE AND RESPONSIBILITY

The Health Products and Food Branch (HPFB) is responsible for the regulatory review process of drugs and food besides other related activities. All drugs can be sold in Canada, once they have successfully passed the review process to ensure their safety, efficacy and quality. The Branch evaluates and monitors thousands of human and veterinary drugs, medical devices, natural health products available to Canadians, as well as the safety and quality of food in Canada. The Branch also contributes to the health and well-being of Canadians in a variety of other ways, such as establishing nutrition policies and standards.

With respect to human drugs, the following organizations are responsible:

1. Therapeutic Products Directorate: Responsible for evaluating the safety, effectiveness and quality of pharmaceutical drugs and medical devices available to Canadians.
2. Biologics and Genetic Therapies Directorate: Responsible for evaluating the safety, effectiveness and quality of biological radiopharmaceutical drugs as well as blood and blood products, viral and bacterial vaccines, genetic therapeutic products, tissues, organs, and xenografts.

3. HPFB Inspectorate: Responsible for delivery of inspection, investigations, and most Establishment Licencing and related laboratory analysis functions.
4. Marketed Health Products Directorate: Responsible for post-market assessment and surveillance of pharmaceutical and biological drugs, medical devices, natural health products and radiopharmaceuticals.
5. Natural Health Products Directorate: Responsible for managing the natural health product program and providing Canadians with access to natural health products that are safe, effective and of high quality, while respecting freedom of choice and philosophical and cultural diversity.

## MANAGEMENT OF DRUG SUBMISSIONS

All drugs sold in Canada must be approved by Health Canada. These include, but are not limited to, drugs imported from other countries, drugs manufactured in Canada, and drugs for export where the exporting company needs Canadian approval in order to enter into the other country. The types of drugs regulated include pharmaceuticals (prescription/nonprescription), innovator and generic products, biological drugs, radiopharmaceuticals, natural health products including homeopathic products and traditional herbal medicine. Disinfectants for use on medical instruments, hospitals and food preparation surfaces are also regulated as drugs. Drugs for animal use are regulated as veterinary drugs.

## DRUG APPROVAL PROCESS

New drugs can be sold in Canada once they have successfully passed a review process to assess their safety, efficacy and quality. Responsibility for this review process rests with Health Canada's Health Products and Food Branch. The HPFB evaluates and monitors the safety, efficacy and quality of thousands of drugs, medical devices and natural health products that are available to Canadians.

### Clinical Trials

As a first step in the drug development, preclinical studies are carried out to evaluate the safety of a drug and its potential use. These studies are carried out in vitro and in vivo to assess the performance of the drug, including the assessment of the existence and extent of its toxicity. Such preclinical studies provide important information on the potential use of the drug prior to its testing on humans in clinical trials. If preclinical studies are promising, sponsors should apply for authorization of clinical trials involving human subjects. Clinical trials are conducted and information is obtained on the product's safety and efficacy. HPFB reviews the information before a clinical trial begins. It is important that the clinical trial application ensures that the proposed trials have been properly designed and that patients are not exposed to undue risk. Good Clinical Practices principles must be followed throughout such studies. Inspections are conducted on clinical trial drugs similar to that of other jurisdictions (8,11).

## New Drugs

A New Drug Submission (NDS), containing scientific information about the product's safety, efficacy and quality, is filed for seeking marketing authorization in CD format (5). The data include the results of both preclinical and clinical studies, details of the method of manufacture, of drug substance and drug products and information on packaging and labeling. This also includes the therapeutic claim and value, as well as condition of use. A typical schematic new drug evaluation process is as follows:

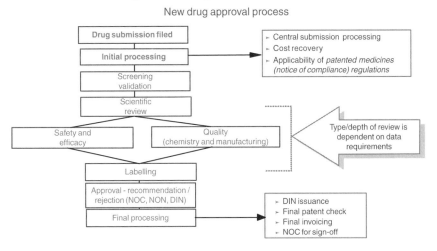

## Generic New Drugs

An Abbreviated New Drug Submission (ANDS) is required for obtaining authorization for a generic product. The submission must have quality standards like an NDS and must show to be as safe and efficacious as the brand-name product. The submission includes scientific information as well as comparative data with the brand-name product. The generic submission must show that the amount of medicinal ingredient is identical as that of the innovator product. The comparison is usually done through comparative bioavailability studies. A typical schematic of the generic new drug evaluation process is given below:

Review of generic new drugs

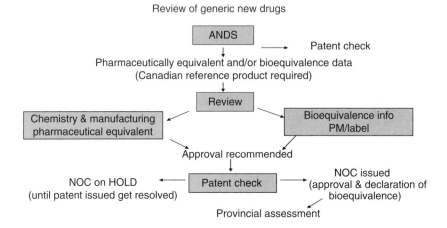

## Patented Medicines Notice of Compliance Regulations

In order to protect the intellectual property while allowing generics to come on the market immediately after patent expiry, Patented Medicines Notice of Compliance (NOC) Regulations must be respected. Brand name companies can file a patent to protect a drug and such a patent is entered into the Patent Register. However, generic companies have to clear all patent issues before being allowed to market. Typical Patent Medicine NOC Regulations are described in the following schematic diagram:

**Patented medicines (NOC) regulations**

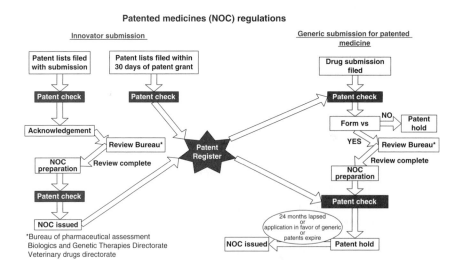

## Drug Identification Number

A DIN application is required to be filed for products that do not meet the definition of a new drug. In such circumstances, the substance for use as a drug has been sold in Canada for a sufficient time and quantity to establish their quality and safety.

### Priority Review

Priority review or expedited approval is performed on drugs with a performance target of 150 days. The priority review policy applies to New Drug Submissions or Supplemental New Drug Submissions for serious life-threatening diseases when there is no drug presently in Canada, or the drug is an improvement over existing therapies. Example of serious conditions includes cancer, Alzheimer and AIDS (6,10).

### Notice of Compliance with Condition

In certain situations, a Notice of Compliance with Condition may be granted to expedite access to potentially life-saving drugs under the Notice of Compliance with Condition policy. It is expected that the review can be completed within the performance target date. These target dates are given below (7,9).

### Performance Targets

| Performance targets | | |
|---|---|---|
| ⌂ The type of data package (safety, efficacy, quality) submitted and whether or not it is accepted for priority review determines the performance target | | |
| Examples: | | |
| ⌂ Processing | | - 10 days* |
| ⌂ Screening | | - 45 days* |
| ⌂ NDS–Review | :priority | - 180 days* |
| | :non-priority | - 300 days* |
| ⌂ ANDS–Review | | - 180 days* |
| | | * Calendar days |

## REFERENCES

1. Innis MQ. An Economic History of Canada. Toronto: The Ryerson Press, 1935: 71.
2. Select Documents, 1783–1885, p. 301–2.
3. Carman HJ. Social and Economic History of the US. New York: D.C. Health & Co., 1934.

4.  Silverman M, Lee, PR. Pill, Profits, and Politics. Los Angeles: University of California Press, 1974; 3–4.
5.  Guidance for Industry: Preparation of New Drug Submissions in the CTD Format. Health Canada, June 2003.
6.  Guidance for Industry: Priority Review of Drug Submissions. Health Canada, November 2002.
7.  Guidance for Industry: Notice of Compliance with Conditions. Health Canada, November 2002.
8.  Health Canada Guidance Document: Guidance for Clinical Trial Sponsors, 2001.
9.  Health Canada Guidance Document, Notice of Compliance with Conditions (NOC/c), 2007.
10. Policy Priority Review of Drug Submissions, November 2005.
11. Health Canada/ICH Guidance Document E6, Good Clinical Practice Consolidated Guideline, 1997.
12. Health Canada, Food and Drug Act and Regulations.

# 38

# Regulating Modified-Release Drug Delivery Technologies in Australia

### Andrew Bartholomaeus

*Drug Safety Evaluation Branch, Therapeutic Goods Administration, Canberra, ACT, Australia*

### Carolyn Rolls

*Mallesons Stephen Jaques, Melbourne, Victoria, Australia*

### Michael S. Roberts

*School of Medicine, University of Queensland, Princess Alexandra Hospital, Brisbane, Queensland, Australia*

## INTRODUCTION

The goal of pharmaceutical scientists has long been to deliver drugs to specific target tissues at the right amount, at and for the right amount of time and with a minimum of side effects. Although these goals remain to a large extent unachieved for many drugs, the tools available with which to attack these goals have become increasingly sophisticated over recent years and offer the promise of truly novel approaches to targeted and controlled drug delivery. These novel approaches presented by emerging new therapeutic modalities, such as those based on nanotechnology and biotechnology, also present increasing challenges to be overcome by the pharmaceutical chemist. Biotechnology products for example may be antigenic, have very short half-lives, or may not distribute effectively to the target tissue compartment. Or perhaps gene therapy products may need to be targeted to specific cells within a single tissue to avoid inappropriate modification of nontarget cells, and as such their delivery mechanism requires the capacity for very precise target differentiation.

Conventional drug delivery systems already offer a wide range of delivery characteristics which can be exploited to achieve specific pharmacodynamic and pharmacokinetic objectives. Oral preparations such as tablets, capsules, powders, syrups, or suspensions, offer patient convenience, generally lower cost, less health care practitioner input and perhaps localized action on the gastrointestinal tract (GIT) where this is desired. Sustained release or enteric coated oral preparations go some way to enhancing these dose forms by reducing side effects in nontarget tissues of the GIT or reducing the dose frequency and perhaps avoiding toxicities associated with peak plasma concentrations for narrow therapeutic range drugs. Even these relatively simple delivery systems however may be enhanced by new technologies and processes. Poorly soluble drugs can now be readily reduced to nanoparticulate size and delivered as a suspension to aid absorption, or perhaps microencapsulated in liposomes or bound to substances targeting specific uptake mechanisms.

Similarly the wide variety of options for topically applied medication allows targeting of specific surface tissues, or avoidance of specific barriers to absorption, with suppositories, pessaries, creams, ointments, dermal patches, medicated bandages, powders, lotions etc. Again, these preparations may be amenable to modifications of varying sophistication which facilitate systemic delivery of drug in a controlled manner, nicotine replacement patches for example.

The difficulty of all of these approaches however is that for systemic targets additional barriers are interposed between the drug application site and the target tissues. These additional barriers (skin, mucosa, liver metabolism, etc.) significantly constrain or confound the options for modifying the characteristics and behavior of a preparation once it reaches the systemic absorption. While considerable progress remains to be made in the development of topical and oral dosage forms, current technologies are offering exciting prospects for significant advances in parenteral preparations which have previously remained somewhat intractable with respect to modified delivery options. Thus iv preparations can now, or will soon, be developed which provide sustained/controlled-release characteristics, target specific cell or tissue types, deliver potent antitumor agents directly to the intracellular compartment of the tumor cell, protect biological drugs from rapid break down and/or mask their immunogenicity, or release a drug in a controlled manner in response to a specific biological signal.

New drug delivery techniques are needed that exploit physiological differences in target versus bystander tissues. Multi-component preparations are one approach to this. Monoclonal antibodies (MAB), targeted to a protein expressed on a specific target cell, attached to a cellular toxin is one approach to this. The intention is that the MAB binds to the target cell and, once internalized by the cell and metabolized, releases the toxin to kill the cell.

Although there is a tendency in the lay and scientific literature to discuss new technological capabilities as discrete entities with labels such as nanotechnology, biotechnology and gene technology, in reality these silos are essentially figmentory. Even apart from the simplistic observation that biological molecules very often fall into the nanometer size range, the increasing convergence of these technologies make it difficult to identify a specific application as being one of a particular "technology." Equally, manufacturers do not market, and governments do not generally regulate "technologies" per se. Pharmaceutical products are the result of multiple technologies being brought to bear on a specific issue.

This chapter will discuss the current regulatory aspects being applied in this area for modified-release systems in Australia, as well as comment on challenges being posed by recently developed drug systems, and explore some possibilities for future development.

## Current Australian Regulatory Approach

The Therapeutic Goods Administration (TGA) is a unit of the Australian Department of Health and Ageing (the Department). The TGA administers the Therapeutic Goods Act 1989 (Act), a national system of controls relating to the quality, safety, efficacy, and timely availability of therapeutic goods that are used in Australia, whether produced in Australia or elsewhere, or exported from Australia (1). All medicines being imported into, manufactured in, supplied in or exported from Australia, must be included in the Australian Register of Therapeutic Goods (the Register) (2). Official standards for medicines under the Act include Therapeutic Goods Orders and the British Pharmacopoeia 2007 (1,3). In special cases, a standard specified by another pharmacopoeia, such as the United States Pharmacopeia (1) or an agreed nonpharmacopoeial standard, may be acceptable. The registration of medicines involves technical data requirements which generally follow the same guidelines as used by the European Union (2,4).

While not all modified-release preparations are prescription medicines the more sophisticated of these will generally fall into this category. Thus, the following discussion is limited to prescription medicines. Similar processes exist in Australia for complimentary medicines and other non-prescription medicines.

When a registered product application is submitted to the TGA, it is first evaluated by the agency and its various committees (5). In all cases however the delegation for decision making rests with officers of the TGA who may or may not concur with the advice of the respective committees. The Australian Drug Evaluation Committee (ADEC), e.g., while legally providing advice to the Minister for Health, in essence provides advice back to the TGA delegate on specific questions asked of it by the delegate and other matters the committee may deem relevant to a specific application.

Generally all applications for prescription products containing a new active ingredient are currently referred to ADEC for advice. In making their determination regarding the approval of a new product the TGA must have regard to (*i*) the quality, safety and efficacy of the product for the requested indication and (*ii*) the timeliness of availability of a new medicine. In providing advice to the TGA delegate the ADEC will give consideration to these issues and base their recommendations on the medical and scientific evaluations of data submitted in support of the application for registration and any other relevant data available to the TGA or to the experts serving on the committee, at the time of consideration. Although not specifically stated in legislation the balance of risk and benefit is a key consideration for the TGA delegate and the advisory committees.

The Pharmaceutical Subcommittee (PSC) makes recommendations to ADEC regarding the pharmaceutical chemistry, quality control, bioavailability and pharmacokinetics of formulations (including modified release) in registration applications (2,5).

## APPLICATION PROCEDURE FOR REGISTRATION

The procedure for submitting an application for marketing approval by the TGA is set out in the Australian Regulatory Guidelines for Prescription Medicines (ARGPM) (2). Similar guidelines exist for nonprescription (OTC) medicines and for complimentary medicines. Section 2.5 of the ARGPM explains that under the Therapeutic Goods Regulations of the Act, there are three categories of applications. Specifically:

- Category 1 applications cover applications for registration of a formulation containing a new active, or changes to a registered formulation if the formulation does not meet the specific requirements of Category 2 or 3.
- Category 2 applications cover formulations previously approved in two acceptable countries (currently Canada, Sweden, the Netherlands, the United Kingdom and the United States).
- Category 3 applications involve changes to the quality data of formulations already registered by the TGA which may or may not render the formulations separate and distinct (and therefore separately registrable) and which, in the opinion of the TGA, do not need to be supported by clinical, nonclinical or bioequivalence data.

Category 2 applications are very rare, partly due to the lack of provision of reports from some agencies to the sponsors, but largely because the TGA tends to receive applications for new drugs at or about the same time as the European Agency for Evaluation of Medicinal Products (EMEA) and FDA. As timeliness of supply is a key agency consideration, waiting for reports to become available from other major agencies is not a practicable option.

## REVIEW BY THE TGA

An application to the TGA for marketing approval of a formulation comprising a new active is usually submitted by a pharmaceutical company, or an organization employed by the pharmaceutical company that specializes in preparing TGA applications. As a new active is involved, this application will be a Category 1 application and is submitted in five "Modules" (2). Australia accepts and encourages the submission of applications in the Common Technical Document Format and is currently working on facilitating electronic submission of data. Modules 2 to 5 correspond to equivalent documents required for approval of new actives in Europe by the EMEA. In summary, Module 1 includes prescribing information for the active such as the product information (PI) sheet, package inserts, proposed labeling and packaging. Module 2 is a three part summary of information extracted from Modules 3, 4, and 5 relating to quality, safety and efficacy of the active. Module 3 comprises a report of studies relating to the quality of the active and its proposed formulation for sale. Module 4 comprises a report of nonclinical studies relating to safety. Module 5 comprises a report of the clinical studies. For Module 3, the pre-clinical investigation should include formulation data relating to: characterization of the active, composition, impurity data, pharmaceutical development and stability data to assess stability. For Module 4, the pre-clinical investigations should include pharmacodynamic, pharmacokinetic, and toxicology studies.

Of particular relevance here are alternative formulations developed for a known active ingredient, for example:

- a modified-release formulation (e.g., a controlled-release, modified-release, extended-release, delayed-release, or a target-directed dosage form);
- formulation suitable for an alternative route of administration (e.g., topical formulation compared with an oral formulation);
- formulation that encourages better patient compliance (e.g., requiring fewer doses, having better taste or easier administration such as oral rather than injectable);
- formulation having improved properties (e.g., improved stability or user safety);
- generic formulation derived from an innovator formulation;
- formulation to maintain a brand premium product.

The most common requirement for regulation of modified-release formulations of an existing active would be a submission consisting of (*i*) the composition of the alternative formulation, (*ii*) quality assurance details on the active, (*iii*) details of the manufacturing process, and (*iv*) pharmacokinetic and biopharmaceutical data and the basis on which the change in formulation was made. As an example, consider a new modified-release formulation that is bioequivalent to a formulation previously approved by the TGA. The new formulation would be submitted as a Category 1, Category 2, or Category 3 application with reference to Section 2.5 of the Australian Regulatory Guidelines for Prescription Medicines (2). If the new formulation has previously been approved by drug authorities overseas, it may be possible to file a Category 2 application based on two independent evaluation reports from two approved countries where the formulation has already been approved. Although as explained previously this is an unusual and rarely practical option. Approved countries are currently Canada, Sweden, Netherlands, the United Kingdom and the United States. The data submitted for approval in the approved countries must be re-presented with the Australian Category 2 marketing approval application. The new formulation could also be a Category 3 application based on its bioequivalence to the formulation previously approved, hence bioequivalence, clinical and nonclinical data may not be required. Nonclinical data is most likely to be required where sophisticated target directed dose form modification is being employed and substantial changes to specific tissue exposures might be anticipated. As stated at Section 4.3, the ARGPM adopts the European Community drug approval guidelines' definition of "essentially similar." The definition provides that a product is essentially similar to another product if it has

- the same qualitative and quantitative composition in terms of active principles/substances;
- the same pharmaceutical form;
- bioequivalency.

A generic medicine is one that is "essentially similar" to an innovator product.

When the new formulation is "essentially similar" to the formulation previously approved, in lieu of safety and efficacy data, a bioavailability study can be submitted to show that the alternative formulation is sufficiently similar in plasma concentration/time profile to the previously registered formulation of the active. Appendix 15: Biopharmaceutic Studies (June 2004) of the Australian Regulatory Guidelines for Prescription Medicines includes the investigation of bioavailability, relative bioavailability and bioequivalence of different dosage forms or formulations, and the effect of food or antacids on their bioavailability (6). As specified in that guidance "The Therapeutic Goods Administration (TGA) has adopted the Committee for Medicinal Products for Human Use (CHMP) Note for Guidance on the Investigation of Bioavailability and Bioequivalence" with the requirement that "application for registration of a generic product in Australia should generally include a bioequivalence study versus a leading brand obtained in Australia" (7). The guidance goes on to state that the "TGA has also adopted the CHMP Note for Guidance on Quality of Modified Release Products: A: Oral Dosage Form. B: Transdermal Dosage

Forms; Section 1 (Quality) (CPMP/QWP/604/96) which provides additional guidance on dissolution and bioavailability aspects of modified-release products" (8). The guideline further emphasizes that

- "More extensive studies are expected to characterize the pharmacokinetics of new drug substance drug substances, even if otherwise excluded below (for example, absolute bioavailability studies are normally required for all new chemical entities except those intended for intravenous administration)."

- "*Dissolution profiles* ... should be generated in a comparative manner as follows: At least six (and preferably 12) dosage units (for example, tablets, capsules) of each batch are tested individually and mean and individual results reported. The stirrer used is normally a paddle at 50 rpm for tablets and a basket at 100 rpm for capsules. However, other systems or speeds may be used if adequately justified and validated. The percentage of nominal content released is measured at a number of suitably spaced time points providing a profile for each batch, for example, at 10, 20, and 30 minutes, or as appropriate to achieve virtually complete dissolution. The batches are tested using the same apparatus and if possible on the same day. Test conditions are normally those used in routine quality control or, if dissolution is not part of routine quality control, any reasonable, validated method. Under some circumstances, insufficient recently manufactured batches may be available. It would then be acceptable to test retention samples, and to explain in the test report why this was done, stating the age and storage history of the samples. If in a particular case the sponsor believes that single point dissolution results would suffice, for example if >85% of the drug is released under acceptable test conditions in 15 minutes, an argument to this effect may be provided."

- "Biopharmaceutic data as indicated below should be submitted, unless otherwise justified, for any new medicinal product which is an oral tablet, capsule or suspension, intramuscular or subcutaneous injection, topical medicine, product for inhalation or transdermal dosage form where the product has a systemic action. Unless otherwise justified, studies should be carried out for each strength of a product."

- Each new innovator medicine containing a new chemical entity requires
  - absolute bioavailability (compared with that of an intravenous injection or infusion);
  - relative bioavailability (with that of an oral solution or suspension of defined particle size) where the absolute bioavailability of the new finished product has not been determined but that of a solution or suspension has been determined;
  - bioavailability studies to determine the relative bioavailabilities of the individual enantiomers in racemic drug substances;

- effect of food study(ies);
- bioequivalence of the market formulation(s) compared with the (different) formulation(s) used in pivotal dose-defining and efficacy studies.
- Relevant biopharmaceutic data for the active moiety in the new salt as compared with the same moiety in the currently registered salt.
- Bioequivalence of the active ingredients in the fixed combination product to the ingredients administered separately in registered formulations.
- Bioequivalence of a new dose form to the currently approved dose form (s), and for racemic drug substances, relative bioavailabilities of the individual enantiomers in the new dose form.
- Bioequivalence of a new strength to the previously registered strength(s) if the formulation is not a direct scale of the previously registered strength(s) and the differences between the formulations of the new and registered strength(s) are such that bioequivalence cannot reasonably be assumed.
- Bioequivalence of a new generic medicine and of changed formulation to the original formulation to the corresponding innovator product as marketed in Australia.

In the ratified recommendations of the 109th (2006/4) meeting of the PSC of the ADEC held 24 July 2006 (9), the PSC reiterated its request for the provision of an absolute bioavailability study for all new chemical entities in keeping with ARGPM Appendix 15.3 (6) and overseas guidelines (e.g., CPMP/EWP/QWP/1401/98 Note for Guidance on the Investigation of Bioavailability and Bioequivalence) (7). The Committee stated that it did not "consider that low aqueous solubility constitutes a justification for not undertaking an absolute bioavailability study given that suitable formulations using additives or nonaqueous solvents are now well established. In some cases it may be appropriate to use a low intravenous dose. As investigative formulations can be prepared immediately before use, solution stability problems should also not preclude a study" (9). Appendix 15 suggests that in relation to new modified-release formulations, in vitro and in vivo studies are needed to establish the release and absorption characteristics of the new product (6). The Appendix refers to CHMP Note for Guidance on Quality of Modified Release Products: A: Oral Dosage Form. B: Transdermal Dosage Forms; Section 1 (Quality) (CPMP/QWP/604/96) (8) for further details. Appendix 15 also situations that may justify not submitting biopharmaceutic data, validation and quality control of assay procedures used in biopharmaceutic studies, choice of the reference product for bioequivalence of generic medicines, replacement of dropouts in bioequivalence studies, sequential (add-on) designs and data requirements for biopharmaceutic studies (6).

Alternatively, the alternative formulation may be registered as an additional brand of its previously registered formulation. Typically, the additional data required to support an application in Category 3, or in Category 1 under the "essentially similar" provisions may include, but not be limited to

- specifications for the active ingredient, finished product or excipients,
- method of manufacture of the active ingredient,
- manufacturing procedure for the finished product,
- site of manufacture of the active ingredient or the finished product,
- shelf life,
- storage conditions,
- labelling,
- packaging, including container type,
- a replacement trade name,
- minor changes in formulation (2,6).

EMEA has raised some additional points to consider in relation to line extensions for modified-release products in 2003 (10). These are considered more fully in the Overview Chapter. Other EMEA guidelines of relevance to modified-release formulations as defined by TGA adopted guidelines include: CPMP/QWP/155/96 Note for Guidance on Development Pharmaceutics (effective in 2000) (11) and, effective in June 2006, EMEA/CHMP/167068/2004 Note for Guidance on Pharmaceutical Development (12).

## Other Delivery Systems

ARGPM Appendix 19: Metered Dose Aerosols (Pressurized and Nonpressurized) point out that much of the TGA original guidance document has been superseded by the CHMP guidelines that have been adopted by the TGA (13). However, a number of issues, not addressed by current CHMP guidance, remain covered by this guidance (13). Other guidances of note are those for orally inhaled products (14), dry powder inhalers (15), and pharmaceutical quality of inhalation and nasal products (16). A number of other device technologies are emerging and will require the development of regulatory guidances in the future. The European regulations associated with these technologies, discussed elsewhere in this book (17), are also generally applicable in Australia.

## TGA Experience with Emerging Modified-Release Technologies—Nanotechnology and Biotechnology

To some extent reference to nanotechnology and biotechnology as "emerging" rather than emergent technologies is misleading, as in reality quite sophisticated applications employing such technology have been available for many decades. Technegas (18) by way of example, a nanoparticulate inhalational diagnostic aid for identification of venous thromboembolism, was developed in Australia in the early 1980s. The gas consists of hexagonal flat crystals of Technetium metal cocooned in multiple layers of graphite sheet which isolate the metal from the external environment. Drug products employing nanotechnology and/or biotechnology have also been registered in all the major regulatory jurisdictions and are presented elsewhere in this book. Liposomes (e.g., Caelyx®, Myocet®), polymer protein conjugates (e.g., PegIntron™, Somavert®), polymeric substances (e.g., Copaxone®) or suspensions (e.g., Rapamune®, Emend®) have already been granted Marketing Authorizations within the European Community, the United States, and Australia, under the existing regulatory frameworks. In the manufacture of these drug products, standard processes have generally been employed, which are well described and understood, such as the formation of mixed micelles (Liposomal doxorubicin) or colloidal dispersions (Sonovue®), the manufacture of large peptides by standard synthetic techniques or the manufacture of large molecules by standard polymerization methods.

Long standing processes and techniques are commonly described in terms of the latest technological jargon. While there are powerful financial and career imperatives for doing so, new definitions, from a regulatory perspective, tend to confuse rather than inform discussion. For instance, large soluble biological molecules produced using long-standing techniques and processes are well regulated under current guidelines. However, being nanometer size by virtue of their molecular weight enables them to be described as nanotechnology with a connotation that new regulatory requirements may be required. Nanotechnology, the manipulation of material at the nanometer scale, is a heterogenous mix of technological capabilities. The ability to reproducibly reduce material to defined nanometer sized particles is perhaps the simplest of these but is nonetheless a potentially powerful means of modifying the release characteristics of an active ingredient within a dosage form. To improve the bioavailability of sirolimus (Rapamune) tablets for example, the active substance has been incorporated in a NanoCrystal Colloidal Dispersion (nanodispersion) in which the drug particle size was reduced to nanometer dimensions in the presence of a stabilizer (poloxamer 188). The Nanodispersion was then added to a sugar coating suspension, used to coat inert tablet cores (19).

Similarly, to enhance the bioavailability of aprepitant (Emend) the active has been reduced to a particle size in the nanoscale through wet-milling with subsequent incorporation onto microcrystalline cellulose beads to maintain dispersion of the active. The manufacturing process is described in the EMA EPAR for Emend (20) as comprising

- production of a slurry of water, hydroxypropyl cellulose and aprepitant,
- pre-milling,
- addition of an aqueous sodium lauryl sulphate dispersion,

- mediamilling to form a colloidal dispersion
- addition of an aqueous sucrose dispersion,
- spray-coating of microcrystalline cellulose beads with the colloidal dispersion,
- sieving of the coated beads,
- blending of coated beads with micronized sodium lauryl sulphate,
- encapsulation of the blended beads.

The capacity to mill active ingredients to predefined nanoscale particle sizes and, just as importantly, to maintain the particles in dispersion, offers many possibilities for modified-release preparations using a variety of routes of administration. Maintaining dispersion of nanomaterials is, however, challenging.

Liposomes, discovered in the early 1960s by Bangham et al. (21), are also spherical lipid bilayers with dimensions in the nanometer scale. The advantage of liposomes as drug carriers is that they sequester the active substance within them thus potentially protecting nontarget tissues from unwanted effects of the drug, shielding the drug from metabolism and acting as a slow release matrix, thus providing an extended half life, and facilitate delivery of the drug to target tissues. In addition, liposomes do not penetrate intact continuous capillaries in healthy tissues but do so in tumors with leaky vasculature enabling liposome delivery of anticancer drugs to tumors (22). Liposomes, as drug delivery systems for breast cancer, has been recently reviewed (23).

One of the limiting characteristics of naked liposomes is that they are recognized by the immune system and tend to be phagocytosed by circulating macrophages. The technique of PEGylation, attachment of a polyethylene glycol polymer, has been employed with a number of biological molecules as a means of reducing their immunogenicity and increasing blood circulation time. This approach has been used in the registered drug Pegvisomant, a 40–50 kDa molecular variant of the human growth hormone, which consists of a recombinant protein component and polyethylene glycol, with 4 and 5 PEG groups per molecule. Pegylation of the protein significantly increases the half-life. Liposomes are also able to be PEGylated achieving a similar reduction in their immunogenicity. This approach has been employed with doxorubicin in the anticancer product Caelyx. Caelyx utilizes a proprietary liposomal delivery system known as Stealth® or sterically stabilized liposomes, with surface-bound methoxypolyethylene glycol distearoylphosphoethanolamine sodium salt. Use of liposomes as the drug delivery vehicle significantly increases the therapeutic ratio of doxorubicin by reducing its cardiotoxicity—a dose limiting side effect (24).

There are many other modified-release dose forms that can be referred to, as well as those involving more specific targeting to various regions of the body. An important aspect to be recognized from a regulatory perspective is that a number of the so-called emerging issues may have been previously addressed for similar products defined differently. However, with an ever increasing sophistication in drug product development, statistical analysis, analytical procedures and improved quality assurance and other quality processes, the regulatory guidelines for products in Australia, will, as elsewhere, need to continue to be developed and refined.

## REFERENCES

1.  Therapeutic Goods Administration website available at http://www.tga.gov.au/docs/html/tga/tgaginfo.htm (last accessed October, 2007)—see outline of their role at 'Regulation of Therapeutic Goods in Australia.'
2.  *Australian Regulatory Guidelines for Prescription Medicines (Guideline)* accessible at http://www.tga.gov.au/pmeds/argpm.pdf (last accessed October, 2007)
3.  http://www.tga.gov.au/legis/frli/bp2007.htm (last accessed October, 2007)
4.  http://www.emea.europa.eu/index/indexh1.htm (last accessed October, 2007)
5.  TGA website, ADEC section accessible at www.tga.gov.au\docs\html\adec\adec.htm#adrac
6.  http://www.tga.gov.au/pmeds/argpmap15.pdf (Accessed 3 Nov 2007)
7.  http://www.tga.gov.au/docs/pdf/euguide/ewp/140198entga.pdf (Accessed 3 Nov 2007)
8.  http://www.tga.gov.au/docs/pdf/euguide/qwp/060496en.pdf (Accessed 3 Nov 2007)
9.  http://www.tga.gov.au/docs/html/adec/psc0109.htm (Accessed 3 Nov 2007)
10. http://emea.europa.eu/pdfs/human/ewp/187503en.pdf (Accessed 3 Nov 2007)
11. http://www.tga.gov.au/docs/pdf/euguide/qwp/015596en.pdf (Accessed 3 Nov 2007)
12. http://www.tga.gov.au/docs/pdf/euguide/emea/16706804en.pdf (Accessed 3 Nov 2007)
13. http://www.tga.health.gov.au/pmeds/argpmap19.pdf (Accessed 3 Nov 2007)
14. http://www.tga.gov.au/docs/pdf/euguide/ewp/415100en2004.pdf (Accessed 3 Nov 2007)
15. http://www.tga.gov.au/docs/pdf/euguide/qwp/015896en.pdf (Accessed 3 Nov 2007)
16. http://www.tga.gov.au/docs/pdf/euguide/qwp/4931305en.pdf (Accessed 3 Nov 2007)
17. Wade G, Keitel S, Korakianiti1 E. Regulatory aspects of delivery systems in the EU. 2007 In: Modified-Release Drug Delivery Technology, 2nd ed. New York: Informa Healthcare USA, 2008.
18. http://jcsmr.anu.edu.au/technegas/home.html
19. http://www.emea.europa.eu/humandocs/PDFs/EPAR/rapamune/420600en6.pdf
20. http://www.emea.europa.eu/humandocs/PDFs/EPAR/emend/452103en6.pdf
21. Bangham AD, Standish MM, Watkins JC. Diffusion of univalent ions across lamellae of swollen phospholipids. J Mol Biol 1965; 13:238–52.
22. Vasey PA, Kaye SB, Morrison R, et al. Phase I clinical and pharmacokinetic study of PK1 (HPMA copolymer doxorubicin): first member of a new class

of chemotherapeutic agents–drug-polymer conjugates. Clin Cancer Res 1999; 5:83–94.

23. Sharma G, Anabousi S, Ehrhardt C, Ravi Kumhar MNV. Liposomes as targeted drug delivery systems in the treatment of breast cancer. J Drug Target 2006; 14(5):301–10.

24. Muggia FM, Young CW, Carter SK. Anthracycline Antibiotics in Cancer Therapy. The Hague, the Netherlands: Martinus Nijhoff Publishers, 1982: 1–567.

# Index

t = location of tables.
f = location of figures.